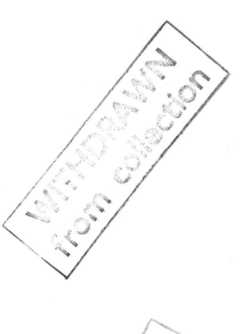
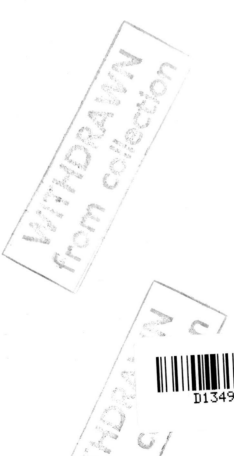

Mental Health and Well-Being in Animals

Mental Health and Well-Being in Animals

Edited by Franklin D. McMillan

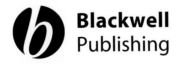

Blackwell
Publishing

Franklin D. McMillan, DVM, is a Diplomate of the American College of Veterinary Internal Medicine, a private practice clinician, and an adjunct clinical faculty member of the Western University of Health Sciences College of Veterinary Medicine.

Blackwell Publishing Professional
2121 State Avenue, Ames, Iowa 50014, USA

Orders:	1-800-862-6657
Office:	1-515-292-0140
Fax:	1-515-292-3348
Web site:	www.blackwellprofessional.com

Blackwell Publishing Ltd
9600 Garsington Road, Oxford OX4 2DQ, UK
Tel.: +44 (0)1865 776868

Blackwell Publishing Asia
550 Swanston Street, Carlton, Victoria 3053, Australia
Tel.: +61 (0)3 8359 1011

First edition, 2005

Library of Congress Cataloging-in-Publication Data

Mental health and well-being in animals / edited by Franklin D. McMillan.—1st ed.
   p. cm.
   Includes index.
   ISBN 0-8138-0489-2 (alk. paper)
   1. Animals—Diseases. 2. Animals—Health. 3. Mental health. 4. Veterinary medicine. I. McMillan, Franklin D.

   SF745.M46 2004
   636.089'3—dc22

                       2004013349

The last digit is the print number: 9 8 7 6 5 4 3 2

Contents

Contributors

Marc Bekoff, PhD
Professor of Biology
Ecology and Evolutionary Biology
University of Colorado
Boulder, Colorado 80309-0334

Michel Cabanac, MD
Professor of Physiology
Laval University Faculty of Medicine
Département d'anatomie et de physiologie
Faculté de médecine
Université Laval
Québec, Canada
G1K 7P4

Marian Stamp Dawkins, BA, D.Phil
Professor of Animal Behaviour
Department of Zoology University of Oxford
South Parks Road, Oxford OX1 3PS UK

Katherine Eckert, MA
UC Davis School of Veterinary Medicine
Class of 2007
One Shields Ave
Davis, CA 95616

Daniel Q. Estep, PhD
Certified Applied Animal Behaviorist
Vice-President, Animal Behavior Associates, Inc.
4994 South Independence Way
Littleton, CO 80123

Michael W. Fox, DSc, PhD, BVet Med, MRCVS
Chief Consultant/Veterinarian, India Project for
Animals and Nature
4912 Sherier Place, NW
Washington, DC 20016

Temple Grandin, PhD
Associate Professor
Department of Animal Sciences
Colorado State University
Fort Collins, CO 80523-1171

Suzanne Hetts, PhD
Certified Applied Animal Behaviorist
Co-Owner, Animal Behavior Associates, Inc.
4994 S. Independence Way
Littleton, CO 80123-1906

Lesley King, D.Phil.
Linacre College
St. Cross Road, Oxford, OX1 3JA

Amy R. Marder, VMD
Director, Behavioral Service at the Animal Rescue
League of Boston
President, New England Veterinary Behavior
Associates
8-A Camellia Place
Lexington, MA 02420

Hal Markowitz, PhD
Biology Department
San Francisco State University
1600 Holloway Avenue
San Francisco, CA 94132

Franklin D. McMillan, DVM
Diplomate, American College of Veterinary Internal
Medicine
Medical Director, VCA Miller-Robertson Animal
Hospital
Adjunct Faculty, Western College of Veterinary
Medicine
8807 Melrose Ave
Los Angeles, CA 90069

Karen L. Overall, MA, VMD, PhD
  Diplomate, American College of Veterinary
    Behaviorists
  ABS Certified Applied Animal Behaviorist
    Research Associate
  Center for Neurobiology and Behavior
  Psychiatry Department
  University of Pennsylvania
  School of Medicine
  50B Clinical Research Bldg
  415 Curie Blvd
  Philadelphia, PA 19104

Jaak Panksepp, PhD
  Distinguished Research Professor, Emeritus
  Department of Psychology
  Bowling Green State University
  Bowling Green, OH 43403
  Head, Affective Neuroscience Program
  Falk Center for Molecular Therapeutics
  Department of Biomedical Engineering
  Northwestern University
  Evanston, IL 60201

J. Michelle Posage, DVM
  New England Veterinary Behavior Associates
  8-A Camellia Place
  Lexington, MA 02420

Pamela J. Reid, PhD
  Certified Applied Animal Behaviorist
  Director, ASPCA Animal Behavior Center
  424 East 92nd Street
  New York, NY 10128

Bernard E. Rollin, PhD
  University Distinguished Professor
  Professor of Philosophy
  Professor of Animal Sciences
  University Bioethicist
  Colorado State University
  Fort Collins, CO 80523

Andrew N. Rowan, PhD
  The Humane Society of the United States
  2100 L Street NW
  Washington, DC 20037

Zack Rozier
  Research Assistant
  Mercer University
  120 Viking Ct. #5
  Athens, GA 30605

Lynne Seibert, DVM, MS, PhD,
  Diplomate, American College of Veterinary
    Behaviorists
  Veterinary Specialty Center
  20115—44th Avenue West
  Lynnwood, WA 98036

Gregory B. Timmel, DVM
  Kamuela Animal Clinic, Ltd.
  67-1161 Mamalahoa Hwy.
  Kamuela, HI 96743

Françoise Wemelsfelder, PhD
  Senior Research Scientist
  Sustainable Livestock Systems Group
  Research and Development Division
  Scottish Agricultural College
  Bush Estate, Penicuik
  Midlothian EH26 0PH
  Scotland, UK

John C. Wright, PhD
  Certified Applied Animal Behaviorist
  Professor of Psychology
  Mercer University
  106 Wiggs Hall
  1400 Coleman Ave
  Macon, GA 31207

Preface

The pebble was tossed into the water by Charles Darwin in 1872 when he declared in his book *The Expression of the Emotions in Man and Animals* that humans are not the only members of the animal kingdom that experience a wide array of emotions and feelings. Despite the reputation of the renowned biologist, the ripples that this tiny rock generated went largely unappreciated at the time. In fact, these ripples remained quite small until the middle of the next century. In the past 40 years alone, the rapid advances of research in the cognitive sciences and related fields have caused the ripples in the water to swell to thunderous Waikiki-size waves. The message these waves carry is that no distinct line separates the human mind from the nonhuman mind. The more science learns about the animal mind, the more difficult it is to believe that the mental lives of nonhuman animals are fundamentally different from ours, that they somehow feel pain differently, feel less pain, feel physical pain but not emotional pain, or they don't feel pain or suffer emotional distress at all. This book is the result of the forces behind these changing beliefs.

Because of its diverse nature, caring for animals is a very complex endeavor. A multitude of issues face those who tend to animals. What are the causes of distress and suffering in animals, and how can we help protect animals from their harm? What causes animals to enjoy life, and how can we help bring that about? When an animal behaves in odd ways, what can that tell us about the way it is feeling? How hard is it on highly social animals like dogs, horses, and primates when they spend their days devoid of social companionship? Do animals experience mental illnesses? If so, what do the illnesses look like, and what can we do about them? Can animals be emotionally abused? If so, how

would we recognize, prevent, and treat that? What is stress, what causes it, and how can we help animals avoid it or better cope with it? Does stress have the same impact on the health of animals as it does for human beings? To whom would an animal caregiver go to seek counsel on how to lessen his or her pet's stress? Does any evidence exist to support the use of positive moods and emotions to enhance health? What has science unearthed about the mental health and well-being of the hundreds of millions of farm animals? How does mental health factor into a pet's quality of life, and how can quality of life be improved? Are there any special mental health considerations for the aging animal? Is it possible to raise the general happiness level of a perfectly healthy animal? If so, how? What can be done during an animal's upbringing to best achieve a lifetime of emotional health and stability?

At present, no unified field of study exists that can supply the answers to these questions. This seems rather puzzling, if not outright incomprehensible. They certainly all seem to be closely related issues—it certainly *looks* like they all should be in one field of study. And the one common factor in all of these issues just happens to be, in my view, the *only* part of life that matters to the animal: its mental life. The animal mind. *Everything* that that animal experiences in life, from the joy of play to the pain of a broken leg to the agony of separation from its mother to the pleasure of a tasty treat—every suffering, delight, stress, thrill, misery, comfort, anguish, and merriment—they all play out on one stage: the animal's mind. With this magnitude of importance, the mind and mental life would be expected to command the most intense, concerted, and focused research efforts. But this is far from the case.

"Do animals have feelings?" This question was answered in the affirmative by Charles Darwin in the mid-1800s. Then how, one might ask, could this question appear in bold headline print on the cover of *US News & World Report* on October 30, 2000? It seems very hard to imagine how in *this* century, a major magazine does a cover story that, if written by virtually any one of the 120 million pet owners in the U.S., would be a *very* short article consisting of the single word "Yes."

Let us look at the issue of animal feelings. Think about the rescues shown on the television news. A horse falls into a deep crevice and can't get out, a whale is beached, a dog falls through the thin ice and is dog-paddling in sub-freezing waters, a kitten falls down an open pipe, an otter is covered in oil from a tanker spill. All of these true incidents required not one, but teams of rescuers, involving great expense and often substantial risk to human life. If animals did not have feelings, every one of these animals could have been simply ignored. No feelings, no sufferings. But we don't ignore them. We go to such expense and jeopardize human lives in these situations for one reason: animal feelings. If the brain of that imperiled animal wasn't generating some very powerful unpleasant feelings, we could all go about our days as we would if a tree were to be blown over by a strong wind.

To be sure, the "intuitiveness" and "obviousness" of animal emotions and feelings do not make them so. An interesting occurrence a few years ago demonstrated this to me first-hand. I was serving as the scientific consultant for the movie *Dr. Dolittle*, starring Eddie Murphy. In this movie we used a lot of live animals and a lot of animitronic animals. Animitronic animals, for those who may not know, are animal robots—with many moving parts and operated by puppetry or remote control. When they are operated, they look and act incredibly realistically. On the first day of filming, we were shooting the scene in which Dr. Dolittle brings his dog, Lucky, to the animal hospital because of a troubling cough. The scene had Lucky on the exam table with Dr. Dolittle looking on as the veterinarian did the examination. The director would frequently call me over and ask how to make the scene look realistic, such as where to place the stethoscope on the dog's chest. In preparation to shoot the scene, the crew lifted Lucky onto the exam table. Right then, the director called me aside to ask me some questions. When I turned back around, we began shooting the scene. My eyes were on Lucky, and I immediately

found myself amazed at Lucky's performance—he responded on cue and did everything perfectly. And when he had to repeat it, he did it perfectly again. But he was not just impressive in his intelligence—he displayed a range of emotions in his face and body motions on cue that would rival the performance of our finest actors. I even felt some twinges of sympathy for him in light of the indignity of having to do the same thing over and over. As I'm standing there in wide-eyed awe of this dog's incredible mental capacities, I happen to glance over to the side of the set, and sitting there is . . . Lucky! It turns out that when I was talking with the director, the crew had switched the real Lucky with the animitronic Lucky. I had been admiring the mental depth and skills of a machine, a nonconscious collection of moving mechanical parts. I had been one-hundred percent fooled. This raises a very obvious question: is it possible that we are *all* being fooled when we look at animals? Are animals just nature's little animitronics?

It is very easy to ascribe feelings and other human mental attributes to animals, especially to those that closely resemble us. Once that occurs, any caring person will experience empathy for that creature. There are even people who feel sorry for the little scraggly tree that nobody wants on the Charlie Brown Christmas special. Some evidence even suggests that ascribing feelings to other beings may be a part of human nature. Primate researcher Daniel J. Povinelli has proposed that humans have evolved an instinctual propensity to attribute emotion to other animals, even to inanimate objects. The robot dog manufactured by Sony, called AIBO (pronounced "eye-bo"), has acquired such a fanatic owner base that AIBO clubs exist all over the country and on the Internet. Club members are very open to admit that they look at their "dogs" as much more than machines, and they proudly talk about them as if they had actual personalities, emotions, and feelings.

So here we are. Many are convinced beyond any doubt that at least some animals—mammals, birds, and maybe others—are fully conscious, thinking, feeling beings. Some do not. If the latter are correct, then the book you are holding right now would have all the legitimacy of a scholarly tome on the spectrophotometric analysis of the various hues of green in the cheese that makes up the moon. You would be holding an expensive doorstop (that a lot of us went to great effort to create for you).

This "problem" of being certain that animals are sentient is not a problem for the public. In America as well as countries the world over, the public is not satisfied to sit and wait while scientists continue to debate this issue. Laws are being passed in rapid fashion, ranging from outlawing gestation crates for sows to banning the declawing of cats. Of course, there would be no reason for any of these laws if animals cannot experience feelings.

Studying the mental realm of animals presents many challenges not encountered in other branches of science. One of the biggest problems we face is the existence of frustratingly confusing and imprecise terminology and definitions for issues of the mind. What is stress? No universally accepted definition exists. Likewise for distress, suffering, welfare, well-being, happiness, quality of life, affect, feeling, discomfort, and even emotion. None of these terms can dependably convey the same information between two individuals as, say, blood pressure or vision can. It is not even clear whether many differently named concepts are not actually the very same thing. Is happiness different from psychological well-being? Is stress different from distress? Even the terms mental health, mental well-being, and mental wellness—are they all referring to positive states or to a continuum that varies from negative to positive? For example, authors frequently write phrases such as, "To achieve mental well-being, the animal's needs must . . . ." But if mental well-being is, as most authors contend, a spectrum, then it would not be possible to "achieve" mental well-being.

In studying mental health in animals, it is important that we examine the course that the mental health field took in humans. As will become apparent, an important mistake was made that we in the animal fields must not repeat.

The field of human psychology, a tiny profession in the early 1940s, grew rapidly after the return of U.S. troops from overseas after World War II. Our soldiers came back with deep emotional scars that needed healing, and the ranks of psychiatrists were much too meager to meet the need. In response, Congress passed the Veterans Administration Act in 1946, which helped create a large new pool of psychologists to tend to our wounded veterans. Understandably, with the need being the healing of mental disorders, that's where the interest, money, and research went. As this attention to suffering continued over the subsequent decades, the fact that the psychological make-up of a human being involved more than disease and suffering, but also included the positive aspects of existence such as happiness, emotional pleasantness, and life satisfaction, took a back seat or was wholly ignored. In fact, at this time, it was generally assumed that happiness was what you had if you were free of psychological disorders. Seen this way, happiness was achieved through treating mental illnesses, making any research on happiness itself appear rather silly and pointless. Over the next half century, the very reason that the field of psychology flourished—to heal mental disorders—remained the focus of every aspect of the profession (Seligman 2002).

Myers and Diener (1995) noted that because of psychology's focus on negative emotions such as depression and anxiety over time, "psychology" became synonymous with "mental illness." Seligman (2003) noted that "In spite of its name and its charter, the National Institute of Mental Health has always been the National Institute of Mental Illness."

To illustrate the effect this emphasis on the negative has had on our thinking, imagine that I had titled this book *Mental Health in Animals*. Give a few moments of thought to this title. Picture yourself coming across this book at a bookstore. As you reach to pull the book off the shelf to look it over, what would you be expecting the content to be? If you think like virtually everyone else, you would think that you are about to peruse a book on the various mental illnesses and disorders that animals suffer from. Would the thought that the book might be about promoting mental well-being, happiness, and enjoyment of life have even entered your mind?

Myers and Diener (1995) state that during the latter half of the twentieth century, the number of articles published in the psychology literature on negative (unpleasant) mental states exceeded those published on positive states by a ratio of 17:1. Not until the last 2 decades of the twentieth century did researchers begin to examine the positive side of the psychological well-being spectrum. The field of "subjective well-being" (the term Diener had to use when he started studying positive mental states because this term would sound more scientific than "happiness" [Richardson 2002]), which examines such topics as life satisfaction, emotional well-being, and happiness, has since grown rapidly.

Because the field of mental health in animals has not yet emerged as a distinct discipline of study, it is both opportune and essential that in the formation of this field, we do not commit the same error. One of the principle objectives of this book is to present a balanced view of mental health so that at the very outset, the positive psychological states—those that have the potential for enhancing the life experience—will be placed on an equal level of importance as the negative states.

Preventing the negative-positive imbalance of the field of mental health is not the only obstacle we face as this new field emerges. We have to first repair the big chunk of damage that can be traced back more than 400 years to the noted philosopher René Descartes. In a story that most readers of this book know well, Descartes's attempts to study the human body did not sit well with the reigning Church, which was the greatest power of the day. When the Church expressed its dissatisfaction with the study of God's handiwork, Descartes struck a deal with the Church officials. He divided human existence into two realms—the physical body and the mental-spiritual realm—and assured the church leaders that if they would allow him to study the physical body unfettered, then he would regard the spiritual part of the human to be the exclusive domain of the Church and something he would not tread on or otherwise disturb. This artificial construct—a firm wall between the mental and physical—has guided scientific and medical thought ever since, much to the detriment of animal *and* human welfare.

Once the body and mind were (conceptually) separate, the animal mind suffered a fatal blow at the beginning of the twentieth century. Early in the century, researchers in psychology and animal behavior were deeply troubled that their field was not being accepted as "real" or "hard" science (Rollin 1989). In a groundbreaking paper, Watson (1913) appealed to the field of psychology to "throw off the yoke of consciousness," for, by concerning itself with such a vague and nonscientific concept, "[psychology] has failed . . . to make its place in the world as an undisputed natural science" like physics and chemistry. Consciousness and its associated notions (mind, emotions, feelings) were not directly observable, measurable, and verifiable and did not behave like objects of a real science. Thus, Watson implored those in the field to "never use the terms consciousness, mental states, mind . . . and the like"(Watson 1913). Watson decreed that the field should instead concentrate on behavior because overt actions could be seen, measured objectively, and verified. Watson was proposing that animal behavior be treated exclusively as a simple stimulus-response reaction; the mechanisms at work in the "black box" of the mind—mental states and cognitions—were nonsci-

entific and hence to be ignored. With this, in the eyes of the scientific community, the animal mind ceased to exist.

The mind remained "lost" for three quarters of a century until it "reappeared" in 1976, with the publication of Donald Griffin's enormously influential book *The Question of Animal Awareness* (Griffin 1976). But a curious thing happened. The animal mind was embraced only by the field of cognitive sciences and flatly ignored by the field that tends to the animal body—veterinary medicine. So although both components of the animal were once again "alive" and under study, they had not actually been rejoined. Instead, in a remarkable development, the animal mind and the animal body began to run parallel, but distinctly separate, courses and have ever since. In the process, two separate literatures have developed—one attends to the animal body (veterinary medicine), and the other to the animal mind (cognitive sciences). This split in the scientific literature between the animal mind and body is so complete that it is almost as if two entirely different types of animal organisms inhabit the earth: mental animals and physical animals.

This divide has left us thus far with no cohesive picture of the animal mind. Each of the various disciplines studying animals—comparative psychology, cognitive ethology, neuroscience, animal science, veterinary medicine, and veterinary clinical behavior—communicates little if at all with the others, and despite its vast importance, the mind, and specifically mental health, of animals has to date not been compiled and structured into an organized field or body of knowledge. Clearly, the now-voluminous and rapidly growing body of research about animal emotions, sufferings, and psychological health comprises a solid scientific foundation for the establishment of the field of mental health and well-being in animals. But for now, this wealth of information remains, for the most part, widely scattered throughout a vast and diverse array of scientific journals, lay magazines, textbooks, and popular books.

All of this has resulted in a different kind of challenge for establishing a field of mental health in animals. We are not faced with the task of simply erecting a new discipline; we have to reassemble our object of study at the same time. With the well-established knowledge of the inseparability of the body and mind, until the animal mind and body are reunited, we face severe limitations in making advancements in the understanding of mental health and well-being in animals. A second objective of this book, then, is to bring together the fields of cognitive sciences and veterinary medicine (which includes the field of clinical animal behavior) to create a comprehensive resource integrating all of the knowledge from the various disciplines. By eliminating the gap that separates these two major fields of animal study and care, we will, in a very real sense, reunite the animal mind and body.

This book is divided into four sections. Part I presents an overview of the most important general concepts of mental health and well-being in animals. Part II deals with the negative—the bad, the unpleasant, the hurting—conditions of the mind and what can be done for them. Part III is a focus on the positive—the good, the pleasurable, the enjoyable—conditions of the mind and how we can promote them. Part IV looks at some special populations of animals for which mental health and well-being issues play an especially prominent role.

An important note must be made before we get started. In 1897, a veterinary textbook entitled *The Veterinary Science: The Anatomy, Diseases and Treatment of Domestic Animals* was published (Hodgins & Haskett 1897). In it are numerous descriptions of pain in animals, including that experienced during what we now consider barbaric surgical procedures. A typical passage reads, "If the wound is torn too much, tie the dog's mouth with a rope or muzzle so he cannot bite you, also tie his legs to hold them firmly, then stitch the wound up with a needle and twine. . . . " Another description about founder in pigs reads, "From the severe pain of the feet and not being able to get around to eat its food it soon falls off in condition and becomes very gaunt." A final example describing the signs of colic in horses reads, "The horse is attacked very suddenly, begins to tremble, paws with one foot and then with the other, and turns the head around to the side, cringes and lies down. . . . The pain keeps on increasing, the symptoms get worse, and he does not get a minute's peace. . . . He sweats freely, and the lining of his eyes becomes very much reddened and angry . . . and the pain keeps on increasing. At this stage his ears begin to lop over and he gets a very haggard look on his face, as if in extreme agony. After a few hours he is a pitying sight to see." The reason this is so important is that even with such graphic evidence of intense suffering, it wasn't until the very end of the *next* century—in the 1990s—that the veterinary profession began a serious effort to relieve pain in its animal patients.

We are now embarking on a new venture—to tend to the animal mind through promoting positive experiences and relieving the emotional pains from which animals can suffer. Let us this time not allow a hundred years to pass before we take action.

Franklin D. McMillan, DVM
Los Angeles
November, 2004

REFERENCES

Griffin D. 1976. The question of animal awareness: Evolutionary continuity of mental experience. New York: Rockefeller University Press.

Hodgins JE, Haskett TH. 1897. *The veterinary science: The anatomy, diseases and treatment of domestic animals.* London, Canada: The Veterinary Science Company.

Myers DG, Diener E. 1995. Who is happy? *Psychol Sci* 6:10–19.

Richardson JH. 2002. Wheee! A special report from the happiness project. *Esquire* June:82–130.

Rollin BE. 1989. *The unheeded cry: Animal consciousness, animal pain and science.* Oxford, UK: Oxford University Press.

Seligman MEP. 2002. *Authentic happiness.* New York: Simon & Schuster.

Seligman MEP. 2003. *TIME* Jan 20:73.

Watson JB. 1913. Psychology as the behaviorist views it. *Psychol Rev* 20:158–164.

Foreword

As a boy I grew up on a farm surrounded by animals; pigs, cows, rabbits, chickens, bees, dogs, and cats. On the farm it was a common occurrence to be faced with animal suffering, emotions, and cognition. To assume they didn't suffer or feel or think would be ludicrous and foolhardy. You had to know the personalities and moods of the cows you milked or you could end up with more than a little milk on your face. We saw joy and depression in our animals just as in ourselves. When an animal was hurt they suffered and we responded immediately to relieve their pain; to do otherwise was unthinkable. Looking back on those days I now realize that my large farm family had unwittingly taken Darwin's notion of continuity seriously without knowing it. It was simply accepted that there was a continuity of mind and emotions, and that although sometimes our fellow animals' joy or pain was expressed differently, it was still joy or pain.

It wasn't until college and my advanced courses in science that my unwitting Darwinian view of our fellow animals was replaced with the accepted and acclaimed Cartesian view. My "hayseed" naiveté was quickly stamped out with opprobrium's like "anthropomorphism" and "sentimentality" and "subjective opinions." I was encouraged to abandon these and replace them with "objectivity." It was as if my abandonment of what I knew to be true was the prerequisite to get into a very special and exclusive club. The attraction catered to our species' greatest weakness: our arrogance. By taking this up I could join a very exclusive priesthood and rise above the common person and especially the ignorant farm boys of the world. Gaining admittance to this revered priesthood would make me feel special and superior... better than most of my fellow humans as well as all the other organic beings on the planet if not the universe. Anthropocentricism is hard to abandon if you happen to be human. I didn't realize at the time that objectivity, while worthwhile in some cases, can also be used as poison to blind scientists to suffering.

This intoxicating arrogance soon dissipated when I entered the graduate program at University of Nevada at Reno to study in Experimental Psychology. I was hired on as a research assistant to Drs. R. Allen Gardner and Beatrice T. Gardner. They were the originators of the now famous Project Washoe. Washoe was an infant chimpanzee who the U.S. Air Force had brought over to participate in their space program. The Gardners obtained her from the U.S. Air Force to begin a cross-fostering study where they, and their students, would raise Washoe as if she were a deaf human child. Project Washoe was a great success and Washoe became the first of our fellow animals to acquire a human language, American Sign Language (ASL) for the Deaf. Washoe is the type of person who has a "presence" about her. She is a very self-confident person as well as being one of the most compassionate and empathic persons I know. But it is her self-confidence that changed me. I came onto the project with my newly acquired sanctimonious Cartesian delusions and Washoe brought me back to Darwinian reality. Not only did she not consider humans to be special, but she also considered herself to certainly outrank the new students on her project. We noted that with new students on the project Washoe would slow down her speed of signing to the novice, which in turn had a very humbling effect on the aspiring scientist. In the normal course of caring for Washoe, she would order me around and demand that things be the way she wanted them to be, and she was strong enough to enforce her wishes. But, like a sibling, she cared for us a great deal. The Gardners caught on film a situation where one of Washoe's favorite human companions, Susan, was crying and Washoe ran to her aid to hug and comfort her. In her run to Susan she would leave her normal comfortable quadrapedal run and change to the awkward bipedal run so she could sign "HUG" to Susan as she ran to her. Over the years this compassion has endured as one of Washoe's most dominant personality characteristics. She always expresses her care for those in need, regardless of whether it's a fellow chimpanzee with a sore foot or a human friend who has miscarried.

This compassion is not limited to Washoe. Today she lives with Tatu and Dar, two other cross-fostered chimpanzees and Loulis, whom she adopted when he was 10 months of age. Loulis has acquired all of his ASL signs from Washoe and the other chimpanzees. The day before yesterday was my 61st birthday and in celebration my wife Debbi and I went out for a movie and dinner. In the movie theatre while making a last minute trip to the restroom I walked into a guardrail pipe that caught my upper thigh with such force that I had to limp to the restroom while trying to work out the muscle bruise to my thigh. Needless to say, it hurt a great deal. The next morning at 7AM Debbi and I greeted the chimpanzees, some still covered in their beds or snuggled in their nests. Tatu was awake and she had her blankets gathered in front of her while doing her typical comforting walk-rock. I went over to the wire separating us and squatted down to wish her a GOOD MORNING in ASL. My thigh was still quite sore and stiff and I must have given a slight grimace when I squatted down, though I didn't realize it. Tatu immediately stopped rocking and asked me "HURT?" holding the ASL sign with the questioning expression on her face. I signed, "YES, HURT THERE," indicating my thigh. Tatu moved her blankets aside, came to the wire, and extended her lips through the wire and I gave her my pronated wrist to kiss. Her kiss did make it better. It is always nice to know that someone is concerned and cares about you. This morning when I came in, the minute Tatu saw me she stopped her usual blanket rock-walk and asked me "HURT?" I answered "YES BUT I BET-TER." This seemed to satisfy her because she went back to her blankets until I squatted down and greeted her. Behavior such as Tatu's is common among all of the chimpanzees at our facility, and I have reported several such instances in my book *Next of Kin*. It is particularly ironic to me that we humans, who consider ourselves demiurges or at minimum the paragon of animals, would so often come in sec-ond to a chimpanzee with regard to empathy, compassion, and caring for another species. They are not blinded to the suffering of others.

Given our personal experiences in academics and with Darwin's theory, which embraces the continuity of the mind as well as the body, the question arises as to how we came to this profoundly flawed Cartesian state. The answer is simple; perhaps our species' greatest weakness is our arrogance and undiscerning acceptance of those who pander to this arrogance and our demiurge pretensions, Plato being one of the earliest examples of this mindset. Plato gave Man a rational soul and a brute soul. The rational soul gave Man rational thought and when he died, this part was permitted entry into heaven. The brute soul was ruled by irrational emotions and died with the body. But only *some* human beings had a rational soul, and everyone else had brute souls, including all of our fellow animals as well as women and slaves. This model justified the exploitation of the "have-nots" as a noble act to improve life for the special few at the top. Plato's student Aristotle picked this up and translated it into a Scala Naturae, which put the sole processor of the rational soul, Man, on top, and then after a difference in kind, ranked those relegated to having only brute souls. Women were with the brutes, and Aristotle felt they were only good for two things: cooking and having children. When the Catholic Church arose they badly needed a hierarchy that displaced women and animals, so the church adopted this pagan worldview as their philosophy of record. Descartes, being a good Catholic subject, adopted and adapted it as well for his philosophy. The big change he made in Plato's model was that Man was still on top with the rational soul, but now women and animals were no longer emotional slaves, but instead machines. The origin of the two schools of Subjective Psychology and Objective Psychology can be traced to this philosophy. By being machines, it simply meant that the yelp of a dog that is struck by its master is no different than the ringing of a bell that is struck by its owner. If the reader is offended by the objectification of subjects such as women, or even when forests are destroyed for monetary profit, you now know whom to blame: Rene Descartes and all those who have embraced this erroneous philosophy. In a pragmatic sense it has done a great deal of harm, not only to those who have been treated like machines, but to those who treated them in this way. The animal, child, or woman suffers, but the abusers suffer as well by committing the act. It slowly chokes any compassion or empathy they might have and makes them less of an organic being than they were before the act.

Times are changing and there are signs that our civilization is beginning to leave the delusional arrogance of Cartesian discontinuity behind and instead embrace the biological reality of Darwinian continuity of mind and body. This book is one such sign, where the minds of our fellow animals are recognized and as a result their mental health is considered a legitimate endeavor to study and treat. This is a remarkable feat when I consider that in my lifetime it was considered perfectly ethical to drive a piston into an unanesthetized chimpanzee's head, or to sew a monkey's eyes shut all in the name of objective science. This first step is very encouraging. Of course it will bring some discomfort to the misguided Cartesians in our midst because it implicitly raises some ethical concerns. Given the reality of the continuity of mind and emotions, doesn't it make sense to abandon Aristotle's Scala Naturae vertical scale and replace it with Darwin's

horizontal gathering of organic beings? And if we do this, is the next step to provide the protection and care to fellow animal beings as we would our fellow human beings? It is my hope that we will embrace the biological reality and its ethical implications.

I look forward to reading the contributions of this noted assemblage of experts in the mental health of our fellow animals. The sheer presence of such a book and the impressive array of noted scientists speaks loudly to the change we are experiencing. If I could I would only change one thing about this book, and that is its title. The title speaks to pervasiveness of our civilizations' assumption that we are outside of nature with the implicit implication that we humans are not "animals." I would change the title to "Mental Health and Well-Being in our Fellow Animals."

Roger S. Fouts, PhD
  Friends of Washoe Chimpanzee and Human
    Communication Institute
  Central Washington University

Part I
Foundations of Animal Mental Health and Well-Being

1
On Understanding Animal Mentation

Bernard E. Rollin

The very idea of a book on mental health and emotional well-being in animals would predictably have brought forth guffaws and ridicule across the scientific community as recently as the late 1980s. In agricultural science, one of the few areas to even talk about animal welfare, the definition of welfare did not include any reference to subjective states of the animal, but instead focused exclusively on productivity. As the CAST report put it,

> The principle [sic] criteria used thus far as indexes of the welfare of animals in production systems have been rate of growth or production, efficiency of feed use, efficiency of reproduction, mortality and morbidity. (CAST 1981)

In other words, the welfare of an animal was to be determined by how well it fulfilled the human purposes to which it was put, not by how it felt.

One might expect such a response from industrialized, post-World War II agriculture, where the supreme values were "efficiency and productivity," industrial values that, in the second half of the twentieth century, tended to supplant the traditional agricultural values of way of life, husbandry, and stewardship. After all, agriculturalists were primarily committed to producing massive amounts of food as cheaply as possible, keeping the cost of food low for consumers, feeding a rapidly burgeoning population, and applying scientific and industrial methods to yet another area that had been largely unchanged for thousands of years. United States Department of Agriculture (USDA) funding drove land grant universities in that direction so that, ironically, the schools that were chartered in part to help sustain small agriculture were instrumental in hastening its demise. But what of other areas of science that did not directly serve an economic function—biomedicine, psychology, biology? Unfortunately,

these areas too exhibited virtually no concern for animal welfare and related concepts.

As we will discuss in detail later in this volume, to generate an account of animal welfare that is of any use, one needs at least two conceptual components: First, one needs some approach to animal subjective experience. To say that an animal is in a state of poor welfare, we mean that it is suffering to some extent—physical pain, fear, anxiety, loneliness, boredom, or other noxious subjective experiences. In the end, animal thought and feeling are constitutive of what we need to worry about when we use an animal for testing, research, or agriculture.

To take a simple example, rodeo bulls show all evidence of enjoying bucking off cowboys; they are typically not experiencing any pain in the process, and certainly no fear. Assuming they are adequately fed and housed, it is reasonable to say that, as far as the bull is concerned, its job does not harm its welfare. (Though people may of course object to such spectacles on other grounds.) In contrast, consider a young calf used for calf roping. Even ranchers are uncomfortable with such an event because the immature animal surely experiences fear and physical pain when jerked at the end of a rope.

Yet another component is essential to making welfare determinations: the ethical judgment as to how much pain or discomfort one *ought* to allow an animal used by humans to experience. This is essentially a moral question. Consider animals—beef cattle—raised by cow-calf producers on western rangelands. It is generally acknowledged that such animals are far better off than animals raised in full confinement, if only because their *telos*, or nature, is largely respected, say as opposed to a sow or veal calf in a crate. Ranchers generally care about their animals a good deal, yet brand them and castrate males without anesthesia. Yet they will claim that the animals enjoy positive welfare, because these economically necessary procedures are of short duration and cause only very short-term pain, whereas the remainder of the animal's ranch life is pleasant. Much of the public, however, considers even short-term pain induced by a third-degree burn in branding to be morally unacceptable and would thus confute the rancher claim about cattle welfare being "acceptable."

Thus, talking of welfare in animals used by humans (i.e., animals whose welfare is in human hands) depends on assuming that we can judge animal subjective experiences and then rate these experiences morally. (This is of course less of a moral problem with "wild animals," whose welfare is far less a function of human treatment and more a function of nature. Nonetheless, *judging* welfare will still depend on assessing animal experience and on having some notion of what an animal in such circumstances *ought* to expect to experience, hence, our debatable but morally laudable tendency to want to feed wild animals during drought and famine.)

The problem that excluded welfare talk from all areas of biomedicine, biology, and psychology is basically one of unexamined assumptions that are highly debatable but were rarely questioned during most of the twentieth century—what I have elsewhere called scientific ideology or the Common Sense of Science. As Aristotle long ago pointed out, every field of human activity, be it art, medicine, law, mathematics, politics, or science rests on making certain assumptions. As in the paradigmatic case of geometry, the assumptions are taken for granted, not proven, because all proof depends on using the assumptions. If the assumptions are capable of being proven, it would have to be on the basis of other assumptions, which would themselves need to be either assumed or proven, etc., *ad infinitum*. Because an infinite regress is impossible, we begin with certain unproven assumptions. Examples of such assumptions are myriad: It was long assumed in Western art that works of art needed to be representational; the legal system assumed that we could coherently distinguish between actions for which people could be held responsible and those for which they could not; medicine assumed the concepts of health and disease; morality assured that our moral concepts applied only to our treatment of (some) humans, etc.

None of this, however, means that assumptions cannot be challenged. Modern art challenged the representational assumption; biological knowledge

can lead us to question the degree to which human action is really "free"; medical community pronouncements about obesity, child abuse, alcoholism, and violence challenge our concepts of disease. Indeed, one useful definition of philosophy is that it exists to challenge assumptions on the basis of reason. Such challenges can in turn yield major conceptual and even scientific revolutions, as when Einstein challenged the accepted concepts of Absolute Space and Time.

When, however, certain assumptions in various fields become insulated from and impervious to rational criticisms, they become ossified into ideologies. The Nazi assumptions about inherently inferior races, the fundamentalist belief in the literal truth of sacred texts, and the Catholic view of the Trinity as being three-in-one despite the inability to reconcile that view with logic all represent clear examples of ideological belief that will be held onto regardless of empirical or logical refutation. Ideologies are pervasive world views, views of a field, or assumptions that resist or even forbid criticism.

Beginning in the late nineteenth century but actually rooted in much earlier scientific thought (e.g., Newton's famous dictum "I do not feign hypotheses"), the scientific community developed a view of science that rapidly hardened into scientific ideology, or, as I have called it, the Common Sense of Science (Rollin 1998), for it was to science and scientists what common sense was to ordinary people in ordinary life. This view was based on the desire to draw a clear line of demarcation between science and nonscience and to exclude from science notions such as *life force* (*élan vital*), entelechies, absolute space and time, and aether that had become adopted illegitimately in biology and physics.

The key to this ideology was that nothing could be admitted into science that was not subject to empirical verification and falsification. Testability (verifiability and falsifiability) became the *sine qua non* for what could legitimately be considered part of science. This was meant to exclude speculative, mystical notions from the domain of science, but soon was far more widely applied and used to exclude value judgments in general, and ethical judgments in particular, from science because they could not be tested. (Wittgenstein once remarked that if you take an inventory of all the *facts* in the universe, you won't find it a fact that killing is wrong.) The slogan for much of the twentieth century was that "science is value-free."

The second mischievous implication of restricting the scientific to the observable was the declaration that science could not deal with mental states, which are inherently subjective in both humans and animals, and what is inherently subjective is not testable. One wit, commenting on the history of psychology, quipped that, after losing its soul, psychology proceeded to lose its mind. What is particularly perplexing about this second component of scientific ideology is that it was radically incompatible with Darwinism, the regnant paradigm in biological science.

It was axiomatic to Darwin that if physiological, morphological, and metabolic traits were phylogenetically continuous, so too were mental and psychological ones. Darwin believed this to be true not only of cognition but also of emotion. One of his all-but-forgotten books details his experiments on the problem-solving ability (intelligence) of earthworms, and the title of his classic work, *The Expression of the Emotions in Man and Animals*, underscores his view of continuity of mentation. Darwin's secretary, George Romanes, was entrusted by Darwin with much of the writing on animal mentation, and he produced two brilliant but barely remembered tomes on this subject, entitled *Animal Intelligence* and *Mental Evolution in Animals*.

Romanes reasoned that though controlled experimentation could provide some knowledge of animal behavior and thought, the vast majority of such knowledge would properly come from anecdotes recounting observations of animal behavior under natural conditions. Acutely conscious of the fact that anecdotal information can be extremely unreliable, Romanes (1898) devised a method for critically sifting or, in his words, "filtering" anecdotes:

> First, never to accept an alleged fact without the authority of some name. Second, in the case of the name being unknown, and the alleged fact of sufficient importance to be entertained, carefully to consider whether, from the circumstances of the case as recorded, there was any considerable opportunity for malobservation; this principle generally demanded that the alleged fact, or action on the part of the animal should be of a particularly marked and unmistakable kind, looking to the end which the action is said to have accomplished. Third, to tabulate all important observations recorded by unknown observers, with the view of ascertaining whether they have ever been corroborated by similar or analogous observations made by other and independent observers. This principle I have found to be of great use in guiding my selection of instances, for where statements of fact which

present nothing intrinsically improbable are found to be unconsciously confirmed by different observers, they have as good a right to be deemed trustworthy as statements which stand on the single authority of a known observer, and I have found the former to be at least as abundant as the latter. Moreover, by getting into the habit of always seeking for corroborative cases, I have frequently been able to substantiate the assertions of known observers by those of other observers as well or better known.

Though part of scientific ideology is having healthy contempt for anecdote, I do not share this view and see Romanes' method as perfectly compatible with the common sense we use in daily life. After all, consider our knowledge of human behavior. How much of this knowledge is derived from laboratory experimentation—virtually none! Virtually all of this knowledge—with the exception of a few social-psychological insights such as those provided by Milgrim's work on obedience or Zimbardo's work on simulating guards and prisoners—comes from interaction with other people in daily life. The same is true of our knowledge of animal behavior. For example, though the cat is one of the most studied animals in twentieth-century physiological psychology, all that has been learned has to do with cats under unusual circumstances (brain lesioning, deprivation, and so on). None of this work produced a single book on normal cat behavior!

In 1985, Morton and Griffiths produced a classic paper on recognizing pain in animals, in response to researchers complaining about new laws mandating the control of pain. These researchers expressed ideology-based agnosticism at knowing how to identify pain in animals. Morton and Griffiths gave two responses: first, they provided a calculus for evaluating pain—2 points for the animals not eating, 4 points for vocalizing, and so on. In this case, Morton and Griffiths said, essentially, that if a scientist is in doubt about animal pain, he or she should ask an animal caretaker, ranch manager, or technician—in short, those who live with the animals. Morton and Griffith's second approach was the one they considered most accurate. In this approach, those who live with animals must know the animals' mental states to survive. In the 1940s, psychologist David Hebb (1946) reported that zookeepers said they could not do their jobs if they were not permitted to use mentalistic locutions about the animals' changes.

My own animal science students some years ago were taking an animal behavior course from a person agnostic about animal consciousness. Most of the students were ranch kids, having grown up with animals, and, having addressed nearly 30,000 ranchers in my career, I know that no ranchers doubt that animals are conscious. I asked the students how they dealt with the professor's agnosticism about animal awareness. "Oh, we give him back what he preaches on tests," they said, "but we forget all that crap when we go back to the ranch. If I can't say 'the bull is in a mean mood today,' I won't live long!"

In a paper I delivered as a keynote speech to the International Society for Applied Animal Behavior (Rollin 2000), I argued that the rejection of anecdote (and anthropomorphism) as a source of information about animal consciousness was misguided. After all, every report of scientific experiment is itself an anecdote, and the scientists reporting it have a strong vested interest in its being accepted. With all we know of data falsification and "publish or perish" pressure, why consider the scientist a more credible source of knowledge than the disinterested lay observer, corroborated across time and space by others?

In any event, returning to the main thread of our discussion, the denial of consciousness was directly incompatible with classical Darwinism, but that did not bother either Behaviorist psychologists (who dominated psychology in Britain and the U.S.) or Ethologists (who dominated Europe). Positivism eclipsed Darwinism. When Ethologists met with Behaviorists for the first time in 1948, as chronicled in the volume *Instinctive Behavior*, they agreed on virtually nothing except the unknowability of animal consciousness (Schiller 1957).

Because Behaviorism dominated U.S. animal psychology for much of the twentieth century, it is worth briefly mentioning how it came to trump Darwinism. J. B. Watson almost single-handedly accomplished this feat, though he was originally a believer that psychology should study consciousness, even complaining in an early book review that the book did not talk enough about consciousness. Later in his life, however, Watson argued that if psychology was to achieve the status of other sciences, it in essence needed to stop dealing with the subjective and consider only observed learned behavior, which to him assured objectivity. Furthermore, from an objective psychology could and would come practical applications—a behavioral technology, as it were, that would allow society to create ideal educational institutions, rehabilitate criminals, and cure psychological and anti-social aberrations. (This pro-

ject was carried on by B. F. Skinner [Kitchener 1972].) Furthermore, Watson had been a founder of modern advertising psychology, had succeeded in the industry, and had sold Behaviorism through the mass media while most other scientists shunned (and still shun) the press.

In any event, Behaviorism denied the studiability of mentation in humans *or* animals, with Watson at one point coming close to affirming that "we don't have thoughts, we only think we do." So dominant was Behaviorism that it occasioned a marvelous speech by Gordon Allport when he was president of the American Psychological Association:

> So it comes about that after the initial take-off we, as psychological investigators, are permanently barred from the benefit and counsel of our ordinary perceptions, feelings, judgments, and intuitions. We are allowed to appeal to them neither for our method nor for our validations. So far as *method* is concerned, we are told that, because the subject is able to make his discriminations only after the alleged experience has departed, any inference of a subjectively unified experience on his part is both anachronistic and unnecessary. If the subject protests that it is evident to him that he had a rich and vivid experience that was not fully represented in his overt discriminations, he is firmly assured that what is vividly self-evident to him is no longer of interest to the scientific psychologist. It has been decided, to quote Boring, that "in any useful meaning of the term existence, private experience does not exist". (1939)

And, commenting on the idea that all human psychology could be modeled in rat learning (i.e., conditioning), Allport produced this gem:

> A colleague, a good friend of mine, recently challenged me to name a single psychological problem not referable to rats for its solution. Considerably startled, I murmured something, I think, about the psychology of reading disability. But to my mind came flooding the historic problems of the aesthetic, humorous, religious, and cultural behavior of men. I thought how men build clavichords and cathedrals, how they write books, and how they laugh uproariously at Mickey Mouse; how they plan their lives five, ten or twenty years ahead; how, by an elaborate metaphysic of their own contrivance, they deny the utility of their own experience, including the utility of the metaphysic that led them to this denial. I thought of poetry and puns, of propaganda and revolution, of stock markets and sui-

cide, and of man's despairing hope for peace. I thought, too, of the elementary fact that human problem-solving, unlike that of the rat, is saturated through and through with verbal function, so that we have no way of knowing whether the delay, the volition, the symbolizing and categorizing typical of human learning are even faintly adumbrated by findings in animal learning. (1939)

In short, Behaviorism combined with Positivism to produce the two components of Scientific Ideology we have discussed. In today's world, where concern for animal treatment is a major social issue across the Western world, the general public would never have permitted the denial of mentation. However, during the period roughly from 1920 to 1970, society did not manifest such concern, so ethics did not choke ideology, and the scientific denial of animal consciousness (indeed, human consciousness) endured.

It should be noted that although one cannot produce a "bible" of scientific ideology, the value-free aspect was literally written in the introductions to biology textbooks at least into the 1990s. Indeed, this view was omnipresent in science. All students were taught that science did not make ethical judgments. Science courses did not engage ethical issues occasioned by the sciences, nor did scientific conferences or science journals. Even when society was highly critical of animal use in research, the scientific/medical community responded by trotting out sick people, threatening to not cure children, and generally responding every bit as emotionally as their anti-vivisectionist critics because, to Positivism, ethical judgments *are* nothing but emotional predilections mistakenly put in propositional form. I have argued that the major reason for societal rejection of biotechnology is the failure of the scientific community to articulate the ethical issues emerging from genetic engineering and cloning. The resulting lacuna in social thought is then filled by doomsayers (such as Jeremy Rifkin) or theologians. George Gaskell (1997) of the London School of Economics demonstrated through survey data that Europeans reject biotechnology not, as common scientific wisdom suggests, out of *fear*, but on moral grounds.

This is well-illustrated in the story of Dolly, the cloned sheep. When scientists failed to articulate any ethical issues associated with cloning, the public raised its own issues. Within a week of the announcement of Dolly's cloning, a *Time* magazine survey showed that fully 75 percent of the general public saw cloning as "violating God's will" (Anonymous 1997).

In one of the most extraordinary incidents bespeaking the pervasiveness of this ideology, James Wyngaarden, then head of National Institutes of Health (NIH) and arguably in that role, the chief spokesman for the biomedical research establishment, affirmed at his alma mater, Michigan State University, that "although scientific advances like genetic engineering are always controversial, science should never be hindered by ethical considerations" (Anonymous, 1989). Tellingly, when I read this statement to my students and ask them to guess its source, they say Hitler.

I would argue that few things have hurt science as badly as removing itself from ethical issues. In addition to hurting biotechnology, science's failure to truly engage the ethical issues in animal research almost led to severe legislative curtailment of biomedical funding. Failure of the scientific community to consider the moral issues of research on humans has led to Draconian federal regulations in that area, and the lack of moral thinking and training has led to the proliferation of fraud and deception in science. (After all, if science has nothing to do with ethics, why not falsify data!)

Animal research is done largely with public money (though the percentage funded privately by drug companies, biotech companies, etc., is increasing). In this case, it is necessary to have public support for research. Much of that public support depends on public perception that animal research is very conscious of its ethical dimensions. Indeed, researchers' actions and statements evidencing lack of ethical awareness led to the crises of confidence in animal research in the late 1970s and early- to mid-1980s. This lack of confidence in turn led to the federal passage in 1985 of laws written over a decade by my colleagues and myself to instill moral concern into science, erode scientific ideology, and assure proper animal treatment. We shall shortly discuss these laws and the fine job they have done to restore public confidence in animal research by eroding scientific ideology.

Just as we have discussed the way in which the belief that science is value-free that is inherent in scientific ideology alienated animal research from public morality and public moral concern for animals, the denial of the knowability of (if not existence of) animal subjective experiences further alienated the scientific community from society, who intuitively always believed in animal consciousness and who, beginning in the 1970s, generated ever-increasing moral concern for animal treatment.

For younger people trained after the late 1980s, it is difficult to fathom the degree to which the denial of consciousness, particularly animal consciousness, was ubiquitous in science. In 1973, the first U.S. textbook of veterinary anesthesia was published, authored by Lumb and Jones. Although the book gave numerous reasons for anesthesia (to keep the animal from hurting you, keep it from injuring itself, allow you to position the limbs for surgery), the control of felt pain was never even mentioned. When I went before Congress in 1982 to defend our laboratory animal legislation, I was advised to demonstrate that such laws were needed. To accomplish this goal, I did a literature search on laboratory animal analgesia and, *mirabile dictu*, found only one or two references, one of which argued that there *should be* such knowledge.

In 1982, the crescendo of concern among the public about animal pain was so great that the scientific community felt compelled to reassure the public that animal pain was indeed an object of study and concern, so they orchestrated a conference on pain and later published a volume entitled *Animal Pain: Perception and Alleviation* (Kitchell & Erickson 1983). Despite the putative purpose of the volume, virtually none of the book was devoted to perception or alleviation of felt pain. As a result of scientific ideology, pain was confused with nociception so that the volume focused on the neurophysiology and electrochemistry of pain, what I at the time called the "plumbing of pain," rather than the morally relevant component of pain, namely that it *hurts*.

Most surprising to members of the general public is the fact that veterinarians were as ignorant and skeptical about animal consciousness, even animal pain, as any scientist. To this day, and certainly in the 1980s, veterinarians called anesthesia "chemical restraint" or "sedation" and performed many procedures (e.g., horse castration) using physical restraint—jocularly called "bruticaine"—or paralytic drugs such as succinyl choline chloride, which is a curariform drug inducing flaccid paralysis, not anesthesia. Indeed, one surgeon told me that until he taught with me, it never dawned on him that the horse being castrated under succinyl choline hurt.

This sort of absurdity also occurred in physiological psychology. I have already mentioned the psychological community's rejection of animal consciousness. Yet the same community regularly performed stereotaxic brain surgery and brain stimulation using succinyl choline without anesthesia, because the psychologists wanted the animals "conscious."

That ideology could triumph logic and even reason was manifest in this area. In the late 1970s, I debated a prominent pain physiologist. His talk expounded the thesis that because the electrochemical activity in the cerebral cortex of the dog (his research model for studying pain) was different from such activity in the human and because the cortex was the seat of processing information, the dog did not feel pain the way humans did. His talk took an hour, and I was expected to rebut his argument. My rebuttal was the shortest public statement I ever made. I said, "As a prominent pain physiologist, you do your work on dogs. You extrapolate the results to people, correct?" He said yes. "Excellent," I said, "then either your speech is false, or your life's work is!"

In a similar vein, I experienced the following incident. In the mid-1980s, I was having dinner with a group of senior veterinary scientists, and the conversation turned to the subject of this chapter: namely, scientific ideology's disavowal of our ability to talk meaningfully about animal consciousness, thought, and awareness. One man, a famous dairy scientist, became quite heated. "It's absurd to deny animal consciousness," he exclaimed loudly. "My dog thinks, makes decisions and plans, etc., etc," all of which he proceeded to exemplify with the kind of anecdotes we all invoke in such common-sense discussions. When he finally stopped, I turned to him and asked, "How about your dairy cows?" "Beg pardon?" he said. "Your dairy cows," I repeated, "do they have conscious awareness and thought?" "Of course not," he snapped before proceeding to redden as he realized the clash between ideology and common sense and what a strange universe this would be if the only conscious beings were humans and dogs, perhaps humans and *his* dog.

A colleague of mine who was doing her PhD in the mid-1980s in anesthesiology was studying anesthesia in horses. The project involved subjecting the animal to painful stimuli and seeing which drugs best controlled the pain response. When she wrote up her results, her committee did not allow her to say that she "hurt" the animals, nor could she say that the drugs controlled the pain—that was ideologically forbidden. She was compelled to say that she subjected the horses to a stimulus and to describe how the drugs changed the response.

One of the best stories covering the ideological denial of consciousness was told by Dr. Robert

Rissler, the USDA/Animal Plant and Health Inspection Service (APHIS) veterinarian in charge of writing the regulations interpreting the 1985 laboratory animal laws. Rissler related that he was particularly worried about one provision of the law, namely the requirement that nonhuman primates be housed in environments that "enhanced their psychological well-being." As a veterinarian, Rissler said, he knew nothing about either primates or psychological well-being. It occurred to him to approach the primatology division of the American Psychological Association. He made an appointment and tendered his queries to some eminent scientists in the field. "Psychological well-being of primates," they said. "Don't worry Dr. Rissler, there is no such thing." Acutely aware of when the new law would take effect, Rissler replied, "Well there will be after January 1, 1987, whether you people help me or not!"

These anecdotes help to buttress my claim early in this chapter that a scientific book on animal mental and emotional health would have been impossible even 15 years ago. It is therefore important to explain why it is now a much more legitimate project, though one that older, die-hard ideologies would doubtless continue to reject.

First and foremost, it is now abundantly clear that the public is displaying significant moral concern for animal treatment in all areas of animal use, from abattoirs to zoos. One major social ethical concern that has developed over the past three decades is a significant emphasis on the treatment of animals used by society for various purposes. It is easy to demonstrate the degree to which these concerns have seized the public imagination. According to two major organizations having no incentive to exaggerate the influence of animal ethics—the U.S. National Cattlemen's Beef Association and the NIH (the latter being the source of funding for the majority of biomedical research in the U.S.)—by the early 1990s, Congress had been consistently receiving more letters, phone calls, faxes, e-mails, and personal contacts on animal-related issues than on any other topic (McCarthy 1988, 1992).

Whereas 25 years ago, one would have found no bills pending in the U.S. Congress relating to animal welfare, the past five to six years have witnessed 50–60 such bills annually, with even more proliferating at the state level. The federal bills range from attempts to prevent duplication in animal research, to saving marine mammals from becoming victims of tuna fishermen, to preventing importation of ivory, to curtailing the parrot trade. State laws passed in large numbers have increasingly prevented the use of live or dead shelter animals for biomedical research and training and have focused on myriad other areas of animal welfare. Numerous states have abolished the steel-jawed leghold trap. When Colorado's politically appointed Wildlife Commission failed to act on a recommendation from the Division of Wildlife to abolish the spring bear hunt (because hunters were liable to shoot lactating mothers, leaving their orphaned cubs to die of starvation), the general public ended the hunt through a popular referendum. Seventy percent of Colorado's population voted for its passage. In Ontario, the environmental minister stopped a similar hunt by executive fiat in response to social ethical concern. California abolished the hunting of mountain lions, and state fishery management agencies have taken a hard look at catch-and-release programs on humane grounds.

In fact, wildlife managers have worried in academic journals about "management by referendum." According to the director of the American Quarter Horse Association, the number of state bills related to horse welfare filled a telephone-book-sized volume in 1998 alone. Public sentiment for equine welfare in California carried a bill through the state legislature, making the slaughter of horses or shipping of horses for slaughter a felony in that state. Municipalities have passed ordinances ranging from the abolition of rodeos, circuses, and zoos to the protection of prairie dogs and, in the case of Cambridge, Massachusetts (a biomedical Mecca), the strictest laws in the world regulating research.

Even more dramatic, perhaps, is the worldwide proliferation of laws to protect laboratory animals. In the United States, for example, as we mentioned, two major pieces of legislation regulating and constraining the use and treatment of animals in research were passed by the U.S. Congress in 1985, despite vigorous opposition from the powerful biomedical research and medical lobbies. This opposition included well-financed, highly visible advertisements and media promotions indicating that human health and medical progress would be harmed by implementation of such legislation.

In 1986, Britain superseded its pioneering act of 1876 with new laws aimed at strengthening public confidence in the welfare of experimental animals. Many other European countries and Australia and New Zealand have moved in a similar direction, despite the fact that some 90 percent of laboratory animals are rats and mice, not generally thought of as the most cuddly and lovable of animals.

Many animal uses seen as frivolous by the public have been abolished without legislation. Toxicological testing of cosmetics on animals has been truncated; companies such as the Body Shop have been wildly successful internationally by totally disavowing such testing, and free-range egg production is a growth industry across the world. Greyhound racing in the U.S. has declined, in part for animal welfare reasons, with the Indiana veterinary community spearheading the effort to prevent greyhound racing from coming into the state. Zoos that are little more than prisons for animals (the state of the art during my youth) have all but disappeared, and the very existence of zoos is being increasingly challenged, despite the public's unabashed love of seeing animals. And, as Gaskell and his associates' work has revealed, genetic engineering has been rejected in Europe not, as commonly believed, for reasons of risk but for reasons of ethics—in part for reasons of animal ethics. Similar reasons (e.g., fear of harming cattle) have, in part, driven European rejection of the use of bovine somatotropin (BST). Rodeos such as the Houston Livestock Show have, in essence, banned jerking of calves in roping, despite opposition from the Professional Rodeo Cowboys Association, who themselves never show the actual roping of a calf on national television.

Inevitably, agriculture has felt the force of social concern with animal treatment; indeed, it is arguable that contemporary concern in society with the treatment of farm animals in modern production systems blazed the trail leading to a new ethic for animals. As early as 1965, British society took notice of what the public saw as an alarming tendency to industrialize animal agriculture by chartering the Brambell Commission, a group of scientists under the leadership of Sir Rogers Brambell, who affirmed that any agricultural system failing to meet the needs and natures of animals was morally unacceptable. Though the Brambell Commission recommendations enjoyed no regulatory status, they served as a moral lighthouse for European social thought. In 1988 the Swedish Parliament passed, virtually unopposed, what the *New York Times* called a "Bill of Rights for farm animals," abolishing in Sweden, in a series of timed steps, the confinement systems still currently dominating North American agriculture. Much of northern Europe has followed suit, and the European Union is moving in a similar direction. Recently, activists in the U.S. have begun to turn their attention to animal agriculture and to pressure chain restaurants and grocery chains, and it is reasonable to expect U.S. society to eventually demand changes similar to those that have occurred in Europe. Unfortunately, the agricultural community did not heed the signs and, as people at the 2002 Reciprocal Meat Conference, the annual meeting of the American Meat Science Association, told me, lost the moral high ground to the activists.

Obviously, in the face of all of this manifest and politically powerful social-ethical concern about animal treatment, Scientific Ideology could not be sustained. Consider a recent editorial (April 2002) in *Nature* contemplating the dramatic rise of ethical concern for animals.

> Whether or not animals have "rights," we should learn more about their capacity for suffering. In Germany, the right of freedom to research is enshrined in the nation's constitution. But that may soon have to be balanced against a new constitutional right of animals to be treated as fellow creatures, and sheltered from avoidable pain. Not surprisingly, biomedical researchers fear that their work will be mired in legal challenges.
>
> The latest moves in Germany are the product of political circumstances, but attempts to give animal rights a legal foundation are quietly gathering momentum worldwide. Three years ago, New Zealand's parliament considered and ultimately rejected a plan to extend basic human rights to the great apes. At a growing number of law schools in the United States, courses in animal law are popular.
>
> Some commentators have already countered that "rights" are only created by beings capable of asserting themselves, therefore very young children, and animals, are properly accorded protection, not rights (see *Nature* 406, 675–676; 2000).
>
> Nevertheless, most experts would agree that we have barely started to understand animal cognition. Even our knowledge of animal welfare is still rudimentary. We can measure levels of hormones that correlate with stress in people. But is a rat with high levels of corticosteroids suffering? We just don't know.
>
> Given the passions raised by animal experimentation, and the importance of biomedical research to human health, the science of animal suffering and cognition should be given a higher priority. We owe it to ourselves, as much as to our fellow creatures, not simply to leave the lawyers to battle it out. (Anonymous 2002)

In other words, it will no longer work for science to deny animal consciousness. Similarly, of course, it is no longer sensible politically, let alone intellectually, for the scientific community to deny that how we treat animals is a moral issue. Society will simply no longer tolerate either component of scientific ideology.

A related point emerges from unending public fascination with animal behavior and mentation. About 18 months ago, I received a phone call from a *New York Times* reporter who had been shocked to learn that the single topic consistently occupying the most time on New York City cable television was animals. I have been told many times by newspaper reporters and television producers that animals sell papers. Some cable systems have two "Animal Planet" channels, and hardly a week goes by without some television or magazine story covering animal thought, emotion, and intelligence. A scientist who fails to acknowledge animal mentation, therefore, grows increasingly non-credible.

The second major reason for the demise of scientific ideology, I would argue, is the powerful influence of the 1985 laboratory animal laws. When my colleagues and I drafted these laws beginning in the 1970s, aside from protecting laboratory animals and science, our agenda was to displace scientific ideology as an impediment to scientists thinking about animals in ethical terms and recognizing animal awareness. By mandating "ethical review" of animal projects by local committees of peers, community members, and nonscientists, we hoped to restore ethical thinking about animal use to scientists and undercut the "science is value-free" ideology. Having sat on such a committee since 1980 and having consulted for the committees of many institutions, I can attest to the fact that they successfully undercut scientific ideology because it is, after all, common-sensical to see laboratory animal use as morally problematic and animals as conscious, feeling beings. These committees and laws, then, help scientists to "reappropriate common sense." I have discussed the mechanism by which this occurs in detail in a recent paper (see Rollin 2002).

As important as ethical discussion was as a dimension of these laws aimed at undercutting scientific ideology, equally important was the way in which the laws solved the denial of consciousness and feeling in animals. For years I had written and lectured on the scientific and conceptual implausibility of denying pain and distress in animals, lectures which fell largely on deaf ears and writings that were dispersed, in the classic phraseology of Frederick Engles, like "so many cabbage leaves." So, quite simply, the laws decreed that animals experienced pain and distress and required the control of such pain and distress. Furthermore, the laws recognized psychological well-being and environmental enrichment by requiring "exercise for dogs" and living environments for primates that "enhanced their psychological well-being," though Congress refused our suggestion of requiring enriched living environments for all laboratory animals. (NIH has, however, pressed the research community in that direction.)

The results have been stellar, particularly in the area of animal pain. From the paltry couple of articles I found in 1982, the literature on animal pain and pain control has exploded to thousands of articles, and the use of pain control has become second nature in research institutions. As an added bonus, because veterinary school faculty are usually veterinary researchers and teachers, the message and knowledge was transmitted to veterinary students who in turn, like the rest of society, were becoming very concerned about animal welfare. When these students graduated, they in turn brought the knowledge to their employers, many, if not most, of whom had been trained in agnosticism about pain. This knowledge expansion was further encouraged as drug companies, notably Pfizer, entered the market with very successful analgesics for dogs—carprofen in the case of Pfizer.

A vivid illustration of the power of the laws to change gestalts can be found in the following anecdote: In 1981, I appeared at an American Association for Laboratory Animal Science (AALAS) meeting to discuss the possibility of federal legislation for laboratory animals. To point the issue, I asked the group of laboratory animal veterinarians on the panel with me what analgesic each of them would use on a rat in a crush experiment. None could respond, and some said they couldn't know an animal felt pain. When the laws passed, I phoned one of the agnostic veterinarians with whom I was friendly and repeated the question. He, in turn, rattled off four or five analgesic regimens. "What happened?" I queried. "In 1981 you were agnostic about pain. Now you have five regimens. What changed?" "Oh," he said, "when pain control was required, we went to the drug companies." "What do you mean?" I asked. "Simple," he said, "all human analgesics are tested on rats." In other words, though he had known all this in 1981, this veterinarian hadn't seen controlling pain in rats as relevant until the laws forced a change in his gestalt.

Though often accused of "foot-dragging," the USDA/APHIS, the agency charged with enforcing and interpreting the Animal Welfare Act, behaved very wisely with regard to pain and distress. Although the laws passed in 1985 and went into effect in 1986, the USDA did not even begin to discuss distress until about 2000. By then, ideologically based opposition to talking about pain had been eclipsed by the flood of research and activity in the area and by the general awareness that uncontrolled pain was biologically devastating and skewed results. Clearly, the same holds true of fear, boredom, loneliness, and anxiety, all of which we have every reason to believe exist in animals. And, equally important, social ethics ever-increasingly demand control of all modes of animal suffering occasioned at human hands.

Our foregoing discussion provides us with a perspective on why a book on animal mental health is so needed and so welcome at this historical juncture. There are in fact a multitude of reasons. In the first place, recall our earlier discussion of growing social concern for animal welfare in all areas of animal use. Although research and agriculture, at least, took some time to realize it, this is indeed a serious global social movement that won't go away. Furthermore, the movement in society largely involves common decency and common sense, for example in rejecting tiny austere cages for zoo animals and absurdly small enclosures for production sows, to name two obvious examples. But as time progresses and the most obvious and egregious affronts to animal welfare are eliminated, more subtle understanding of animal welfare will need to occur, as indicated in the *Nature* editorial cited earlier. Consider one example—environmental enrichment: It seems (and seemed) intuitively obvious that laboratory animals need far more natural environments than we provide. Yet in some cases, cage enrichment counter-intuitively raises the stress level for the animals rather than lowers it, perhaps because, it has been suggested, they now *care more* about their surroundings.

The point is that animal welfare science is required to answer a variety of questions that emerge as society looks at animal use in terms of animal welfare. We have already seen that animal subjective experience is pivotal to animal welfare and animal happiness, and thus an understanding of animal distress and what McMillan (2002b) has called "emotional pain" depends on study of animal thought and feeling. This is precisely the subject dealt with in this volume.

We have learned much about animal mental well-being serendipitously from research with no such aim. For example, John Mason, in studying stress in mice in the 1970s, found that the traditional dogma that stress is a nonspecific response to noxious circumstances is simply not true (Mason 1971). One can raise mice's ambient temperature out of the comfort zone and get a radically different stress response depending on whether they are given time to acclimate. Though in good ideology of science fashion, Mason hated to admit that the animals' cognitive grasp of the situation controlled the stress response, he did precisely say this, while placating ideology by affirming that eventually, cognitive states will be expressible in neuro-physiological terms.

Mental health concepts are not only pivotal to animal welfare but are just as important to successful animal management for human purposes. Human-animal interactions have an enormous effect on agricultural animal production and reproduction, as Hemsworth has elegantly shown (Hemsworth and Coleman 1998). Seabrook and common sense both recognize that a (if not *the*) essential variable in getting high milk production from cattle is personality of the herdsman (Seabrook 1980). Far ahead of his time, Ron Kilgore (1978) showed that moving cattle to a new environment evokes a greater stress response than electro-shock does. Temple Grandin has made a career of showing the livestock industry how to profit more by taking cognizance of animals' mental health and well-being (see Grandin, this volume).

Animal research is a bent reed without taking cognizance of animal thought and feeling. Uncontrolled pain in animals results in greater levels of infection, slower healing of wounds, and even metastatic spread of tumors. Eloquent experiments by Gartner showed that simply moving a cage in which rats are housed or uncorking a bottle of ether in an environment in which animals are housed can generate physiological stress responses that persist for 45 minutes (Gartner et al. 1980). Animal pain and stress can affect learning and toxicity. Environmental quality, as already mentioned, can affect stress in animals unpredictably, which can in turn affect a host of physiological, reproductive, and metabolic variables. In short, failure to pay attention to animal thought and feeling can totally vitiate animal research by introducing countless variables that distort results (see Markowitz & Timmel, this volume).

Without an understanding of animal mental health, we cannot rationally revise our agricultural production systems as society demands. Interestingly enough, "cow comfort" is a major buzz word in the dairy industry, and much more attention is indeed being paid to improving cow comfort. Yet, to my knowledge, the dairy industry has yet to admit—as indeed the entire agriculture industry, particularly animal scientists, has yet to admit—that what need to be studied are thought and feeling, happiness and unhappiness, and mental and physical well-being.

Finally, as McMillan has pioneered in pointing out, veterinary medicine can benefit immeasurably from the study of animal mental health and well-being (McMillan 2002a). Despite an enormous literature clearly evidencing psychogenic and psychosomatic dimensions of sickness in animals and psychological modulators of both pain and disease (for example, chronic pain in animals seems to be best modulated by psychological means, just as is the case in humans), veterinary medicine remains pretty much blind to and ignorant of animal mentation and mental health. The one exception is perhaps in the area of animal behavior, where pathology is being treated pharmacologically with human drugs. But to treat animal behavior chemically without understanding the nature and proper function of the animal mind in the life of the animal is to bandage symptoms, not deal with the root of the problem, just as in food animal medicine, we do not get to the root of so-called production diseases (i.e., that the production methods are pathological and pathogenic) working against animals' physical and mental health. Cribbing and weaving in horses, stereotypical behavior in captive species, bar- and tail-biting, and cannibalism and feather-pecking in pigs and chickens are not vices—badness displayed by the animals—as the industry calls them, but tragic and costly results of not understanding the animals' physical and mental natures and of failing to attend to the fact that these animals have minds and mental lives in the first place.

In a popular new book entitled *The New Work of Dogs*, journalist Jon Katz (2003) enumerates, even as I have done elsewhere, the many new roles our companion animals are expected to perform in a society where neighbors avoid neighbors, half of marriages end in divorce, nuclear and extended families have disintegrated, terminal illness isolates people from other people, and old people are an embarrassment to be warehoused. Katz relates that animals are supposed to provide human-like friendship, love, comfort, self-esteem, even a reason for living. If this is the case, do we not have a strong and profound moral obligation to reciprocate? Clearly, this would be an impossible task unless we understand the animals' psychological needs, not our selfish projections thereon. Euthanasia or abandonment for behavior problems is still a major cause of death for companion animals; this alone should serve as a clarion call to understanding animal minds and animal mental health.

There is probably a very deep, almost mystical sense in which we will never fully understand an animal's mind, though this is indeed also true of our fellow humans—there is no way I can begin to understand a marathon runner's pleasure at "breaking the pain barrier" or an accountant's claim that he or she loves his or her work, or what a member of the opposite sex feels in the throes of sexual pleasure. All other minds, are, in a profound sense, "other." This is one of the great mysteries in life, even when we communicate with other humans through the gift of language.

I have felt this mystery with an orangutan during a brief communication when I momentarily shared a thought with her when she questioningly traced a scar on my arm with her finger; with my 150-pound Rottweiler while wrestling with him, knowing full well he could tear my throat out at will; with my horse when I watched him walk on eggs when I put a paralyzed child on his back; with the junkyard attack dog I adopted at the end of his life as I watched him sleep with my wife's pet turkey napping on his head; with my friend's horses when my horse was stricken with moon blindness and her subordinate gelding, much abused by her dominant gelding, suddenly stood up to his tormentor to assure that the blind animal would be able to eat without harassment; with my cat as we share a moment of mutual affection; with cows as they lovingly mother their calves. These incidents bespeak and tease us with mysteries that tantalize and entice but which, in the end, we will probably never fathom. Perhaps this strange combination of kinship and chasm separating us helps us stand in awe: "Tiger tiger burning bright . . . ."

But even as we acknowledge this, we are not exonerated from an obligation to understand animals as best we can before we hit that wall. Scientific ideology has done us great mischief by its failure to try. We may all hope that this book establishes a beachhead from which we can make ever-increasingly successful forays into what we can know of animal minds and mental health.

REFERENCES

Allport G. 1939. The psychologist's frame of reference. In: Hilgard ER (ed), *1978 American psychology in historical perspective*. Washington, DC, American Psychological Association:371-399.

Anonymous. 1997. CNN/Time Poll: Most Americans say cloning is wrong. Retrieved March 1, 1997, from http://www.cnn.com/TECH/9703/01/clone.poll/

Anonymous. 2002. Rights, wrongs, and ignorance. *Nature* 416:351.

CAST (Council for Agricultural Science and Technology). 1981. *Scientific aspects of the welfare of food animals*. Ames, Iowa: Council for Agricultural Science and Technology, Report No. 91.

Director addresses health care issues. 1989. *Michigan State news* 27:8.

Gartner K, Buttner D, Dohler K, et al. 1980. Stress response of rats to handling and experimental procedures. *Lab Anim* 14:267–274.

Gaskell G. 1997. Europe ambivalent on biotechnology. *Nature* 387:845ff.

Hebb DO. 1946. Emotion in man and animal. *Am Psychol* 15:735–745.

Hemsworth PH, Coleman GJ. 1998. *Human-livestock interactions: The stockperson and the productivity and welfare of intensively farmed animals*. Oxford: CAB International.

Katz J. 2003. *The new work of dogs*. New York: Villard.

Kilgore R. 1978. The application of animal behavior and the humane care of farm animals. *J Anim Sci* 46:1478–1486.

Kitchell RL, Erickson HH (eds). 1983. *Animal pain: Perception and alleviation*. Bethesda, MD: American Physiological Society.

Kitchener RF. 1972. B.F. Skinner—the butcher, the baker, the behavior shaper. *Boston studies in the philosophy of science*, Vol. 20. Boston: D. Reidel.

Lumb WV, Jones EW. 1973. *Veterinary anesthesia*. Philadelphia: Lea and Febiger.

Mason JW. 1971. A re-evaluation of the concept of 'non-specificity' in stress theory. *J Psychiat Res* 8:323–333.

McCarthy C. 1988, 1992. Personal communication. NCBA, Denver Office.

McMillan FD. 2002a. Development of a mental wellness program for animals. *J Am Vet Med Assoc* 220:965–972.

McMillan FD. 2002b. Emotional pain management. *Vet Med* 97:822–834.

Morton DB, Griffiths PHM. 1985. Guidelines on the recognition of pain, distress and discomfort in experimental animals and an hypothesis for assessment. *Vet Rec* 20:432–436.

Rollin BE. 1998. *The unheeded cry: Animal consciousness, animal pain and science*, 2nd ed. Ames: Iowa State University Press.

Rollin BE. 2000. Scientific ideology, anthropomorphism, anecdote, and ethics. *New Ideas Psychol* 18:109–118.

Rollin BE. 2002. Ethics, animal welfare, and ACUCs. In: Gluck JP, DiPasquale T, Orlans FB, et al. (eds), *Applied ethics in animal research*. West Lafayette, IN, Purdue University Press:113-131

Romanes G. 1898. *Animal intelligence*. London: Kegan Paul, Trench, Trubner.

Schiller CH. 1957. *Instinctive behavior*. New York: International Universities Press.

Seabrook MF. 1980. The psychological relationship between dairy cows and dairy cowmen and its implications for animal welfare. *Int J Stud Anim Prob* 1:295–298.

2

The Question of Animal Emotions: An Ethological Perspective

Marc Bekoff

SCIENCE SENSE, COMMON SENSE, AND HUNCHES: ON KNOWING AND BEING CERTAIN

It is hard to watch elephants' remarkable behavior during a family or bond group greeting ceremony, the birth of a new family member, a playful interaction, the mating of a relative, the rescue of a family member, or the arrival of a musth male, and not imagine that they feel very strong emotions which could be best described by words such as joy, happiness, love, feelings of friendship, exuberance, amusement, pleasure, compassion, relief, and respect. (Poole 1998)

Sometimes I read about someone saying with great authority that animals have no intentions and no feelings, and I wonder, "Doesn't this guy have a dog?" (de Waal 2001)

Anyone who has ever lived with a dog or cat intuitively *knows* that these mammals have rich emotional lives. They also know that when their companions are not feeling well physically or psychologically, the animals show clear changes in behavior and temperament that mirror their well-being. What do I mean by the word *know*? This is a fair question, for most scientists claim that we never can really *know* anything with certainty. Rather, the data we collect support or refute what we believe to be the case, to be a fact of the matter, with greater or lesser certainty. This is as close to knowing as we can get. Often we can falsify a claim but not prove it or know it with certainty.

Studies of animal cognition and emotions are usually motivated by the question "What is it like to be a ____?" where the blank is filled in with one's animal of choice. As humans who study other animals, we can only describe and explain their behavior using words we are familiar with from an anthropocentric point of view. But in trying to understand the workings of a nonhuman mind, our goal should be to approach the task from the animal's point of view.

Those who harbor doubts that dogs have emotions, that they can experience joy, fear, depression, and anxiety, would do well to ask people who return to homes that are strewn with garbage and valued possessions when their canine companions have been left alone all day. They should watch dogs play with one another. And if dogs do not have emotional experiences, why do veterinarians routinely treat them with psychoactive drugs such as Prozac (see Marder & Posage, this volume)? Furthermore, recent research on empathy in other species has shown it to be much more widespread in nonhuman animals than had been appreciated (Preston & de Waal 2002).

When it comes to the study of animal emotions, we still have much to learn. Certainly, Poole's quote at the beginning of this chapter contains some speculation. Neither she nor anyone else *knows* whether animals experience this wide array of emotions. We still have few detailed studies of the emotional lives of animals, and we need to remain open to the idea that their emotions are just as central to their lives as our emotions are to our lives.

When considering the emotional lives of animals, skeptics can be rather sanguine concerning the notions of proof or what is actually known, often employing a double-standard. In practice, this means that they require greater evidence for the existence of animal emotions than they do in other areas of science. But because subjective experiences are private matters, residing in the brains (and hearts) of individuals and inaccessible in their entirety to others, it is easy for skeptics to claim that we can never be sure about animal emotions and declare the case closed. Nonetheless, a cursory glance at many studies in animal behavior, behavioral ecology, neurobiology, and disease research shows clearly that only rarely do we ever come to know everything about the questions at hand, yet this does not stop us from making accurate predictions concerning what an individual is likely to do in a given situation or from suggesting the use of a wide variety of treatments to help alleviate different diseases. This is all in the patent absence of incontrovertible proof—in the absence of total certainty.

In this chapter, I will discuss some aspects of animal emotions from which the presence or absence of emotions can clearly be used as a reliable indicator of individual well-being (for example, Désiré et al. [2002], in which the authors take a similar approach in a project in applied ethology for farm animals). There is no doubt that animal feelings are the primary focus in our care of animals (Dawkins 1990). To this end, I discuss various aspects of animal emotions, provide examples in which researchers unequivocally claim that animals feel different emotions, and suggest that researchers revise their agenda concerning how they go about studying the passionate nature of animals. In particular I suggest that scientists pay closer attention to anecdotes along with empirical data, evolutionary biology, and philosophical arguments as heuristics for future research. I agree with Panksepp (1998), who claims that all points of view must be given fair consideration as long as they lead to new approaches that lead to a greater understanding of animal emotions.

EMOTIONS IN ANIMAL LIFE

Dolan (2002) has claimed that "More than any other species, we are beneficiaries and victims of a wealth of emotional experience." Surely this is a premature assertion and ignores much of what we already know about the nature of animal emotions. A few clear examples of animal emotions make it obvious that some animals experience a wide range of emotions some of the time.

FLINT AND FLO: DYING OF GRIEF

The following is an account by Jane Goodall (1990) of a chimpanzee family in Gombe, in which Flo and Flint—mother and son—had been close companions all of Flint's life. When Flo died, Dr. Goodall recorded these observations of Flo's son:

> Never shall I forget watching as, three days after Flo's death, Flint climbed slowly into a tall tree near the stream. He walked along one of the

branches, then stopped and stood motionless, staring down at an empty nest. After about two minutes he turned away and, with the movements of an old man, climbed down, walked a few steps, then lay, wide eyes staring ahead. The nest was one which he and Flo had shared a short while before Flo died . . . in the presence of his big brother [Figan], [Flint] had seemed to shake off a little of his depression. But then he suddenly left the group and raced back to the place where Flo had died and there sank into ever deeper depression . . . Flint became increasingly lethargic, refused food and, with his immune system thus weakened, fell sick. The last time I saw him alive, he was hollow-eyed, gaunt and utterly depressed, huddled in the vegetation close to where Flo had died . . . the last short journey he made, pausing to rest every few feet, was to the very place where Flo's body had lain. There he stayed for several hours, sometimes staring and staring into the water. He struggled on a little further, then curled up—and never moved again.

ECHO, ENID, AND ELY: A MOTHER'S DEVOTION

Cynthia Moss, who has studied the behavior of wild African elephants for more than three decades, relates the following story of a mother's devotion (Moss 2000): The gestation period for elephants is 22 months, and a female gives birth to a single calf every four to five years. Mothers also lactate to provide food for about four years. In 1990, Dr. Moss made a film about a family of elephants called the EBs, whose leader, Echo, was a "beautiful matriarch." Echo gave birth in late February to a male, Ely, who could not stand up because his front legs were bent. Ely's carpal joints were rigid. Echo continuously tried to lift Ely by reaching her trunk under and around him. Once Ely stood, he shuffled around on his carpi for a short while and then collapsed to the ground.

When other clan members left, Echo and her nine-year-old daughter, Enid, stayed with Ely. Echo would not let Enid try to lift Ely. Eventually, the three elephants moved to a water hole, and Echo and Enid splashed themselves and Ely. Despite the fact that Echo and Enid were hungry and thirsty, they would not leave an exhausted Ely. Echo and Enid then made low rumbling calls to the rest of their family. After three days, Ely finally was able to stand.

Echo's devotion paid off. But there is more to this story, details of which could only be gathered by conducting long-term research on known individuals. When Ely was seven years old, he suffered a serious wound from a spear that was embedded about one foot into his back. Although Echo now had another calf, she remained strongly bonded to Ely and would not allow a team of veterinarians to tend to him. When Ely fell down after being tranquilized, Echo and other clan members tried to lift him. Echo, Enid, and another of Echo' daughters, Eliot, remained near Ely, despite attempts by the veterinarians to disperse the elephants so they could help Ely. The elephants refused to leave, despite gunshots being fired over their heads. Finally, Ely was treated and survived the injury. Echo had been there to attend to Ely when he was a newborn and later when he was juvenile.

SHIRLEY AND JENNY: LIFE-LONG FRIENDS

Elephants live in matriarchal societies in which strong social bonds among individuals endure for decades. Their memory is legendary. Shirley and Jenny, two female elephants who were brought together by happenstance, demonstrated a profoundly emotional encounter. At different times, each was brought to the Elephant Sanctuary in Hohenwald, Tennessee—founded and run by Carol Buckley—so they could live out their lives in peace, absent the isolation and abuse they had suffered in the entertainment industry. With video cameras rolling, Shirley was introduced to Jenny. When Jenny first met Shirley, there was an urgency in Jenny's behavior. She wanted to get into the same stall with Shirley. Loud roars emanated from deep in each elephant's heart as if they were old friends. Rather than being cautious and uncertain about one another, they touched each other through the bars separating them and maintained very close contact. Their keepers were intrigued by how outgoing each elephant was and suspected that this was more than two elephants meeting one another for the first time. Sure enough, while searching their records, the keepers discovered that Shirley and Jenny had lived together in the same circus 22 years earlier. After such an extended time apart, the elephants' memories of each other remained strong, and ever since their emotional reunion, they have been inseparable.

A DARWINIAN INFLUENCE

It is remarkable how often the sounds that birds make suggest the emotions that we might feel in similar circumstances: soft notes like lullabies while calmly warming their eggs or nestlings; mournful cries while helplessly watching an intruder at their nests; harsh or grating sounds while threatening or attacking an enemy. . . . Birds so frequently respond to events in tones such as we might use that we suspect their emotions are similar to our own. (Skutch 1996)

As long as some creature experienced joy, then the condition for all other creatures included a fragment of joy. (Dick 1996)

Current research, especially in ethology, neurobiology, endocrinology, psychology, and philosophy, provides compelling evidence that at least some animals likely feel a full range of emotions, including fear, joy, happiness, shame, embarrassment, resentment, jealousy, rage, anger, love, pleasure, compassion, respect, relief, disgust, sadness, despair, and grief (Skutch 1996; Panksepp 1998; Poole 1998; Archer 1999; Cabanac 1999; Bekoff 2000a, 2000b, 2002a). Popular accounts (for example, Masson & McCarthy 1995) have raised awareness of animal emotions, especially among nonscientists, and provided scientists with much useful information for further research. Such books also have raised hackles among many scientists for being "too soft"—that is, too anecdotal, misleading, or sloppy (Fraser 1996). Burghardt (1997a), however, despite finding some areas of concern in Masson and McCarthy's book, writes: "I predict that in a few years the phenomena described here will be confirmed, qualified, and extended." Fraser (1996) also noted that the book could well serve as a useful source for motivating future systematic empirical research.

Researchers interested in exploring animal passions ask such questions as: Do animals experience emotions? What, if anything, do they feel? Can we draw a line that clearly separates those species that experience emotions from those that do not?

Charles Darwin is usually given credit for being the first scientist to give serious and systematic attention to the study of animal emotions. Darwin applied the comparative method to the study of emotional expression. He used six methods to study emotional expression: observations of infants; observations of the mentally ill who, when compared to normal adults, were less able to hide their emotions; judgments of facial expressions created by electrical stimulation of facial muscles; analyses of paintings and sculptures; cross-cultural comparisons of expressions and gestures, especially of people distant from Europeans; and observations of animal expressions, especially those of domestic dogs.

In his books *On the Origin of Species* (1859), *The Descent of Man and Selection in Relation to Sex*

(1871), and *The Expression of the Emotions in Man and Animals* (1872), Darwin argued that there is continuity between humans and other animals in their emotional (and cognitive) lives, that there are transitional stages, not large gaps, among species. In *The Descent of Man and Selection in Relation to Sex*, Darwin claimed that "the lower animals, like man, manifestly feel pleasure and pain, happiness, and misery." The differences among many animals, he claimed, are differences in degree rather than in kind.

The continuity that Darwin first proposed is now being confirmed by a series of elegant studies by Michel Cabanac and his colleagues. Cabanac postulated that the first mental event to emerge into consciousness was the ability of an individual to experience the sensations of pleasure or displeasure. Cabanac's research suggests that reptiles experience basic emotional states and that the ability to have an emotional life emerged between amphibians and early reptiles (see Cabanac, this volume). In separate studies, Cabanac and his colleagues have elucidated remarkable similarities between feeling-based behaviors in humans and nonhuman animals, offering strong evidence that animals have feelings that operate virtually identically to human feelings (Cabanac 1979, 1992; Cabanac & Johnson 1983; Balasko & Cabanac 1998).

WHAT ARE EMOTIONS?

Emotions can be broadly defined as psychological phenomena that help in behavioral management and control, yet a concise and universally accepted definition of emotion has thus far not been achieved. Some researchers feel that the word "emotion" is so general that it defies any single definition. Indeed, the lack of agreement on a definition may well have hampered progress in our understanding of emotions.

To date, no single theory has captured the complexity of the phenomena we call emotions (Griffiths 1997; Panksepp 1998). Panksepp's (1998) suggestion that emotions be defined in terms of their adaptive and integrative functions rather than their general input and output characteristics is consistent with the view taken here. Panksepp (1998) claims, "To understand the basic emotional operating systems of the brain, we have to begin relating incomplete sets of neurological facts to poorly understood psychological phenomena that emerge from many interacting brain activities." There is no doubt that there is, as Darwin proposed, continuity between the neurobehavioral systems that underlie human

and nonhuman emotions, that the differences between human and animal emotions are, in many instances, differences in degree rather than in kind.

Most researchers now believe that emotions are not simply the result of some bodily state that leads to an action (i.e., that the conscious component of an emotion *follows* the bodily reactions to a stimulus), as postulated in the late 1800s by William James and Carl Lange (Panksepp 1998). James and Lange argued that fear, for example, *results from* an awareness of the bodily changes (heart rate, temperature) that were stimulated by a fearful stimulus.

Following Walter Cannon's criticisms of the James-Lange theory, researchers today believe that a mental component exists that need not follow a bodily reaction (Panksepp 1998). Experiments have shown that drugs producing physiologic changes accompanying an emotional experience—for example, fear—do not produce the same type of conscious experience of fear (Damasio 1994). Also, some emotional reactions occur faster than would be predicted if they depended on a prior bodily change communicated via the nervous system to appropriate areas of the brain.

THE NATURE AND NEURAL BASES OF ANIMAL PASSIONS: PRIMARY AND SECONDARY EMOTIONS

The emotional states of many animals are easily recognizable. Their faces, their eyes, and the ways in which they carry themselves can be used to make strong inferences about what they are feeling. Changes in muscle tone, posture, gait, facial expression, eye size and gaze, vocalizations, and odors (pheromones), singly and together, indicate emotional responses to certain situations. Even people with little experience observing animals usually agree with one another on what an animal is most likely feeling (Wemelsfelder & Lawrence 2001). Their intuitions are borne out because their characterizations of animal emotional states predict future behavior quite accurately. To be sure, this predictive value offers one of the strongest arguments for the existence of emotions and feelings in nonhuman species (Bekoff 2004).

Primary emotions, considered to be basic inborn emotions, include generalized rapid, reflex-like ("automatic" or hard-wired) fear and fight-or-flight responses to stimuli that represent danger. Animals can perform a primary fear response such as avoiding an object, but need not be consciously aware of the object eliciting this reaction. Loud raucous sounds, certain odors, and objects flying overhead often lead to an inborn avoidance reaction to all such stimuli that indicate danger. It is well-accepted that natural selection has guided the development of innate reactions that are crucial to individual survival. Because there is little or no room for delay or error when confronted by danger, these reactions are automatic, unconscious, and instantaneous.

Primary emotions are wired into the evolutionary old limbic system (especially the amygdala), considered by many to be the "emotional" part of the brain, so named by Paul MacLean in 1952 (MacLean 1970, Panksepp 1998). Structures in the limbic system and similar emotional circuits are shared among many different species and provide a neural substrate for primary emotions. In his triune brain theory, MacLean (1970) suggested that the brains of higher animals actually consist of three brains: the reptilian or primitive brain (possessed by fish, amphibians, reptiles, birds, and mammals); the limbic or paleomammalian brain (possessed by mammals); and the neocortical, or "rational," neomammalian brain (possessed by a few mammals, such as primates). Each brain is connected to the other two but also has its own capacities. Although the limbic system seems to be the main area of the brain in which many emotions reside, current research (LeDoux 1996) indicates that all emotions are not packaged into a single system and that more than one emotional system may exist in the brain.

Secondary emotions are those that are experienced or felt, those that are evaluated and reflected on. Secondary emotions involve higher brain centers in the cerebral cortex. Thought and action allow for flexibility of response in changing situations after evaluating which of a variety of actions would be the most appropriate to perform in the specific context. Although most emotional responses appear to be generated unconsciously, consciousness allows an individual to make connections between feelings and action and allows for variability and flexibility in behavior (Damasio 1994).

Perhaps the most difficult of unanswered questions concerning animal emotions concerns how emotions and cognition are linked and how emotions are felt, or reflected on, by humans and other animals. We do not know which species have the capacities to engage in conscious reflection about emotions and which might not. Damasio (1999a, 1999b) provides a biological explanation for how emotions might be felt in humans. His explanation might also apply to some animals. Damasio sug-gests that various brain structures map both the organism and external objects to create what he calls a second-order representation. The mapping of the organism and the object most likely occurs in the thalamus and cingulate cortices. A sense of self in the act of knowing is created, and the individual knows "to whom this is happening." The "see-er" and the "seen," the "thought" and the "thinker," are one in the same.

EMOTIONS IN ANIMALS— AN ETHOLOGIST'S VIEW

As I mentioned above, examples of animal emotions are abundant in popular and scientific literature (Masson & McCarthy 1995; Panksepp 1998; Bekoff 2000a, 2000b, 2002a, 2002b). The following observations illustrate specific emotions in animals.

JOY, HAPPINESS, AND PLAY

Social play is an excellent example of a cooperative behavior in which many animals partake, and one that they seem to enjoy immensely. Individuals become immersed in the activity, and there seems to be no goal other than to play. As Groos (1898) pointed out, a feeling of incredible freedom exists in the flow of play. The cooperation needed for animals to engage in social play and the emotions experienced while playing might also be important in the evolution of social morality and fairness (Bekoff 2002a, 2002b), or what I call "wild justice" (Bekoff 2004).

Animals seek play out relentlessly, and when a potential partner does not respond to a play invitation, they often turn to another individual (Bekoff 1972, Fagen 1981, Bekoff & Byers 1998). Specific play signals also are used to initiate and maintain play (Bekoff 1977, 1995; Allen & Bekoff 1997). If all potential partners refuse his or her invitation, an individual will play with objects or chase its own tail. The play mood is also contagious; just seeing animals playing can stimulate play in others. Animals seek out play because it is fun. Consider my field notes of two dogs playing:

> Jethro runs toward Zeke, stops immediately in front of him, crouches or bows on his forelimbs, wags his tail, barks, and immediately lunges at him, bites his scruff and shakes his head rapidly from side to side, works his way around to his backside and mounts him, jumps off, does a rapid bow, lunges at his side and slams him with his hips, leaps up and bites his neck, and runs away. Zeke takes wild pursuit of Jethro and leaps on his back and bites his muzzle and then

his scruff, and shakes his head rapidly from side to side. They then wrestle with one another and part, only for a few minutes. Jethro walks slowly over to Zeke, extends his paw toward Zeke's head, and nips at his ears. Zeke gets up and jumps on Jethro's back, bites him, and grasps him around his waist. They then fall to the ground and wrestle with their mouths. Then they chase one another and roll over and play.

I once observed a young elk in Rocky Mountain National Park, Colorado, running across a snow field, jumping in the air and twisting his body while in flight, stopping, catching his breath, and doing it again and again. There was plenty of grassy terrain around, but he chose the snow field. Buffaloes will also follow one another and playfully run onto and slide across ice, excitedly bellowing "gwaaa" as they do so (Canfield et al. 1998).

It seems more difficult to deny than accept that the animals were having fun and enjoying themselves. Neurobiological data support inferences based on behavioral observations. Studies of the chemistry of play support the idea that play is fun. Siviy (1998; for extensive summaries, see Panksepp 1998) has shown that dopamine (and perhaps serotonin and norepinephrine) are important in the regulation of play and that large regions of the brain are active during play. Rats show an increase in dopamine activity when anticipating the opportunity to play (Siviy 1998). Panksepp (1998) has also found a close association between opiates and play and also claims that rats enjoy being playfully tickled.

Neurobiological data are essential for learning more about whether play truly is a subjectively pleasurable activity for animals as it seems to be for humans. Siviy's and Panksepp's findings suggest that it is. These neurobiological data concerning possible neurochemical bases for various moods, in this case joy and pleasure, offer convincing evidence that enjoyment is a powerful motivator for play behavior.

GRIEF

Many animals display grief at the loss or absence of a close friend or loved one. One vivid description of the expression of grief is offered earlier—Jane Goodall (1990) observing Flint, an eight-and-a-half-year-old chimpanzee, withdraw from his group, stop feeding, and finally die shortly after his mother, Flo, died. The Nobel laureate Konrad Lorenz (1991) observed grief in geese that was similar to grief in young children. He provided the following account of goose grief: "A greylag goose that has lost its partner shows all the symptoms that John Bowlby has described in young human children in his famous book *Infant Grief* . . . the eyes sink deep into their sockets, and the individual has an overall drooping experience, literally letting the head hang. . . ."

Other examples of grief are offered in *The Smile of a Dolphin: Remarkable Accounts of Animal Emotions* (Bekoff 2000a). Sea lion mothers, watching their babies being eaten by killer whales, squeal eerily and wail pitifully, anguishing their loss. Dolphins have been observed struggling to save a dead infant. Elephants have been observed standing guard over a stillborn baby for days with their heads and ears hung down, quiet and moving slowly as if they are depressed. Orphan elephants who have seen their mothers being killed often wake up screaming. Poole (1998) claims that grief and depression in orphan elephants is a real phenomenon. Judy McConnery (quoted in McRae 2000) notes of traumatized orphaned gorillas: "The light in their eyes simply goes out, and they die."

ROMANTIC LOVE

Courtship and mating are two activities in which numerous animals regularly engage. Many animals seem to fall in love with one another, as do humans. Heinrich (1999) is of the opinion that ravens fall in love. He writes, "Since ravens have long-term mates, I suspect that they fall in love like us, simply because some internal reward is required to maintain a long-term pair bond." In many species, romantic love slowly develops between potential mates. It is as if one or both need to prove their worths to the other before they consummate their relationship.

Würsig (2000) has described courtship in southern right whales off Peninsula Valdis, Argentina. While courting, Aphro (female) and Butch (male) continuously touched flippers and began a slow caressing motion with them, rolled toward each other, briefly locked both sets of flippers as in a hug, and then rolled back up, lying side-by-side. They then swam off, side-by-side, touching, surfacing, and diving in unison. Würsig followed Butch and Aphro for about an hour, during which the whales continued their closely connected travel. Würsig believes that Aphro and Butch became powerfully attracted to each other and had at least a feeling of "after-glow" as they swam off. He asks, could this not be leviathan love?

Many things pass for love in humans, yet we do not deny its existence, nor are we hesitant to say that humans are capable of falling in love. It is unlikely that romantic love (or any emotion) first appeared in humans with no evolutionary precursors in animals. Indeed, common brain systems and homologous chemicals that underlie love (and other emotions) are shared among humans and animals (Panksepp 1998). The presence of these neural pathways suggests that if humans can feel romantic love, then at least some other animals also experience this emotion.

HOW TO THINK ABOUT ANIMAL MINDS

THE ANTHROPOMORPHISM DEBATE

The way we describe and explain the behavior of other animals is limited by the constraints inherent in our language. By engaging in anthropomorphism—using human terms to explain animals' emotions or feelings—we are making other animals' worlds accessible to ourselves (Allen & Bekoff 1997, Bekoff & Allen 1997, Crist 1999), but this is not to say that other animals are happy or sad in the same ways in which humans (or even other conspecifics) are happy or sad. Of course, I cannot be absolutely certain that Jethro, my companion dog, was happy, sad, angry, upset, or in love, but these words serve to explain what he might be feeling. However, merely referring acontextually to the firing of different neurons or to the activity of different muscles in the absence of behavioral information and context is insufficiently informative, for we do not know anything about the social milieu in which the animals were interacting. The following quotations capture the essence of my argument.

> We are obliged to acknowledge that *all psychic interpretation of animal behavior must be on the analogy of human experience. . . .* Whether we will or not, we must be anthropomorphic in the notions we form of what takes place in the mind of an animal. (Washburn 1909)

> To affirm, for example, that scallops "are conscious of nothing", that they get out of the way of potential predators without experiencing them as such and when they fail to do so, get eaten alive without (quite possibly) experiencing pain . . . is to leap the bounds of rigorous scholarship into a maze of unwarranted assumptions, mistaking human ignorance for human knowledge. (Sheets-Johnstone 1998)

> In my estimate, what we should fear more than anthropomorphism is an anthropocentrism that

wishes to deny that core cross-species principles are to be found at the very foundation of human existence, or a zoocentrism that sees animals as being so distinct from humans that they will shed no light on many aspects of our psychological nature. (Panksepp 2003)

Using anthropomorphic language does not have to discount the animal's point of view. On the contrary, anthropomorphism allows other animals' behavior and emotions to be accessible to us. Thus, I maintain that we can be *biocentrically anthropomorphic* and do rigorous science. With respect to understanding the dog's mind, taking a *caninocentric* view and trying to be *caninomorphic* should be the goal, as true understanding can only be derived from the animal's point of view.

To make the use of anthropomorphism and anecdote more acceptable to those who feel uncomfortable describing animals with such words as happy, sad, depressed, or jealous, or those who do not think that mere stories about animals truly provide much useful information, Burghardt (1991) suggested the notion of "critical anthropomorphism," in which various sources of information are used to generate ideas that may be useful in future research. These sources include natural history, individuals' perceptions, intuitions, feelings, careful descriptions of behavior, identifying with the animal, optimization models, and previous studies. Timberlake (1999) suggested a new term, "theomorphism," to lead us away from the potential pitfalls of anthropomorphism. Theomorphism is animal-centered and "is based on convergent information from behavior, physiology, and the results of experimental manipulations" (Timberlake 1999). Theomorphism is essentially "critical anthropomorphism" and does not help us overcome the ultimate necessity for using human terms to explain animal behavior and emotions.

THE EXISTENCE OF ANIMAL EMOTIONS: OPPOSING VIEWS

Generally, scientists and nonscientists alike seem to agree that emotions are real and are extremely important, at least to humans and some other animals. People also generally agree on the attribution of different mental states to animals. Wemelsfelder and Lawrence (2001) discovered that when humans were asked to judge the behavior of pigs using subjective words, they used similar judgments.

Although not much consensus exists on the nature of animal emotions, there is no shortage of views on the subject. Some people, following René

Descartes and B. F. Skinner, believe that animals are merely unconscious, unfeeling robots that become conditioned to respond automatically to stimuli to which they are exposed. The view of animals as machines—lacking mental experiences—can successfully explain so much of animal behavior that it is easy to understand why many people have adopted it.

Not everyone accepts that animals are merely automatons, unfeeling creatures of habit, however (Panksepp 1998). Why are there competing views on the existence of animal emotions? This may be attributed in part to the belief held by many that humans are unique and special animals. According to this view, humans were created in the image of God and are the only rational beings, able to engage in self-reflection. This view excludes animals from the realm of "minded" beings, and Rollin (1990) notes that, at the end of the 1800s, animals "lost their minds." In other words, in attempting to emulate the up-and-coming "hard sciences" such as physics and chemistry, researchers studying animal behavior came to the conclusion that too little in studies of animal emotions and minds was directly observable, measurable, and verifiable, so it was best to omit them from consideration. Instead, studies were to concentrate solely on observable behavior because overt actions could be seen, measured objectively, and verified (see also Dror 1999).

The most resolute adherents of the view that consideration of animal (and in some cases human) emotions or mental states is unscientific are the *behaviorists*. Their historical leaders were John B. Watson and, later, Skinner. For behaviorists, following the logical positivists, only observable behavior constitutes legitimate scientific data. Mental processes and contents were considered irrelevant for the understanding of behavior, so they were to be ignored. In contrast to behaviorists, other researchers have faced up to the challenge of learning more about animal emotions and animal minds and believe that it is possible to study animal emotions and minds (including consciousness) objectively (Allen & Bekoff 1997; Bekoff & Allen 1997; Panksepp 1998; Bekoff 2000a, 2000b, 2002a; Hauser 2000).

In the specific case of emotions, there seem to be no avenues of inquiry or scientific data strong enough to convince some skeptics that other animals possess more than some basic primary emotions. Even if future research were to demonstrate that similar (or analogous) areas of a chimpanzee's or dog's brain showed the same activity as a human brain when a person reports that the chimpanzee or dog is happy or sad, some skeptics will continue to hold tightly to the view that we simply cannot know what individuals are truly feeling so these studies are useless. They claim that just because an animal acts "as if" it is happy or sad, we cannot say more than that, and such "as if" statements provide insufficient evidence. The renowned evolutionary biologist George Williams (1992) claimed, "I am inclined merely to delete [the mental realm] from biological explanation, because it is an entirely private phenomenon, and biology must deal with the publicly demonstrable." (See also Williams [1997] for a stronger dismissal of the possibility of learning about mental phenomena from biological research, and Allen & Bekoff, 1997 for a criticism of Williams' logic.)

It is important to stress that emotions clearly drive humans to action, so why can it not be so that at least some other animals are also driven by their emotions? Many people, especially researchers studying animal emotions, are of the opinion that humans cannot be the only animals that experience emotions (Bekoff 2000a, 2000b). Indeed, it is unlikely that secondary emotions evolved only in humans with no precursors in other animals. Poole (1998), who has studied elephants for many years, notes, "While I feel confident that elephants feel some emotions that we do not, and vice versa, I also believe that we experience many emotions in common."

It is very difficult to substantiate the categorical assertion that no other animals enjoy themselves when playing, are happy when reuniting, or become sad over the loss of a close friend. Consider wolves when they reunite, their tails wagging loosely to-and-fro and individuals whining and jumping about. Consider also elephants reuniting in a greeting celebration, flapping their ears and spinning about and emitting a vocalization known as a "greeting rumble." Likewise, consider what animals are feeling when they remove themselves from their social group, sulk at the death of a friend, stop eating, and die.

SELECTIVE ATTRIBUTION

Burghardt (1997b) and others feel comfortable expanding science carefully to gain a better understanding of other animals. However, Burghardt and other scientists who openly support the usefulness of anthropomorphism are not alone (see Crist 1999). Some scientists, as Rollin (1989) points out, feel very comfortable attributing human emotions to, for example, the companion animals with whom they share their homes. These researchers tell stories of how happy the family dog is when they arrive at home, how sad he looks when they leave him at home or take away a chew bone, how he misses his canine friends, or how smart he is for figuring out how to get around an obstacle. Yet, when the same scientists enter their laboratories, dogs (and other animals) become objects, and talking about their emotional lives or intelligence is taboo.

THINKING AHEAD

Clearly, much disagreement exists about the emotional lives of other animals. I argue that we already have ample evidence (and that data are continually accumulating) to support the contention that at least some animals have deep, rich, and complex emotional lives. I also believe that those who claim that few if any animals have such emotional lives—that animals cannot feel such emotions as joy, love, or grief—should share the burden of proof with those who argue otherwise. Why can't we posit that some animals do experience emotions and then have to "prove" that they don't, rather than vice versa?

Categorically denying emotions to animals because we cannot study them directly does not constitute a strong or reasonable argument against their existence. The same concerns could be mounted against evolutionary explanations of a wide variety of behavior patterns, stories that rely on facts that are impossible to verify precisely. Even if joy and grief in dogs are not the same as joy and grief in chimpanzees, elephants, or humans, this does not mean that there are no such things as dog-joy, dog-grief, chimpanzee-joy, or elephant-grief. Even wild animals and their domesticated relatives may differ in the nature of their emotional lives.

The following questions can be used to set the stage for thinking about the evolution and expression of animal emotions: Our moods move us, so why not other animals? Emotions help us manage and regulate our relationships with others, so why not for other animals? Emotions are important for humans to adapt to specific circumstances, so why not for other animals? Emotions are an integral part of human life, so why not for other animals?

By remaining open to the idea that many animals have rich emotional lives, even if we are wrong in some cases, little is truly lost. By closing the door on the possibility that many animals have emotional experiences, even if they are very different from our own or from those of animals with whom we are most familiar, we will forfeit great opportunities to fully understand nonhuman minds.

HOW TO STUDY ANIMAL EMOTIONS

A broad and intensive approach to the study of animal emotions will require that researchers in various fields—ethology, neurobiology, endocrinology, psychology, and philosophy—coordinate their efforts. No one discipline will be able to answer all of the important questions that remain to be answered. Laboratory-bound scientists, field researchers, and philosophers must share data and ideas. Indeed, a few biologists have entered into serious dialogue with philosophers, and some philosophers have engaged in field work (Allen & Bekoff 1997). As a result of these collaborations, each has experienced the others' views and the bases for the sorts of arguments that are offered concerning animal emotions and cognitive abilities. Interdisciplinary research is the rule rather than the exception in numerous scientific disciplines, and there is every reason to believe that these sorts of efforts will also help us learn considerably more about the emotional lives of animals.

The rigorous study of animal emotions is in its infancy, and research will benefit greatly from pluralistic perspectives. A combination of evolutionary, comparative, and developmental approaches set forth by Tinbergen and Burghardt, combined with comparative studies of the neurobiological and endocrinological bases of emotions in various animals, including humans, carries much promise for future work concerned with relationships between cognition and individuals' experiences of various emotions.

Future research must focus on a broad array of taxa, and give attention to not only those animals with whom we are familiar (for example, companion animals) or those with whom we are closely related (non-human primates)—animals to whom many of us freely attribute secondary emotions and a wide variety of moods. Much information can be collected on companion animals due to the familiarity and the close relationship we share with them (Sheldrake 1995, 1999). Species' differences in the expression of emotions and perhaps what they feel like also need to be taken into account.

An example of a study that may serve as a model for future empirical research concerns how the eye white of cows' eyes might be an indicator of their emotional states (Sandem et al. 2002). These researchers discovered that the percentage of eye white was positively correlated with the number of aggressive butts in cows that had been food deprived. They argue that eye white might be a measurable indicator of frustration or contendedness in cows.

Some recent research using functional magnetic resonance imaging (fMRI) on humans by Princeton University's James Rilling and his colleagues (Rilling et al. 2002) might be useful in the study of animal emotions. Rilling, et al. discovered that the brain's pleasure centers are strongly activated when people cooperate with one another and that humans might be neurologically wired to be nice to one another. The importance of this research is that it demonstrates a strong neural basis for human cooperation and that it feels good to cooperate, and that being nice is rewarding in social interactions and might be a stimulus for fostering cooperation and fairness. (For an application of this line of reasoning to the evolution of social morality in animals in which emotional experiences play a central role, see Bekoff 2002b, 2004.) This sort of noninvasive research is precisely what is needed on other animals. We really do not know much about the neural bases of feeling joy or grief in animals, even in our primate relatives. Rilling, et al. (2000) have used fMRI to study mother-infant interactions and other types of social behavior in primates.

ETHOLOGICAL STUDY

Many researchers believe that experimental studies in such areas as neurobiology constitutes more reliable work and generates more useful ("hard") data than, say, ethological studies in which animals are "merely" observed. However, research that reduces and minimizes animal behavior and animal emotions to neural firings, muscle movements, and hormonal changes will not, by itself, lead us to a full understanding of animal emotions. Concluding that we will know most, if not all, that we can ever learn about animal emotions when we have figured out the neural circuitry or hormonal bases of specific emotions will produce incomplete and perhaps misleading views concerning the true nature of animal and human emotions. It is important to extend our research beyond the underlying physiological mechanisms that mask the complexity of the emotional lives of many animals and learn more about how emotions serve them as they go about their daily activities. A combination of "hard" and "soft" interdisciplinary research is necessary to make progress on the study of animal emotions.

It is essential that researchers have direct experience with the animals being studied. There are no substitutes for ethological studies. Field research on behavior is of paramount importance for learning more about animal emotions, for emotions have evolved in specific contexts. Naturalizing the study of animal emotions will provide for more reliable data because emotions have evolved just as have other behavioral phenotypes (Panksepp 1998). Although neurobiological data (including brain imaging) are very useful for understanding the underlying mechanisms of the behavior patterns from which inferences about emotions are made, behavior is primary, whereas neural systems subserve behavior (Allen & Bekoff 1997). In the absence of detailed information on behavior, especially the behavior of wild animals living in the environments in which they have evolved or in which they now reside, any theory of animal emotions will be incomplete. Without detailed information on behavior and a deep appreciation of the complexities and nuances of the myriad ways in which animals express what they feel, we will never come to terms with the challenge of understanding animal emotions.

The Nobel laureate Niko Tinbergen (1951, 1963) identified four areas with which ethological investigations should be concerned, namely, evolution, adaptation (function), causation, and development. His framework is also useful for studying cognition (Jamieson & Bekoff 1993, Allen & Bekoff 1997) and emotions in animals.

Cognitive ethologists want to know how brains and mental abilities evolved—how they contributed to survival—and what selective forces resulted in the wide variety of brains and mental abilities that are observed in various animal species. In essence, cognitive ethologists want to know what it is like to *be* another animal, an approach that seeks the goal of realizing the animal's point of view. In an attempt to expand Tinbergen's framework to include the study of animal emotions and animal cognition, Burghardt (1997b) suggested adding a fifth area that he called *private experience*. This aim is a deliberate attempt to understand the perceptual worlds and mental states of other animals, research that Tinbergen thought was fruitless because we could never know about the subjective or private experiences of animals.

PROBLEM AREAS IN RESEARCH

One problem that plagues studies of animal emotions and cognition is that others' minds are private entities (for detailed discussion of what the privacy of other minds entails, see Allen & Bekoff 1997). Thus, we do not have direct access to the minds of other individuals, including other humans.

Although it is true that it is very difficult, perhaps impossible, to know *all* there is to know about the personal or subjective states of other individuals, this does not mean that systematic studies of behavior and neurobiology cannot help us learn more about others' minds. These include comparative and evolutionary analyses (Allen & Bekoff 1997, Bekoff & Allen 1997).

As mentioned, it is important that we try to learn how animals live in their own worlds, to understand their perspectives (Allen & Bekoff 1997, Hughes 1999). Animals evolved in specific and unique situations, and it undermines progress if we try to understand them from only our own perspective. To be sure, gaining this kind of knowledge is difficult, but it is not impossible. Perhaps the reason so little headway has been made in the study of animal emotions is a fear of being "nonscientific." In response to my invitation to contribute an essay to a book that I edited dealing with animal emotions (Bekoff 2000a), one colleague wrote: "I'm not sure what I can produce, but it certainly won't be scientific. And I'm just not sure what I can say. I've not studied animals in natural circumstances and, though interested in emotions, I've 'noticed' few. Let me think about this." Many other scientists, however, were very eager to contribute. They believed we can be scientific and at the same time use other types of data to learn about animal emotions. It is permissible for scientists to write about matters of the heart (although at least one prominent biologist has had trouble publishing such material [Heinrich 1999]).

All research involves leaps of faith from available data to the conclusions we draw when trying to understand the complexities of animal emotions, and each has its benefits and shortcomings. Often, studies of the behavior of captive animals and neurobiological research are so controlled as to produce spurious results concerning social behavior and emotions because animals are being studied in artificial and impoverished social and physical environments. The study itself might put individuals in thoroughly unnatural situations. Indeed, some researchers have discovered that many laboratory animals are so stressed from living in captivity that data on emotions and other aspects of behavioral physiology are tainted from the start (Poole 1996).

Field work also can be problematic. It can be too uncontrolled to allow for reliable conclusions to be drawn. It is difficult to follow known individuals, and much of what they do cannot be seen. However, it is possible to fit free-ranging animals with devices that can transmit information on individual identity, heart rate, body temperature, and eye movements as the animals go about their daily activities. This information is helping researchers learn more about the close relationship between animals' emotional lives and the behavioral and physiological factors that are correlated with the emotions.

Clearly, an understanding of behavior and neurobiology is necessary if we are ever to understand how emotions and cognition are linked. It is essential that we learn as much as we can about individuals' private experiences, feelings, and mental states. How animals' emotions are experienced is a fertile and important challenge for future research.

ACKNOWLEDGMENTS

Much of this chapter is used, with permission, from Bekoff 2000b (Copyright (c), American Institute of Biological Sciences). I thank Frank McMillan for offering innumerable helpful suggestions on an earlier draft of this essay.

REFERENCES

Allen C, Bekoff M. 1997. Species of mind: The philosophy and biology of cognitive ethology. Cambridge, MS: MIT Press.

Archer J. 1999. The nature of grief: The evolution and psychology of reactions to loss. New York: Routledge.

Balasko M, Cabanac M. 1998. Motivational conflict among water need, palatability, and cold discomfort in rats. Physiol Behav 65:35–41.

Bekoff M. 1972. The development of social interaction, play, and metacommunication in mammals: An ethological perspective. Q Rev Biol 47:412–434.

Bekoff M. 1977. Social communication in canids: Evidence for the evolution of a stereotyped mammalian display. Science 197:1097–1099.

Bekoff M. 1995. Play signals as punctuation: The structure of social play in canids. Behaviour 132:419–429.

Bekoff M (ed). 2000a. The smile of a dolphin: Remarkable accounts of animal emotions. New York: Random House/Discovery Books.

Bekoff M. 2000b. Animal emotions: Exploring passionate natures. BioScience 50:861–870.

Bekoff M. 2002a. Minding animals: Awareness, emotions, and heart. New York: Oxford University Press.

Bekoff M. 2002b. Virtuous nature. *New Sci* 13 July:34–37.

Bekoff M. 2004. Wild justice and fair play: Cooperation, forgiveness, and morality in animals. *Biol Philos.* Manuscript submitted.

Bekoff M, Allen C. 1997. Cognitive ethology: Slayers, skeptics, and proponents. In: Mitchell RW et al. (eds), *Anthropomorphism, anecdote, and animals: The emperor's new clothes?* Albany, NY, SUNY Press:313–343.

Bekoff M, Byers JA (eds). 1998. *Animal play: Evolutionary, comparative, and ecological approaches.* New York: Cambridge University Press.

Burghardt GM. 1991. Cognitive ethology and critical anthropomorphism: A snake with two heads and hognose snakes that play dead. In: Ristau CA (ed), *Cognitive ethology: The minds of other animals— Essays in honor of Donald R. Griffin.* Hillsdale, NJ, Lawrence Earlbaum:53–90.

Burghardt GM. 1997a. Would Darwin weep? Review of Masson and McCarthy's *When elephants weep: The emotional lives of animals. Contemp Psychol* 42:21–23.

Burghardt GM. 1997b. Amending Tinbergen: A fifth aim for ethology. In: Mitchell RW, Thompson N, Miles L (eds), *Anthropomorphism, anecdote, and animals: The emperor's new clothes?* Albany, NY, SUNY Press:254–276.

Cabanac M. 1979. Sensory pleasure. *Q Rev Biol* 52:1–29.

Cabanac M. 1992. Pleasure: The common currency. *J Theor Biol* 155:173–200.

Cabanac M. 1999. Emotion and phylogeny. *J Consciousness Stud* 6:176–190.

Cabanac M, Johnson KG. 1983. Analysis of a conflict between palatability and cold exposure in rats. *Physiol Behav* 31:249–253.

Canfield J, Hansen MV, Becker M, et al. 1998. *Chicken soup for the pet lover's soul.* Deerfield, FL: Health Communications.

Crist E. 1999. *Images of animals: Anthropomorphism and animal mind.* Philadelphia: Temple University Press.

Damasio A. 1994. *Descartes' error: Emotion, reason, and the human brain.* New York: Avon.

Damasio A. 1999a. How the brain creates the mind. *Sci Am* 281:112–117.

Damasio A. 1999b. The feeling of what happens: Body and emotion in the making of consciousness. New York: Harcourt Brace.

Darwin C. 1859. On the origin of species by means of natural selection. London: Murray.

Darwin C. 1871. The descent of man and selection in relation to sex. New York: Random House.

Darwin C. 1872. The expression of the emotions in man and animals, 3rd ed. New York: Oxford University Press.

Dawkins MS. 1990. From an animal's point of view: Motivation, fitness, and animal welfare. Behav Brain Sci 13:1–61.

Désiré L, Boissy A, Veissier I. 2002. Emotions in farm animals: A new approach to animal welfare in applied ethology. Behav Process 60:165–180.

Dick PK. 1968. Do androids dream of electric sheep? New York: Ballantine Books.

Dolan RJ. 2002. Emotion, cognition, and behavior. Science 298:1191–1194.

Dreifus C. 2001. *A conversation with Frans de Waal; Observing the behavior of apes, up close. New York Times* June 26, p. F3.

Dror OE. 1999. The affect of experiment: The turn to emotions in Anglo-American physiology, 1900–1940. Isis 90:205–237.

Fagen RM. 1981. *Animal play behavior.* New York: Oxford University Press.

Fraser D. 1996. Review of Masson and McCarthy's *When Elephants Weep: The Emotional Lives of Animals. Anim Behav* 51:1190–1193.

Goodall J. 1990. *Through a window.* Boston, MA: Houghton-Mifflin.

Griffiths P. 1997. *What emotions really are: The problem of psychological categories.* Chicago: University of Chicago Press.

Groos K. 1898. *The play of animals.* London: D. Appleton.

Hauser M. 2000. *Wild minds.* New York: Henry Holt.

Heinrich B. 1999. *Mind of the raven: Investigations and adventures with wolf-birds.* New York: Cliff Street Books.

Hughes H. 1999. *Sensory exotica: A world beyond human experience.* Cambridge, MA: MIT Press.

Jamieson D, Bekoff M. 1993. On aims and methods of cognitive ethology. *Philos Sci* 2:110–124.

LeDoux J. 1996. *The emotional brain: The mysterious underpinnings of emotional life.* New York: Touchstone.

Lorenz KZ. 1991. *Here I am—where are you?* New York: Harcourt Brace Jovanovich.

MacLean P. 1970. *The triune brain in evolution: Role in paleocerebral functions.* New York: Plenum.

Masson J, McCarthy S. 1995. *When elephants weep: The emotional lives of animals.* New York: Delacorte Press.

McRae M. 2000. Central Africa's orphaned gorillas: Will they survive the wild? *Natl Geogr* February:86–97.

Moss C. 2000. A passionate devotion. In: Bekoff M (ed), *The smile of a dolphin: Remarkable accounts of animal emotions.* New York, Random House/Discovery Books:135–137.

Panksepp J. 1998. *Affective neuroscience.* New York: Oxford University Press.

Panksepp J. 2003. Can anthropomorphic analyses of separation cries in other animals inform us about the emotional nature of social loss in humans? Comment on Blumberg and Sokoloff, 2001. *Psychol Rev* 110:376–388.

Poole J. 1996. Coming of age with elephants: A memoir. New York: Hyperion.

Poole J. 1998. An exploration of a commonality between ourselves and elephants. *Etica & Animali* 9/98:85–110.

Preston SD, de Waal FBM. 2002. Empathy: Its ultimate and proximate basis. *Behav Brain Sci* 25:1–74.

Rilling JK, Gutman DA, Zeh TR, et al. 2002. A neural basis for cooperation. *Neuron* 35:395–405.

Rilling J, Kilts C, Williams S, et al. 2000. A comparative PET study of linguistic processing in humans and language-competent chimpanzees. *Am J Phys Anthropol* Suppl 30:263.

Rollin B. 1989. *The unheeded cry: Animal consciousness, animal pain, and science.* New York: Oxford University Press.

Rollin B. 1990. How the animals lost their minds: Animal mentation and scientific ideology. In: Bekoff M, Jamieson D (eds), *Interpretation and explanation in the study of animal behavior: Vol. I, interpretation, intentionality, and communication.* Boulder, CO, Westview Press:375–393.

Sandem AI, Braastad BO, Boe KE. 2002. Eye white may indicate emotional state on a frustration-con-tentedness axis in dairy cows. *Appl Anim Behav Sci* 79:1–10.

Sheets-Johnstone M. 1998. Consciousness: A natural history. *J Consciousness Stud* 5:260–294.

Sheldrake R. 1995. *Seven experiments that could change the world.* New York: Riverhead Books.

Sheldrake R. 1999. *Dogs that know when their owners are coming home—and other unexplained powers of animals.* New York: Crown Publishers.

Skutch A. 1996. *The minds of birds.* College Station: Texas A&M University Press.

Siviy S. 1998. Neurobiological substrates of play behavior: Glimpses into the structure and function of mammalian playfulness. In: Bekoff M, Byers JA (eds), *Animal play: Evolutionary, comparative, and ecological perspectives.* New York, Cambridge University Press:221–242.

Timberlake W. 1999. Biological behaviorism. In: O'Donohue W, Kitchener R (eds), *Handbook of behaviorism.* New York, Academic Press:243–284.

Tinbergen N. 1951. *The study of instinct.* New York: Oxford University Press.

Tinbergen N. 1963 On aims and methods of ethology. *Zeitschrift für Tierpsychologie* 20:410–433.

Washburn MF. 1909. *The animal mind: A text-book of comparative psychology.* London: Macmillan.

Wemelsfelder F, Lawrence AB. 2001. Qualitative assessment of animal behaviour as an on-farm welfare-monitoring tool. *Acta Agr Scand* A–An. 51:21–25.

Williams GC. 1992. *Natural selection: Domains, levels, and challenges.* New York: Oxford University Press.

Williams GC. 1997. *The pony fish's glow.* New York: Basic Books.

Würsig B. 2000. Leviathan lust and love. In: Bekoff M (ed), *The smile of a dolphin: Remarkable accounts of animal emotions.* New York, Random House/Discovery Books:62–65.

3

The Experience of Pleasure in Animals

Michel Cabanac

There is indeed in them (the animals) pleasure and pain. . . . the animal possesses senses not for being but for well-being . . . taste that is agreeable and distressing, in order for the animal to perceive these qualities in food, desire them and moves itself. (Aristotle 284–322 Ante)

In no case may we interpret an action as the outcome of the exercise of a higher psychological faculty, if it can be interpreted as the outcome of the exercise of one which stands lower in the psychological scale. (Morgan 1894)

Although animal experiments provide a colossal amount of information showing that associating neutral stimuli with reinforcing alimentary stimuli renders rewarding the previously neutral stimuli and, reciprocally, renders these neutral stimuli aversive if associated with negative reinforcements (Miller 1944, Young 1959, Berridge 2000), it is not prudent to extrapolate from animal behavior to cognition as humans know it and to conclude that animals experience pleasure. However, when experimentation is undertaken specifically to study a given aspect of animal consciousness, such as sensory pleasure, it is possible to explore cognition in animals. Do animals experience pleasure? If that is the case, where on the phylogenetic scale did this mental dimension emerge? I shall try to answer both questions.

THE THRESHOLD OF CONSCIOUSNESS

After Descartes, who considered animal behavior purely reflexive, innumerable authors have attempted to answer experimentally, as well as theoretically, the question of animal consciousness.

Griffin (1992) and Dawkins (1993) accept animal consciousness on the basis of ethological observation. Yet if one may consider the existence of a mental space in mammals as obvious, the question of the evolutionary threshold of consciousness remains open. With consciousness, motivated behavior took place that allowed flexible behavioral responses to environmental and internal constraints.

What is the evidence for the presence of consciousness in various phyla and classes? Let us examine the evidence as we move downward on the phylogenetic scale, accepting that humans occupy the highest position and possess the most advanced mental capacities.

The mental performance of anthropoids is impressive. Chimpanzees recognize the family relations between non-familiar individuals on photographs of conspecifics, therefore utilizing purely cognitive information without any other signal such as odor or vocalization (Parr & de Waal 1999). The same method shows that chimpanzees are able to recognize what Parr (2000) considered signs of emotions—e.g., joy, surprise, sadness, fear, and disgust—on conspecifics which they see for the first time. Humans are also able to guess what the chimpanzees see or do not see (Hare et al. 2000). Nobody can deny them a level of cognition close to that of humans, at least qualitatively. Non-anthropoid monkeys also give objective signs of consciousness, which allow their use for studies on human psychopathology and its therapy, as in anxiety disorders (Barros & Tomaz 2002).

Other mammals also show flexible and adaptable behavior. Such a flexibility evokes a mental capacity, as the above exergue from Aristotle reminds us. Yet mammals are not alone in possessing flexible behavior; for example, turtles, probably the modern reptiles closest to the reptilian ancestors of modern mammals, display ludic behaviors. In an enriched environment they spend more than 30 percent of their time playing with useless objects (Burghardt 1998). Iguanas are often kept as pets because they display similar behaviors, and on that basis their owners are usually convinced that the iguanas possess a mental capacity (Krughoff 2000). Using Morgan's canon, cited at the beginning of this chapter, we may move beyond anecdotal evidence to use objective signs of consciousness in animals to be able to discern the threshold of consciousness in zoology. The response to stress provides such a tool.

EMOTIONAL FEVER

The British physiologist E.T. Renbourn showed that the rectal temperature of young human competitors before a boxing match was 1°F higher than normal. Renbourn considered this temperature rise emotional in origin because it was also present in some veteran boxing spectators (Renbourn 1960). Similar observations were made on students in the hours before their academic examinations. Rectal temperatures were elevated up to 1.5°C above normal in 1 percent of these students, and slightly above normal (37.5–37.7°C) for the majority of them. Core temperature returned to normal in the hours after the examinations. The core temperature rise was a fever because no warm discomfort was present in the subjects, as is the case in hyperthermia (Gotsev & Ivanov 1962).

A similar observation was made in rats. Mere handling of a rat by an unfamiliar human is sufficient for the animal to shiver and raise its core temperature by more than 1°C. The elevation is emotional because the response disappears on repeated days if the experimenter becomes familiar to the rat, but returns if the experimenter is changed (Briese & deQuijada 1970). The response is a true fever, i.e., a transient rise of the core temperature set-point, as can be seen from the coordinated physiological responses: shivering and vasoconstriction during the initial period until core temperature rises, then muscular relaxation and vaso-dilatation once core temperature reaches the set-point plateau. At that point if the cause of stress is still present, core temperature and skin temperature oscillate symmetrically (mirror like), a pathognomonic sign of a regulatory process (Figure 3.1).

A similar experiment with chickens (*Gallus domesticus*) yielded similar results (Figure 3.1). As emotional fever is present in mammals and birds that share common reptilian ancestors, one may expect to find it also in modern reptiles because they share common ancestors with modern mammals and birds. This was the case; lizards (Figure 3.1) and turtles, *Clemys insculpta* (Cabanac & Bernieri 2000), responded to handling with a fever. Because reptiles do not possess autonomic temperature regulation, the rise in cloacal temperature was produced behaviorally by the reptiles seeking external infrared heat.

However, the same type of stress produced no fever in amphibians or fish. These animals thermoregulate behaviorally if their environments are equipped with a gradient of temperature. They regulate their core temperature at a higher feverish set-point by moving toward a warmer environment after various pyrogenic injections (prostaglandin, vaccine, etc.), but they never do so after mere handling or control injection (Figure 3.2).

Emotional fever does not seem to exist in animals below reptiles on the phylogenetic scale, although fever is a well-developed defense response to bacterial invasion. It may be hypothesized, therefore, that emotion—and consciousness—started in the animal kingdom with reptiles. Such a hypothesis would be reinforced with the results of the recording of another sign of emotion: tachycardia.

EMOTIONAL TACHYCARDIA

Aside from descriptions of emotional tachycardia in innumerable literary works, this response was scientifically studied by Cannon, who showed it to be one of the most reliable signs of emotion in animals and humans (Cannon 1929). Tachycardia takes place not only when an animal is manipulated by an experimenter, but also when it faces a dominant conspecific (Sgoifo et al. 1994). Heart rate may be recorded and counted telemetrically without perturbation with the aid of a radio transmitter implanted intra-abdominally or simply glued on the animal's back. Handling of a rat or mere touching of a bird so equipped immediately triggers tachycardia (Figure 3.3). Heart rates in lizards and tortoises are also accelerated when the animals are handled. It may be concluded that this is a truly emotional response when the animals are at rest and no muscular activity could have elicited the rise in heart rate.

Handling did not, however, influence the heart rates of two different anuran species—*Rana catesbeiana* and *R. pipiens*—(Cabanac & Cabanac 2000). Thus, amphibians did not display the signs of emotion common to reptiles, birds, and mammals. It may therefore be hypothesized that emotion does not exist in amphibians and other animals lower on

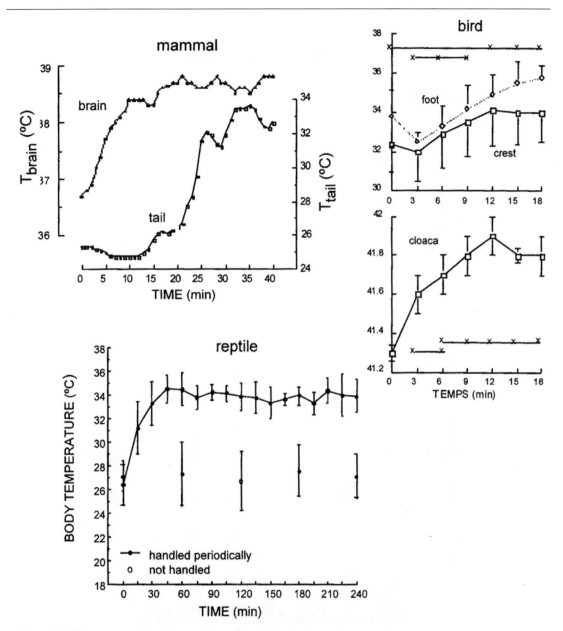

Figure 3.1. Time course of body temperature of several animals.
Mammal: brain and tail-skin temperature of a rat receiving no other treatment than repeated gentle handling. Due to intense peripheral vasoconstriction and shivering, core temperature rose from about 36.8°C to a plateau of approximately 38.5°C. The vertical dashed line shows that vasodilatation occurred only once the core temperature had risen to at least 38.2°C. Then, peripheral vasomotor responses were produced so as to mirror the core temperature, thus showing that the plateau of high level of core temperature was being regulated. This fever had no other cause than emotion (from Briese & Cabanac 1991).
Bird: mean results obtained on three cocks handled every third minute. It can be seen that response was similar to that of the rat: first peripheral vasoconstriction, then vasodilation once core temperature had risen in order to maintain a stable plateau of emotional fever (from Cabanac & Aizawa 2000).
Reptile: mean results of six sessions with the same lizard *Callopistes maculatus* that was manipulated every 15 minutes for 4 hours to record cloacal temperature. The lizard raised its body temperature behaviorally by moving beneath an infrared heating lamp. Such a behavior indicates the resetting of the temperature set-point at an emotional feverish level. The control core temperatures were obtained once daily. Each dot is the mean (± sem) of six measurements on different days (from Cabanac & Gosselin 1993).

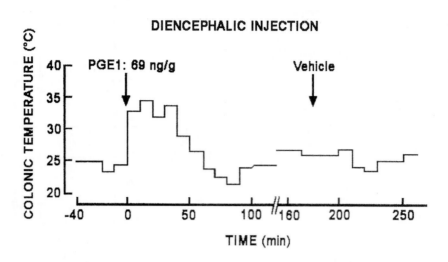

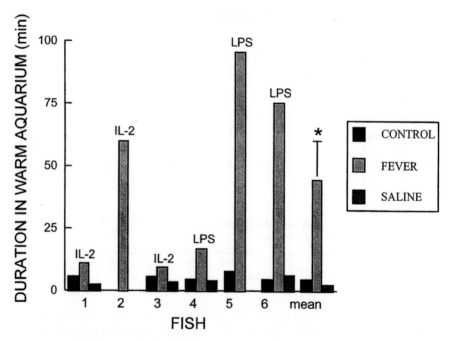

Figure 3.2. Above: Time course of the colonic temperature of one frog before and after injections at time zero of 2.5 µg Prostaglandin E_1, a potent pyrogen (left) and at time 180 min of the same volume of 0.9% sterile saline into the diencephalon. The frog was swimming in a 2-m long water temperature gradient in which it selected its preferred temperature. The animal was taken out of the tank and immobilized manually for the injections. It can be seen that the prostaglandin aroused a transient fever, as seen in the frog swimming toward warmer water. The control session, however, aroused no emotional fever, although the animal had been manipulated, immobilized, and injected before being put back in the water tank (from Myhre et al. 1977).

Below: Duration of stay in the warm half of a two-chamber aquarium by six red fish, *Carassius auratus*, each taken three times: once after saline injection, once after pyrogen injection, and once without treatment. It can be seen that pyrogens were followed by a behavioral fever but that mere handling produced no fever (IL-2 = Interleukin-2; LPS = lipoprotein saccharide) (from Cabanac & Laberge 1998).

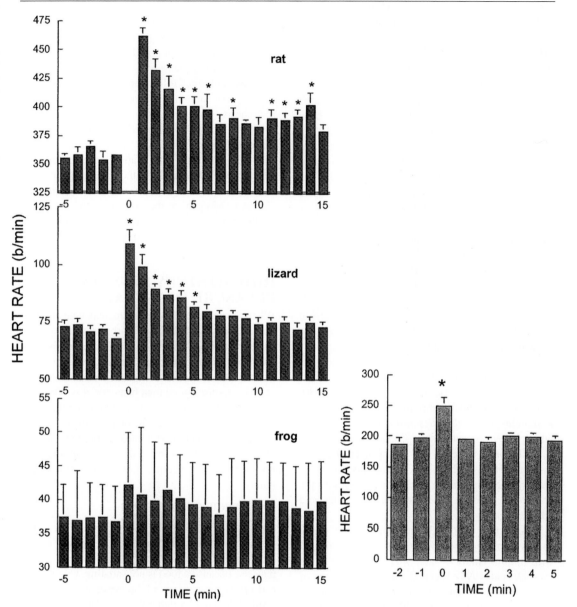

Figure 3.3. Mean heart rate (+sem) of three birds (*Gallus domesticus*), one rat, two lizards (*Iguana iguana*), and four frogs (*Rana catesbeiana*) before and after a one-minute gentle handling of the animals by the experimenter at time zero (mammal data, on left side; bird data, light gray on right). Heart rate was counted electronically from a telemetric EKG signal produced by an emitter implanted surgically in the animals' bodies. Each animal was tested over five sessions. Asterisks indicate a frequency significantly different from the data obtained before handling (ANOVA and post hoc tests, p<0.05). It can be seen that mammals, birds, and reptiles, but not amphibians, responded with tachycardia, a sign of emotion, to the gentle handling (from Cabanac & Cabanac 2000, Cabanac & Bernieri 2000).

the phylogenetic scale. It is possible that during the transition from amphibians to amniotic vertebrates, a qualitative step took place, perhaps due to a complexification of the central nervous system: the emergence of consciousness. According to Michael Lyons (1999), such a change might have been linked

to the passage to aerial life and a more complex environment, especially temperature changes and a greater demand on thermoregulatory processes. Such a hypothesis would explain the fact that reptiles are able to rapidly modify their behavior according to operant conditioning (Holtzman et al.

1999), to display ludic behavior (Burghardt 1998), and most likely to experience sensory pleasure.

ACQUIRED TASTE AVERSION: THE GARCIA EFFECT

Studying the effects of nuclear radiation, Garcia discovered a new mechanism of learning: Irradiated rats rejected some foods that seemed to have acquired aversive properties (Garcia et al. 1974). Systematic study of this new learning mechanism showed that the acquired aversion was due to digestive malaise (nausea, diarrhea) taking place in the hours following the ingestion of a new flavor. Taste aversion learning has been described in a variety of mammals, including rats (Garcia et al. 1955, Rusiniak et al. 1976), coyotes, horses, bats, ferrets, and guinea pigs (Kalat 1975, Gustavson et al. 1976, Terk & Green 1980, Houpt et al. 1990). Experiments on quails and hawks have also shown taste aversion learning in birds (Wilcoxon et al. 1971, Brett et al. 1976). In humans, taste aversion learning consists in a modification of the hedonic value of a flavor associated with a visceral illness. A flavor initially perceived as pleasant becomes unpleasant once aversion has been acquired (Garb & Stunkard 1974, Bernstein & Webster 1980, Berridge 2001). Such a shift in the hedonic value of a stimulus is called *alliesthesia* and, in humans, takes place in consciousness (Cabanac 1971, 1996). I shall come back to this point later. For the moment, let us see the results of attempts to explore the phylogenetic frontier of consciousness with the attempt to produce taste aversion in reptiles and amphibians.

Burghardt *et al* (1973) have shown that garter snakes displayed taste aversion after being injected with lithium chloride—i.e., after digestive disease (Terrick et al. 1995). Figure 3.4 shows the results of an experiment conducted to produce taste aversion in various reptiles and amphibians (Paradis & Cabanac 2002). It can be seen that *i.p.* lithium chloride was followed with taste aversion for the new baits offered to lizards and skinks (which confirms the known results in snakes) but produced no taste aversion in toads and newts. It is likely, therefore, that taste aversion learning is present in reptiles but not in amphibians.

In light of the results obtained with emotional fever, emotional tachycardia, and taste aversion, each of which were present in reptiles and absent in amphibians, it is tempting to conclude that consciousness is present in the reptiles but not in the amphibians, and thus, reptiles but not amphibians would experience sensory pleasure. Such a conclusion implies, of course, that higher vertebrates, such as reptiles, birds, and mammals, possess consciousness and pleasure. Is it possible to obtain direct evidence of sensory pleasure?

Many authors, following Aristotle, take for granted that animals experience pleasure. Such a hypothesis is most often implicitly included in the mentalistic vocabulary used to describe animal behavior. Words such as "motivation," "pain," "hedonic," "hunger," and "satiety" can be found in many papers without the authors being aware of—or intending—their implications of consciousness. However, Morgan, in the exergue at the beginning of the chapter, reminds us to be prudent in arriving at such conclusions. Yet, direct evidence can be obtained.

HOW TO STUDY SENSORY PLEASURE IN ANIMALS

When an experimenter studies mental states in non-human animals, the lack of verbal communication necessitates that the experimenter's conclusions rely solely on behavioral responses. When an experimenter studies mental states in humans and trusts verbal responses more than behavior, it is often forgotten that they also are behavior and that they provide only indirect access to other humans' mental space. Animal behavior is measurable but 1) lacks the precision allowed by verbal response and 2) is not necessarily specific. Let us examine these points.

NON-SPECIFIC RESPONSE

Food intake provides obvious examples of nonspecific sign of pleasure. Food intake does not necessarily reflect the palatability of a given food. Intake may rise because a food is not satiating. Conversely, a decrease or absence of ingestive behavior may result from apraxia rather than aversion, or a small ingestion may be the result of a strong satiating power of the food.

NON-MOTIVATION

The choice of a given food does not necessarily reflect the experience of pleasure by the animal. The selected stimulus may be the less aversive; if we take the example of intra-cranial self stimulation (ICSS) discovered by Olds and Milner (Olds 1955), this becomes apparent. Repeated self-stimulation was understood initially as due to the excitation of a "pleasure center." However, let us imagine that the electrode tip were in a reverberating structure: The

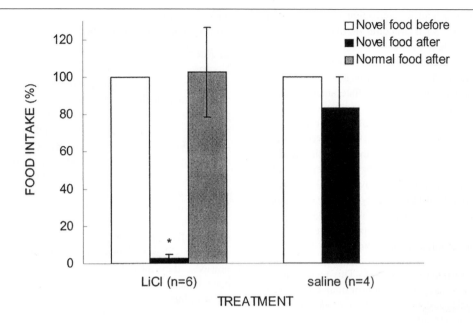

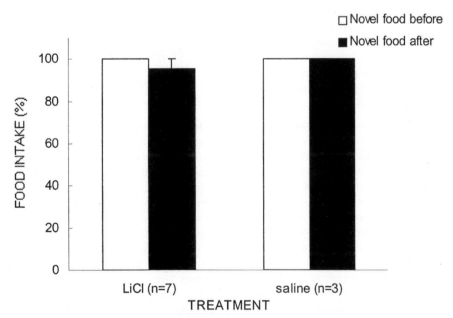

Figure 3.4. Influence of *i.p.* injection of LiCl (0.15 M, 190 mg/kg) on food intake, in % control food intake before treatment. The baits offered before lithium had never been given to the animals before.
Above: Pooled results from reptiles of four species: lizards (*Basiliscus basiliscus* and *B. vittatus*) and skinks (*Eucemes schneideri* and *Mabuya multifasciata*) offered caterpillars. *Left*: Intake of novel food before and after *i.p.* injection of LiCl (0.15 M, 190 mg/kg) and of previous normal food after LiCl ($P < 0.01$). LiCl reduced the intake of the novel food with which it was paired, but not the ingested amount of normal food. This response indicates the specificity of the influence of LiCl and, thus, the presence of taste aversion learning. *Right*: control experiment; injection of isotonic saline had no significant effect.
Below: Pooled results from amphibians. *Left*: Intake of novel food (lombricus worms) before and after *i.p.* injection of LiCl (0.15 M, 190 mg/kg). LiCl had no significant effect ($P > 0.10$). This response suggests an absence of taste aversion learning. *Right*: control experiment; injection of isotonic saline had no significant effect. (from Paradis & Cabanac 2004).

stimulation would be equivalent to the instruction "do it again." Such structures do exist in the central nervous system to facilitate repetitive behaviors without having to concentrate our attention on the command, such as the processes governing walking. If an animal would self-stimulate such a center, it would repeatedly restimulate the same structure, a behavior that could be mistaken for pleasure. We shall see below that Shizgal (1997) solved that problem. I present, nevertheless, this objection to underline the necessary prudence before accepting animal cognition when interpreting animal behavioral responses. At least three methods allow a reasonable degree of certainty regarding animal pleasure. None of the three is 100 percent proof, but the convergence of the three is convincing.

1) *The obstruction method.* This technique does not allow direct insight into animal cognition but allows us to compare attracting foods against one another or against an aversive reference. Initially, the method consisted of offering a food to a rat which had to cross an electric floor to reach the food (Warden 1931). This method permits the ranking of the animals' priorities (food or drink, reaching an offspring by the mother, reproductive partner, etc.) between the given motivation studied and the electrical floor that serves as a standard reference. Nothing forces the animal to cross the electrified floor. What is estimated is its own decision between competing motivating forces.

This method allows us to estimate sensory pleasure when an additional choice is offered to the animal in a situation in which the motivation can be satisfied without crossing the aversive barrier. In this case what is offered on the other side of the obstacle is an additional, but non-vital, reward. This is the case, for example, when a rat has regular chow and water in a heated home nest and more highly palatable foods are then offered at some distance in a lethally cold environment (Cabanac & Johnson 1983). Because the rat has access to all necessary items for survival in its nest, if it leaves the nest to venture into the −15°C environment, it may be assumed that the rat left for the pleasure of enjoying the more-palatable food.

Shizgal uses the same principle when he offers rats the choice between intracranial electrical self-stimulation and gustatory palatable stimuli. He gives rats access to two levers; one lever provides the sweet reward, the other, the electrical intracerebral stimulus. According to the intensity of one stimulus or the other, the rat orients its preference to the given lever (Shizgal 1997). Such a choice is necessarily made utilizing the hedonic experience.

2) *Rat's facial reflexes and postures.* Grill and Norgren (1978) have made a discovery that may seem minor on first examination but is quite important because of the window it opened on the rat's gustatory pleasure. They noticed that the rat responds to taste stimuli with a whole pattern of facial reflexes and postural responses characteristic of the tasted substance. Sweet stimuli elicit tongue and lip movements, lickings, paws-to-mouth motions, and head nodding. Bitter stimuli are followed with a triangle-shaped mouth, dribbling, chin-to-floor movement, and treading of forelimbs (Grill & Norgren 1978). These responses are pure reflexes, as they take place also in decerebrate rats; however, they most likely reflect hedonic experience in these animals, for when similar reflexes take place in human subjects, the reflexes are accompanied by self-reports of pleasure (Steiner 1977). In the human responses, nobody denies the presence of consciousness and pleasure. In addition, these responses in rats follow the same determinism as the hedonic experience that can be experimentally studied in humans (Cabanac & Lafrance 1990). This method permits, with a reasonable degree of certainty, the ability to study the hedonic qualities of taste sensation in rats. Similar results have been published on birds (Gentle & Harkin 1979) but the data are not as extensive as in rats.

3) *Verbal communication.* Pepperberg communicates verbally in English with African Gray parrots (*Psittacus erythacus*). Her birds are able to understand and use abstract concepts such as shape, color, hollow, larger, smaller, or different (Pepperberg 1990). After receiving appropriate verbal instructions, the birds express these concepts either verbally or with their behavior. Thinking that it should be possible to have parrots express fundamental concepts such as "good" and "bad," I acquired an African Gray parrot, a female named Aristotle, taught her the appropriate vocabulary, and attempted to answer the question of avian sensory pleasure. Carefully following Pepperberg's method, I trained Aristotle to speak to allow verbal communication. After the first step of gaining Aristotle's affection, the bird was then taught to speak by following Pepperberg's triangular method in which another person and I would speak together and would look at Aristotle only when it used understandable French words. Thus, Aristotle learned to say a few words for obtaining toys or getting my attention, e.g., "*donne bouchon*" (give cork) or "*donne gratte*" (give tickle), to obtain the appropriate reward. Lastly, the word *bon* (good) was added to the short list of words used by Aristotle. I said "*bon*" when Aristotle obtained the stimuli she had requested, e.g., "*gratte bon*" (tickle good). Aristotle started to use short expressions such as "*yaourt bon*" (yogurt good). Finally, Aristotle transferred the word *bon* to new stimuli such as *raisin* (grape), an expression I had never used myself. Such a transfer likely shows that this bird experienced sensory pleasure (Cabanac 2001). A similar method with anthropoid apes consists of using a computer to exchange concepts and ideas with the animals.

Do these methods allow, beyond a reasonable doubt, to accept that animals experience sensory pleasure? Let us look at the results they provide from various sensory modalities.

GUSTATORY PLEASURE IN RATS

It is commonly accepted that in animals, the seeking and ingesting of food is motivated by pleasure; however, invertebrates behave similarly, and it would be adventurous to accept that they experience pleasure. How can we know, then, that rats differ from invertebrates?

Richter demonstrated that adrenalectomized rats would die within 11 days after surgery but survive indefinitely if they have access to salted water (Richter 1936). Knowing that Addisonian patients also survive with a similar salt-water ingestion because salt gives them pleasure, it is tempting to accept that rats also experience ingested salt as pleasurable, but when the same adrenalectomized and salt-provided rats have their peripheral taste nerves severed, they die (Richter 1939). Also, if salted water is provided to these rats intragastrically rather than orally, the rats are less interested (LeMagnen 1955), although the biological influence of sodium chloride would remain. Finally, rats with a gastric fistula that prevents any postingestive effects drink endlessly (Bedard & Weingarten 1989). These observations, similar to those obtained in humans who report pleasure, lead to the conclusion that the sensation of taste, with its hedonic dimension, is present in rats.

Rats are also capable of quantitatively nuancing their preference of sweet molecules: polycose > maltose > saccharose > glucose (Sclafani & Clyne 1987). In addition, rats reverse their preference from sweet to pure water when dehydrated (Cohen & Tokieda 1972), a change that likely shows positive alliesthesia for water. Positive alliesthesia takes place also with initially aversive stimuli if the stimuli are yoked with sugar or a nutritive load (Mehiel & Bolles 1988, Breslin et al. 1990). In rats, as in humans (Cabanac & Fantino 1977), the internal signal for post-ingestive alliesthesia in gustatory sensation is the intraduodenal concentration of the ingested load (Kenney 1974, Cabanac & Lafrance 1990, 1992). The pattern of stimuli and responses is thus superimposed in rats and humans, with the latter reporting hedonic qualities. Animal experimentation allows further analysis of the determinism of gustatory alliesthesia. The hormonal signal involved is probably cholecystokinin (Waldbillig & O'Callaghan 1980, Ettinger et al. 1986, Mehiel & Bolles 1988). Afferent nervous pathways and centers activated during the rat's gustatory—and presumably hedonic—experience have been analyzed (Norgren & Grill 1982, Giza & Scott 1983, Berridge & Fentress 1985, Berridge & Cromwell 1990, Shizgal & Conover 1996, Shizgal 1997).

As briefly described above, the rat's facial and gestural responses bring precision—albeit indirect—to our understanding of the rat's gustatory pleasure (Norgren & Grill 1982, Berridge 2000). Figure 3.5 gives an example of such a response. When a fasted rat receives a sweet stimulus directly in its mouth, it displays an appetitive response that becomes aversive after concentrated glucose is injected into its stomach or, more effectively, in its duodenum (Cabanac & Lafrance 1992, Sederholm & Södersten 2001). Such an identical response to sweet stimuli with human alliesthesia and rat facial responses is found also with salt sensation; salted water arouses appetitive responses in salt-deprived rats and aversive ones in control rats fed normally. Such a change, therefore, looks like a positive alliesthesia for salt (Berridge et al. 1984). Rats' orofacial and gestural responses to tastes are not rigidly linked to the stimuli but, on the contrary, are flexible and also depend on the animal's internal physiological state.

Grill's method reveals other cases of positive alliesthesia after various tastes, provided these new tastes are "rewarded" with a satiating gastric load (Myers & Sclafani 2001).

The similarity of rats' reflex responses and human alliesthesia is not limited to the above variables but also extends to the influence of body weight set-point. When rats are underfed to lower their body weights, their aversive responses to sweet stimuli after a gastric load disappear until they are allowed to recover their initial body weight (Cabanac & Lafrance 1991). This is also true if a gastric fistula

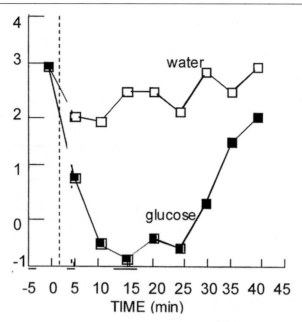

Figure 3.5. Gustatory alliesthesia in rat. Median of the responses in a group of six rats. Every five minutes, a minute sample of sucrose is injected on the rat's tongue, and its gestual and facial responses are recorded. Ordinates indicate the ratings given by a naïve observer who ignores whether the rat receives intragastric glucose or control water load. Positive = ingestive and negative = aversive responses. After the first taste stimulus, 1 g glucose in 5 ml, or 5 ml water (control session), is injected directly into the rat's stomach (vertical dashed line). After intragastric glucose, the sweet stimulus that aroused ingestive responses evolved into indifferent, then aversive, response. Gustatory alliesthesia therefore exists in rats, and in them, the same hedonic laws as in humans are likely to exist (from Cabanac & Lafrance 1990).

prevents ingestion to modify the animal's internal state (Bedard & Weingarten 1989). The influence of body weight set-point on the rat's facial reflex response can be found also in two other cases: ovarian cycle and pharmacology.

The female's ovarian state modulates facial responses to sweet stimuli (Clarke & Ossenkopp 1998); indeed, the hoarding method shows that the female rat's body weight set-point is lower under a follicular than progestative state (Fantino & Brinnel 1986).

The drug *d-fenfluramine*, which was used for some time to lower the body-weight set-point of obese human patients, reduces the appetitive response to sugar (Gray & Cooper 1996), yet this drug was demonstrated to lower the rats' body weight set-point (Fantino et al. 1986).

The rat's reflex facial and gestural responses and the human hedonic responses to alimentary stimuli are strikingly similar. Because the similarity was found valid each time it was investigated (Sclafani 1991, Shulkin 1991, Berridge 2001), these responses were proposed as a criterion of satiety—

i.e., of a mental state—to identify the neural structures responsible for that mental experience (Sawchenko 1998). On that basis, it was proposed that the *nucleus accumbens* is both the locus for the hedonic gustatory sensation and for the motivation to ingest (Peciña & Berridge 2000). The conclusion that rats experience sensory pleasure is reinforced by the behavior of Shizgal's rats. They are equipped with intra-cerebral electrodes allowing bar-pressing self-stimulation and are given access at the same time to a second lever that provides sweet water. These rats alternate their presses on both levers, but if the intensity of one of the two rewards is raised, the rats spend all of their time on the *ad hoc* lever (Shizgal 1997). A similar experiment in which rats could electrically autostimulate their brains showed that body weight loss from undernutrition lowered the threshold of self-stimulation, as if rats replaced one pleasure with another (Carr & Wolinsky 1993). All together, these results lead to the logical conclusion that rats experience gustatory pleasure. Do we find similar evidence in other orders of sensation?

THERMAL PLEASURE IN RATS

In humans, thermal sensation originates in the skin, but the pleasures and displeasures of that sensation are determined by internal signals from deep body temperature within the thermal core. However, these internal signals are also responsible for the thermoregulatory autonomic responses, especially shivering, the main defense reaction against hypothermia. Because shivering always takes place during hypothermia and because shivering gives a conscious sensation, the question remains open as to the real source of thermal cold discomfort. Is it a skin displeasure or a muscular sensation of shivering? Animal experiments answer that question. A curarized animal cannot shiver. If, while curarized, it requests heat, that means that displeasure is aroused from its cold skin and pleasure is produced by warming its skin. In experimental studies, that is what actually occurred. Because a curarized rat is paralyzed and cannot bar-press for heat, the command of the infrared heating lamp must be rendered available to it with Miller's technique (Miller 1969). This consists of recording the rat's electrocardiogram and rendering the infrared heating lamp responsive to a heart rate monitor. Thus, the rat can obtain heat by accelerating or slowing its heart rate. Results showed that, indeed, rats requested heat in the absence of shivering (Figure 3.6). Such a result allows two main conclusions:

- shivering is not necessary to produce cold discomfort; skin sensation is sufficient to motivate the animal, and
- rats experience thermal pleasure and displeasure elicited from their skin temperature.

KINESTHESIC PLEASURE IN THE RAT

Panksepp and Burgdorf (2000) have shown that rats vocalize in the ultrasonic range in response to various stimuli. These investigators found that one of the most efficacious stimuli that rats never hesitate to accept, and even seek, from a human is stroking that resembles tickling. With due caution and prudence, the authors equate the rat's vocalization to laughter. Such responses thus probably indicate the experience of pleasure in the rats.

CONFLICTS OF MOTIVATIONS IN THE RAT

When humans are placed experimentally in conflict situations, they solve their problems and optimize their behavior simply by maximizing the algebraic sum of their pleasures (sensory as well as other pleasures) (Cabanac 1992). Does the same mechanism take place when animals face a conflict of motivations?

If rats are permitted to work for water at 12°C and 36°C, they choose the cool one and drink 12°C water. However, if they have access to only one bottle and various temperatures are alternated, they drink more warm water, with the following decreasing order of volumes ingested: 36.7°C > 26°C > 14°C. It may be concluded that warm water is less rewarding, as more is needed to reach satiety (Ramsauer et al. 1974); therefore, the mere measurement of ingested volume is not the best indicator of pleasure. The following experiment was devised especially to answer the question of the rat's sensory pleasure.

Rats are located in a climatic chamber regulated at ambient temperature –15°C. In this deadly environment, the rat stays in a heated house provided with water and food (regular chow). Although there is no need for the rat to venture into the cold, it does so because during training sessions, it learned that highly palatable foods were available at the end of a 16-m zigzag maze. The palatable foods are meat paté, shortbread, and CocaCola®, offered either separately or together in various sessions. In spite of the extreme cold, the rats ventured to the end of the maze. If they found regular rat chow there, they quickly returned home and stayed there for the remainder of the session. If they found one of the more palatable foods there, however, they consumed it before returning home, then returned to the food repeatedly (Figure 3.7) (Cabanac & Johnson 1983). In a similar experiment in which the cost of food was adjusted by altering the number of bar presses, rats bar-pressed more to obtain a food when it was more palatable (Ackroff & Sclafani 1999).

Such behaviors likely indicate that rats "decided" to obtain the pleasure of ingesting the highly palatable foods. Indeed, there was no need for them to venture out in the freezing cold or to work bar-pressing; their behavior was neither stereotyped nor unavoidable. It is only after discovering the nature of the bait that the rats could compare the pleasure of ingesting the palatable bait with the displeasure of cold discomfort or muscular fatigue. Their situation was the same as that of humans who, placed in a conflict of motivations, maximize their multidimensional pleasure (Cabanac 1992).

This conclusion was also reached by Spruijt et al. (2001), who studied anticipatory behaviors in rats. Their rats displayed unequivocal signs of anticipated pleasure before any contact with a palatable food or reproductive partner. The authors accepted for animals the concept of pleasure as the common

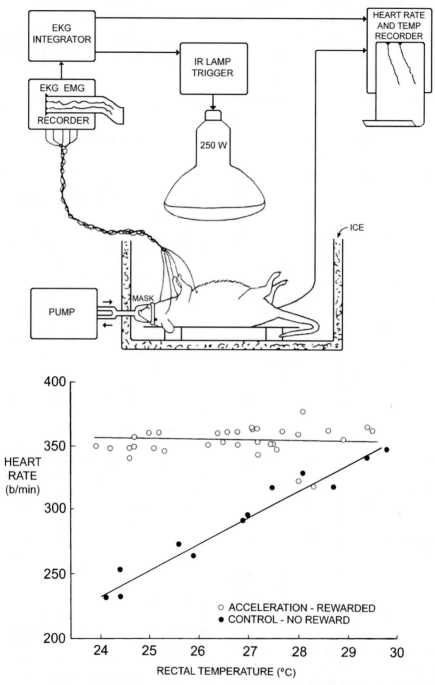

Figure 3.6. *Above*: the experimental setting. A curarized rat is unable to shiver and is kept alive with the respiratory pump. Its heart rate is recorded and integrated from its electrocardiogram (EKG). The integrated heart rate is used to trigger the infrared (IR) lamp. Heart rate and rectal temperature are continuously recorded. The unanesthetized rat can open the infrared lamp for a short burst of heat by accelerating its heart. In control sessions, the reward was obtained with a slowing of the heart rate.

Below: a sample of results. When infrared heat was yoked to accelerated heart rate, the rat maintained its heart rate steady and independent from core temperature. Such results show that heat was rewarding in the absence of shivering; it is therefore likely that rats experience skin temperature pleasure (from Cabanac & Serres 1976).

currency for tradeoffs among various motivations to optimize the resulting behavior.

REPTILES

Figures 3.3 and 3.4 demonstrate that reptile behavior is flexible and that these animals are likely to experience emotion. Is it possible to reach the conviction that they, too, experience sensory pleasure? Such a conclusion is allowed on the basis of the results of experimental conflicts of motivations sim-

ilar to those just described with rats, in which palatability was pitted against cold discomfort.

The paradigm is the same. Reptiles were placed in situations in which they had no need to venture into a cold environment because everything they needed was available under an infrared heating lamp: heat, food and water *ad libitum*. As with the rats of Figure 3.7, a bait was offered in the cold corner of the reptiles' terrarium, away from the infrared lamp. The cost is potentially dangerous, as reptiles have no

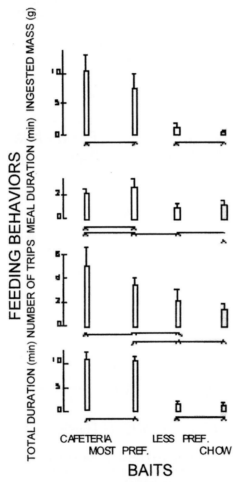

Figure 3.7. Rats are placed in a 16-m long zigzag maze. At one end they have a warm shelter with water and regular chow, *ad lib*. At the other end they can reach a bait, but ambient temperature is −15°C. Thus, they can trade cold discomfort for palatability. In CAFETERIA condition, they find not only their preferred bait but also a variety of other foods. This figure shows that they adjust the various parameters of their foraging trips according to the palatability of the bait they find on arrival to the cold end of the maze. Lines (x____x) are placed between nonsignificantly different columns. All columns on the left side of the figure are significantly higher than those on the right. This shows that palatability provided a reward that matched the discomfort arising from the cold environment (from Cabanac & Johnson 1983).

autonomic defense against hypothermia and must rely only on their behavior to thermoregulate. Three iguanas (*Iguana iguana*) lived in such a terrarium equipped with an infrared lamp, water, and regular pet chow available; the highly palatable food in the cold corner of the terrarium was fresh lettuce. On repeated sessions, the ambient temperature of the climatic chamber was varied so as to produce a wide range of ambient temperatures in the cold corner of the terrarium where the lettuce stood, while the warm corner was kept at a constant warmth.

Figure 3.8 (right) shows that several trips were made to the lettuce when its environmental temperature was lukewarm but that the number of trips to the lettuce decreased with a decrease in ambient temperature. Eventually, the iguanas remained in the warm corner and ingested only regular chow.

Figure 3.8 (left) shows the results of another experiment. The number of trips to the food by other lizards (*Tupinambis teguixin*) when no food was available in the warm corner kept rising when ambient temperature dropped. The reason for this was that the feeding bouts had to be shorter when ambient temperature was low in order for the reptiles to prevent hypothermia. Therefore, to acquire sufficient food, the Tupinambis lizards had to increase the number of short eating bouts. The difference in behavior relative to ambient temperature was striking in both experiments. It is likely that it was out of displeasure that the iguanas did not go to the lettuce when ambient temperature was low, because the behavior of Teguixin showed that they could have.

It is likely, therefore, that reptiles experience sensory pleasure in the modalities of taste and temperature sen-

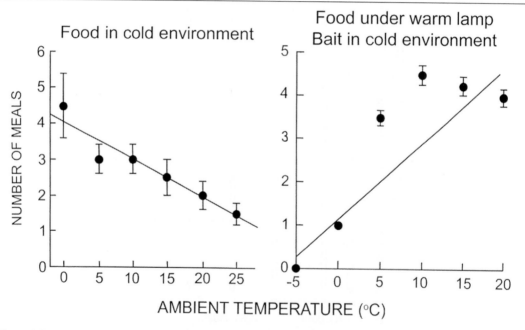

Figure 3.8. *Left:* Mean number of foraging trips (meals) of lizards placed in a situation of conflict: the food is located in a cold environment, away from the heated corner of their terrarium (from Cabanac 1985).

Right: Mean number of foraging trips (meals) of iguanas placed in a situation of conflict: the palatable bait (lettuce) is located in a cold environment, away from the heated corner of their terrarium, where regular iguana chow is available (from Balask— & Cabanac 1998).

Thus, when no alternative is left, reptiles are able to forage in the cold. The rising number of meals with decreasing ambient temperature indicates that the duration of meals was shorter in cold environment, thus preventing hypothermia. However, when the reptiles are not forced to venture into the cold because regular food is available in the warm corner, they decrease the number of trips toward the palatable bait and eventually reject it. The opposite patterns obtained in the two situations likely indicate that on the right, the conflict was between palatability and cold discomfort—two motivations indicative, therefore, of a mental space in reptiles.

sation. This conclusion casts light on the reptiles' capacity to "learn." Holtzman et al. (1999) have shown that snakes quickly learn a behavioral response when they are in an operant conditioning situation. It may be proposed that the reinforcement is a pleasant "sensation."

CONCLUSION

The evidence reviewed in this chapter leads to the following conclusions:

- As shown by signs of emotion and by learned taste aversion, it is likely that consciousness emerged in the reptilian common ancestors of present-day reptiles, birds, and mammals. The advantage conferred to the first animals that possessed consciousness was such that natural selection operated to perennialize it in their descendants. The emergence of consciousness with reptiles implies that lower animals on the phylogenetic scale do not possess it; they operate reflexively only along the program written in their nervous systems. This does not necessarily mean that the lower animals' behavior is inflexible; robots can be programmed so as to be flexible (Johnston 1999). There is no reason why amphibians and fish would not possess reflexive flexibility. Such a flexibility of behavior, however, remains elementary compared to the quasi-infinite possibilities permitted by consciousness.
- It is the hedonic dimension of sensation and consciousness that allows the optimization of behavior in reptiles and the more phylogenetically advanced animals. Maximization of pleasure produces useful behaviors.
- The pleasure of animals is probably not limited to sensory pleasure. Richard Schuster (2002) showed convincingly that mere cooperation in itself was rewarding in addition to the optimization that it might also bring. Pleasure is therefore much older than young humankind. Such remote origin is another, indirect, Darwinian indication of its usefulness. Pleasure provides an explanation for anticipatory behaviors that escape the laws of operant conditioning when foraging behavior does not provide an immediate reward (Cohen & Keasar 2000).

REFERENCES

Ackroff K, Sclafani A. 1999. Palatability and foraging cost interact to control caloric intake. *J Exp Psychol Anim B* 25:28–36.

Aristotle. 284–322 Ante. *Éthique de Nicomaque 10.* Paris: Flammarion.

Balaskó M, Cabanac M. 1998. Behavior of juvenile lizards (*Iguana iguana*) in a conflict between temperature regulation and palatable food. *Brain Behav Evolut* 52:257–262.

Barros M, Tomaz C. 2002. Non-human primate models for investigating fear and anxiety. *Neurosci Biobehav R* 26:187–201.

Bedard M, Weingarten HP. 1989. Postabsorptive glucose decreases excitatory effects of taste on ingestion. *Am J Physiol* 256:R1142–R1147.

Bernstein IL, Webster MM. 1980. Learned taste aversions in humans. *Physiol Behav* 25:363–366.

Berridge KC. 2000. Measuring hedonic impact in animals and infants microstructure of affective taste reactivity patterns. *Neurosci Biobehav R* 24:173–198.

Berridge KC. 2001. Reward learning: Reinforcement, incentives, and expectations. In: Medlin DL (ed), *The psychology of learning and motivation*. New York, Academic Press:223–278.

Berridge KC, Cromwell HC. 1990. Motivational-sensorimotor interaction controls aphagia and exaggerated treading after striatopallidal lesions. *Behav Neurosci* 104:778–785.

Berridge KC, Fentress JC. 1985. Trigeminal-taste interaction in palatability processing. *Science* 228:747–750.

Berridge KC, Flynn FW, Schulkin J, *et al.* 1984. Sodium depletion enhances salt palatability in rats. *Behav Neurosci* 98:652–661.

Breslin PAS, Davidson TL, Grill HJ. 1990. Conditioned reversal of reactions to normally avoided tates. *Physiol Behav* 47:533–538.

Brett LP, Hankins WG, Garcia J. 1976. Prey-lithium aversions. III. Buteo hawks. *Behav Biol* 17:87–98.

Briese E, Cabanac M. 1991. Stress hyperthermia: Physiological arguments that it is a fever. *Physiol Behav* 49:1153–1157.

Briese E, deQuijada MG. 1970. Colonic temperature of rats during handling. *Acta Physiol Lat Am* 20:97–102.

Burghardt GM. 1998. The evolutionary origins of play revisited: Lessons from turtles. In: Bekoff M, Byers JA (eds), *Animal play: Evolutionary, comparative, and ecological perspectives*. New York, Cambridge University Press:1–26.

Burghardt GM, Wilcoxon HC, Czaplicki JA. 1973. Conditioning in garter snakes: Aversion to palatable prey induced by delayed illness. *Anim Learn Behav* 1:317–320.

Cabanac A, Cabanac M. 2000. Heart rate response to gentle handling of frog and lizard. *Behav Process* 52:89–95.

Cabanac M. 1971. Physiological role of pleasure. *Science* 173:1103–1107.

Cabanac M. 1985. Strategies adopted by juvenile lizards foraging in a cold environment. *Physiol Zool* 58:262–271.

Cabanac M. 1992. Pleasure: The common currency. *J Theor Biol* 155:173–200.

Cabanac M. 1996. On the origin of consciousness, a postulate and its corrollary. *Neurosci Biobehav R* 20:33–40.

Cabanac M. 2001. Do birds experience sensory pleasure? *Abstr Psychonomic Soc* 6:25.

Cabanac M, Aizawa S. 2000. Fever and tachycardia in a bird (*Gallus domesticus*) after simple handling. *Physiol Behav* 69:541–545.

Cabanac M, Bernieri C. 2000. Behavioral rise in body temperature and tachycardia by handling of a turtle (*Clemys insculpta*). *Behav Process* 49:61–68.

Cabanac M, Fantino M. 1977. Origin of olfacto-gustatory alliesthesia: Intestinal sensitivity to carbohydrate concentration? *Physiol Behav* 18:1039–1045.

Cabanac M, Gosselin F. 1993. Emotional fever in the lizard *Callopistes maculatus*. *Anim Behav* 46:200–202.

Cabanac M, Johnson KG. 1983. Analysis of a conflict between palatability and cold exposure in rats. *Physiol Behav* 31:249–253.

Cabanac M, Laberge F. 1998. Fever in goldfish is induced by pyrogens but not by handling. *Physiol Behav* 63:377–379.

Cabanac M, Lafrance L. 1990. Postingestive alliesthesia: The rat tells the same story. *Physiol Behav* 47:539–543.

Cabanac M, Lafrance L. 1991. Facial consummatory responses in rats support the ponderostat hypothesis. *Physiol Behav* 50:179–183.

Cabanac M, Lafrance L. 1992. Duodenal preabsorptive origin of gustatory alliesthesia in rats. *Am J Physiol* 263:R1013–R1017.

Cabanac M, Serres P. 1976. Peripheral heat as a reward for heart rate response in the curarized rat. *J Comp Physiol Psychol* 90:435–441.

Cannon WB. 1929. *Bodily changes in pain, hunger, fear, and rage*. New York: Appleton.

Carr KD, Wolinsky TD. 1993. Chronic food restriction and weight loss produce opioid facilitation of perifornical hypothalamic self-stimulation. *Brain Res* 607:141–148.

Clarke SNDA, Ossenkopp KP. 1998. Taste reactivity responses in rats: Influence of sex and the estrous cycle. *Am J Physiol—Reg I* 43:R718–R724.

Cohen D, Keasar T. 2000. Anticipation and prediction of the future profitability of unfamiliar food sources after learning: A necessary component of sampling and learning in foraging. Proceedings of the Conference of the International Society for Behavioral Ecology, Zürich.

Cohen PS, Tokieda FK. 1972. Sucrose water preference reversal in the water deprived rat. *J Comp Physiol Psychol* 79:254–258.

Dawkins MS. 1993. *Through our eyes only? The search for animal consciousness*. Oxford: W. H. Freeman & Co.

Ettinger RH, Thompson S, Staddon JER. 1986. Cholecystokinin, diet palatability, and feeding regulation in rats. *Physiol Behav* 36:801–809.

Fantino M, Brinnel H. 1986. Body weight set-point changes during the ovarian cycle: Experimental study of rats during hoarding behavior. *Physiol Behav* 36:991–996.

Fantino M, Faion F, Rolland Y. 1986. Effect of dexfenfluramine on body weight set-point: Study in the rat with hoarding behaviour. *Appetite* 7 Suppl.:115–126.

Garb JL, Stunkard AJ. 1974. Taste aversions in man. *Am J Psychiat* 131:1204–1207.

Garcia J, Hankins WG, Rusiniak KW. 1974. Behavioral regulation of the milieu interne in man and rat. *Science* 184:824–831.

Garcia J, Kimerdorf DJ, Koelling RA. 1955. Conditioned aversion to saccharin resulting from exposure to gamma radiation. *Science* 122:157–158.

Gentle MJ, Harkin C. 1979. The effect of sweet stimuli on oral behaviour in the chicken. *Chem Sens Flav* 4:183–190.

Giza BK, Scott TR. 1983. Blood glucose selectively affects taste-evoked activity in rat *Nucleus tractus solitarius*. *Physiol Behav* 31:643–650.

Gotsev T, Ivanov A. 1962. Psychogenic elevation of body temperature. *Proc Int Union Physiol Sci* 2:501.

Gray RW, Cooper SJ. 1996. d-Fenfluramine's effects on normal ingestion assessed with taste reactivity measures. *Physiol Behav* 59:1129–1135.

Griffin DR. 1992. *Animal minds*. Chicago: University of Chicago Press.

Grill HJ, Norgren R. 1978. Chronically decerebrate rats demonstrate satiation but not bait shyness. *Science* 201:267–269.

Gustavson CR, Kelly DJ, Sweeney M. 1976. Prey-lithium aversions. I: Coyotes and wolves. *Behav Biol* 17:61–72.

Hare B, Call J, Agnetta B, *et al.* 2000. Chimpanzees know what conspecifics do and do not see. *Anim Behav* 59:771–785.

Holtzman DA, Harris TW, Aranguren G, *et al.* 1999. Spatial learning of an escape task by young corn snakes, *Elaphe guttata guttata*. *Anim Behav* 57:51–60.

Houpt KA, Zahorik DM, Swartzman-Andert JA. 1990. Taste aversion learning in horses. *J Anim Sci* 68:2340–2344.

Johnston VS. 1999. *Why we feel: The science of human emotions*. Reading, MA: Perseus Books.

Kalat JW. 1975. Taste-aversion learning in infant guinea pigs. *Dev Psychobiol* 8:383–187.

Kenney NJ. 1974. Postingestive factors in the control of glucose intake by satiated rats. *Physiol Psychol* 2:433–434.

Krughoff DA. 2000. *Anna my green friend. A journey of discovery love and healing*. Hoyleton, IL: Myiguana.com.

LeMagnen J. 1955. Le role de la réceptivité gustative au chlorure de sodium dans le mécanisme de régulation de la prise d'eau chez le rat blanc. *J Physiol Pathol génér* 47:405–418.

Lyons M. 1999. Personal communication. ATR Media Integration and Communication Research Laboratory, Kyoto, Japan.

Mehiel R, Bolles RC. 1988. Hedonic shift learning based on calories. *B Psychonomic Soc* 26:459–462.

Miller NE. 1944. Experimental studies of conflict. In: Hunt JM (ed), *Personality and the behavior disorders*. New York, Ronald Press:431–465.

Miller NE. 1969. Learning of visceral and glandular responses. *Science* 163:434–445.

Morgan CL. 1894. *An introduction to comparative psychology*. London: Walter Scott.

Myers KP, Sclafani A. 2001. Conditioned enhancement of flavor evaluation reinforced by intragastric glucose II. Taste reactivity analysis. *Physiol Behav* 74:495–505.

Myhre K, Cabanac M, Myhre G. 1977. Fever and behavioural temperature regulation in the frog *Rana esculenta*. *Acta Physiol Scand* 101:219–229.

Norgren R, Grill HJ. 1982. Brain-stem control of ingestive behavior. In: Pfaff DW (ed), *The physiological mechanisms of motivation*. New York, Springer-Verlag:99–131.

Olds J. 1955. Physiological mechanism of reward. In: Jones MR (ed), *Nebraska symposium on motivation*. Lincoln: University of Nebraska Press.

Panksepp J, Burgdorf J. 2000. 50-kHz chirping (laughter?) in response to conditioned and unconditioned tickle-induced reward in rats: Effects of social housing and genetic variables. *Behav Brain Res* 115:25–38.

Paradis S, Cabanac M. 2003. Taste aversion learning in reptiles but not in amphibians. Manuscript submitted.

Paradis S, Cabanac M 2004. Flavor aversion learning induced by lithium chloride in reptiles but not in amphibians. *Behavioural Processes*, 67:11–18.

Parr LA. 2000. Measuring emotion in chimpanzees. Atlanta, GA: Emory University. Doctoral dissertation.

Parr LA, deWaal BM. 1999. Visual kin recognition in chimpanzees. *Nature* 399:647–648.

Peciña S, Berridge KC. 2000. Opioid site in nucleus accumbens shell mediates eating and hedonic 'liking' for food: Map based on microinjection Fos plumes. *Brain Res* 863:71–86.

Pepperberg IM. 1990. Some cognitive capacities of an African Grey Parrot (*Psittacus erithacus*). In: Slater PJB, Rosenblatt JS, Beer C (eds), *Advances in the study of behavior*, Vol. 19. New York, Academic Press:357–409.

Ramsauer S, Mendelson J, Freed WJ. 1974. Effects of water temperature on the reward value and satiating capacity of water in water-deprived rats. *Behav Biol* 11:381–393.

Renbourn ET. 1960. Body temperature and the emotions. *Lancet* 2:475–476.

Richter CP. 1936. Increased salt appetite in adrenalectomized rats. *Am J Physiol* 115:155–161.

Richter CP. 1939. Transmission of taste sensation in animals. *T Am Neurol Assoc* 65:49–50.

Rusiniak KW, Gustavson CR, Hankins WG, *et al.* 1976. Prey-lithium aversions. II. laboratory rats and ferrets. *Behav Biol* 17:73–85.

Sawchenko PE. 1998. Toward a new neurobiology of energy balance, appetite, and obesity: The anatomists weigh in. *J Comp Neurol* 402:435–441.

Schuster R. 2002. Cooperative coordination as a social behavior: Experiments with an animal model. *Hum Nature* 13:47–83.

Sclafani A. 1991. The hedonics of sugar and starch. In: Bolles RC (ed), *The hedonics of taste*. Hillsdale, NJ, Lawrence Earlbaum Associates:59–87.

Sclafani A, Clyne AE. 1987. Hedonic response of rats to polysaccharide and sugar solutions. *Neurosci Biobehav R* 11:173–180.

Sederholm F, Södersten P. 2001. Aversive behavior during intraoral intake in male rats. *Physiol Behav* 74:153–168.

Sgoifo A, Stilli D, Aimi B, *et al.* 1994. Behavioral and electrocardiographic responses to social stress in male rats. *Physiol Behav* 55:209–216.

Shizgal P. 1997. Neural basis of utility estimation. *Curr Opin Neurobiol* 7:198–208.

Shizgal P, Conover K. 1996. On the neural computation of utility. *Curr Dir Psychol Sci* 5:37–43.

Shulkin J. 1991. Hedonic consequences of salt hunger. In: Bolles RC (ed), *The hedonics of taste*. Hillsdale, NJ, Lawrence Earlbaum Associates:89–105.

Spruijt M, vandenBos R, Pijlman FTA. 2001. A concept of welfare based on reward evaluating mechanisms in the brain: Anticipatory behaviour as an indicator for the state of reward systems. *Appl Anim Behav Sci* 72:145–171.

Steiner JE. 1977. Facial expressions of the neonate infant indicating the hedonics of food related chemical stimuli. In: Weiffenbach JE (ed), *Taste and development*. Bethesda, MD, US Dept HEW:173–189.

Terk MP, Green L. 1980. Taste aversion learning in the bat, *Carollia perspicillata*. *Behav Neural Biol* 28:236–242.

Terrick TD, Mumme RL, Burghardt GM. 1995. Aposematic coloration enhances chemorecognition of noxious prey in the garter snake. *Anim Behav* 49:857–866.

Waldbillig RJ, O'Callaghan M. 1980. Hormones and hedonics cholecystokinin and taste: A possible behavioral mechanism of action. *Physiol Behav* 25:25–30.

Warden CS. 1931. *Animal motivation, experimental studies on the albino rat*. New York: Columbia University Press.

Wilcoxon HC, Dragoin WB, Kral PA. 1971. Illness-induced aversions in rat and quail: Relative salience of visual and gustatory cues. *Science* 171:826–828.

Young PT. 1959. The role of affective processes in learning and motivation. *Psychol Rev* 66:104–112.

4

The Science of Suffering

Marian Stamp Dawkins

INTRODUCTION

The most exciting and, at the same time, the most inaccessible, feature of animal life is that of conscious experience. So elusive is it that thoughtful, knowledgeable people can hold diametrically opposite views about its presence in other species. Many dog owners, for example, assume without any doubt that their pets experience pleasure, pain, and suffering much as we do. Many scientists, however, adopt a skeptical "well, we can never know" attitude and regard the question as unanswerable and unscientific to investigate further.

That leaves us with a problem. If we are seriously concerned with suffering in nonhuman animals, we have to be prepared to tackle the issue of conscious experience head-on. When applied to human beings, we use the word suffering to cover a multitude of negative emotional states such as fear, boredom, and frustration, but we also imply *conscious experience* of these states. To talk about suffering in nonhuman animals is to assume that there is a conscious being there to do the suffering. Consciousness thus grabs center stage and refuses to go away. Wrong would be the comfortable way out by just saying that it is too difficult or unscientific, or assuming the luxury of being able to get on with our core research and push the "deep problem" to one side while we do so. For those of us who work in the field of animal welfare research, suffering, with its implications of conscious experience, is the day job, our mainstream concern. If it were not, we could regard sick or injured animals in the same light as we do sick or injured plants. Veterinarians would be in the same business as tree doctors—concerned to save the lives of deteriorating organic beings without having to worry about the possibility that the beings might be feeling anything

in the process. The very real possibility that, in addition to damaged physical health, animals might experience terrifying or painful emotions is what gives animal suffering its moral and ethical importance.

But how can the study of something as private and unobservable as animal consciousness be made scientific when science is, by definition, concerned with what is public and observable? How can we have a science of suffering when the central subject matter itself relies on assumptions that we can see no way of putting to critical test? For every claim that an animal is consciously experiencing fear or pain, someone else can make a counter-claim that it is simply going through the motions but without the accompanying feelings that humans would have. No critical test exists that separates claim and counter-claim. They are stuck together like an object and its shadow—where one goes, the other goes; when one moves, the other moves.

I am not claiming to have any magic solutions to the very real problems of studying animal suffering in a scientific way, but I will try to sketch out a road map of what we have achieved to date. By acknowledging the problems and facing the limitations of our own methods, we can find working solutions even if complete certainty still eludes us. I want to begin, however, by explaining exactly why a scientific approach to consciousness remains such a problem. The revolution started by the late Don Griffin (1981, 1992) that gave rise to a wealth of recent studies in animal cognition may have left the impression that the problems with studying the mental lives of animals have all but disappeared. Recent books on animal emotions (e.g., Masson & McCarthy 1996, Bekoff 2000) may have implied that scientists have now thrown off all their inhibitions about studying what animals feel. In fact, the floodgates were opened, but some regaining of control is now needed. The discipline of studying what is testable and observable is still as necessary as ever, and the last thing a science of suffering should be is a free-for-all in which untested speculation is allowed to go unchecked.

WHY IS ANIMAL CONSCIOUSNESS (STILL) SUCH A PROBLEM?

For all our recent understanding of how the brain works and our increasingly sophisticated methods for monitoring brain activity, we still do not understand a basic fact about ourselves: how does a lump of nervous tissue give rise to conscious experience? An "explanatory gap" still exists between cause (neuronal activity) and effect (what we subjectively feel). As T. H. Huxley (1866) put it nearly one-and-a-half centuries ago, the fact that anything so remarkable as a state of consciousness comes about as a result of the activation of a lump of nervous tissue is just as mysterious as a magic carpet or a genie coming out of a lamp. Anatomical and physiological facts do not tell us what it feels like to be in pain (Young & Block 1998).

This ignorance about the causal origins of our own consciousness severely limits the extent to which we can study its existence in other species. We cannot, from scientific evidence, decide whether other animals are "like us" in the relevant respects that would lead them to suffer "like us" because we don't know what those relevant respects are. Is it the possession of a particular brain structure? The ability to use language? Is it evolutionarily old and therefore likely to be present in many animal species? Or is it a recent development, confined to ourselves and possibly the great apes? There have, of course, been hundreds, if not thousands, of books and papers published in the past ten years claiming to have explained consciousness in some way or another or to have demonstrated consciousness in other species, but it is important that we recognize that the explanatory gap still exists. On one side of the gap we have our feet on the ground in the familiar territory of observable physiology and behavior. On the other side of the gap is the mysterious land of subjective experience, a land whose existence we can each, separately, be sure of because we live in it inside our own skulls, but whose connection to the observable world of science is still essentially unknown. To bridge that gap, we each have to make what amounts to a leap of faith and make some sort of assumption that this or that animal is "like us" in

having brain structures or behavior that leads it to suffer like us. Different people use different bridges (Dawkins 2001). Some put their faith in brain structures, others in behavioral similarities; some argue that the evolution of language was a defining moment in the evolution of consciousness (Dennett 1996).

The situation is further complicated by recent research that has indicated that even for human beings, many actions may be guided unconsciously. We may even have *unconscious* emotions, that is, emotional states in ourselves of which we appear not to be consciously aware but which have a major effect on what we do (Damasio 1999, Berridge & Winkielman 2003). For example, drug addicts will press one of two levers to give themselves a shot of stimulant or morphine even when the dose difference between the levers is so low that there is no autonomic response difference and the addicts report detecting no difference subjectively. In other words, they continue to press the lever that gives the very slightly higher dose even though they are not consciously aware of it being higher (Fischman & Foltin 1992). In people who are not drug addicts, a briefly presented image of a person with a happy face causes the people to consume more fruit juice immediately after seeing the face and to say that the fruit juice tasted better, even though they have no conscious awareness of having seen the face (Berridge & Robinson 2003).

People with brain injuries have provided even more convincing evidence that our behavior can be controlled by pathways in the brain that do not necessarily lead to conscious experience. Patients with damage to the orbito-frontal cortex have particular difficulty with reversal tasks—that is, learning to do the opposite of what they have just learned to do, such as learning that they will get a reward by touching a white panel, and not a black one, when previously it was the black one that delivered the reward. The odd thing is that the patients can often rationalize and say that they know (consciously) which panel they should now press but that they can't help themselves pressing the wrong one—the unconscious pathway seems to take them over (Rolls 1999).

The phenomenon of "blindsight" again illustrates that alternative routes may exist by which our behavior can be controlled, which may or may not be reported to consciousness. Weiskrantz (1997) described a patient, DB, who had a visual field deficit caused by the surgical removal of a small non-malignant tumor in area V1 if his visual cortex that rendered him incapable of seeing in a particular portion of his visual field. (His eyes were receiving information correctly, but the part of his visual cortex that received messages from the relevant part of the retina was damaged.) Weiskrantz discovered, however, that if he asked DB to perform some action that involved the use of the "blind" area of his visual field, such as reaching out and touching it or naming it or saying how it was oriented, DB performed well above chance. He was apparently "seeing" in his blind area but had no conscious awareness of seeing anything at all. In fact, at times, he would become quite angry with Wieskrantz for asking him to comment on things he couldn't see and was genuinely astonished when told that he was answering correctly.

Even in ourselves, then, we are not always conscious of what we are doing or feeling. We, the archetypically conscious animals, do much without being conscious of what we are doing. We largely discover this mismatch between conscious awareness and action by using language and asking people what they are experiencing, a route that is obviously unavailable when studying other species. However, there are ways of getting around the language barrier if we are prepared to be ingenious enough about it. For example, rhesus monkeys have been shown to exhibit "blindsight" by being given a key to press when they know they can see a stimulus but still have to touch a particular part of a screen to get a reward. Monkeys with orbito-frontal damage press the correct part of the screen and the key indicating that they can see the stimulus when it is presented to an area of normal vision, but when the stimulus is presented in their "blind" areas, the monkeys press the key indicating that they can't see anything but continue to press the screen in the correct place for a reward (Cowey & Stoerig 1995). They are behaving as though they can see the stimulus on the screen (because they touch it) but press a key that indicates that they can't see the stimulus in a way that is remarkably similar to Weiskrantz's patients.

All this emphasizes that attributing conscious experiences to nonhuman animals is still a major scientific and a philosophical problem. We may decide for ourselves that many nonhumans are conscious and that animal care legislation should be based on this assumption on the grounds that it is better to give them the benefit of the doubt than to risk inflicting pain and suffering on conscious crea-

tures. But we should not make the mistake of thinking that the problems have gone away. The element of something magical remains, which is distinctly embarrassing for any science. The genie comes out of the lamp, but we haven't a clue how he does it. To make any progress at all in the face of this appalling ignorance, we have to avoid two opposite dangers. On the one hand, we must avoid thinking that there is no problem with discussing the conscious experience of suffering in animals—that there is no explanatory gap, in other words, and that scientists are just being difficult and narrow-minded in insisting that there is. As I hope I have shown, the explanatory gap is huge, more like a wide river than a ditch that can be hopped over. And on the other hand, we must avoid being completely put off by the difficulties of understanding what other species might experience. I am urging caution in developing a science of suffering and of trying to cross the gap, not giving up altogether. For whatever it is and whatever its still-mysterious relationship with nervous tissue turns out to be, consciousness is a biological phenomenon. It arises in ways we don't yet understand from the laws of physics and chemistry. It has evolved by natural selection, either because it was under direct selection pressure and conferred an evolutionary advantage of its own or because it was linked to something else that did. The fact that we don't yet understand how it arises does not mean that trying to make some sort of headway can't be scientific. If consciousness is a biological phenomenon (and how could it not be?), biology without it is incomplete. We have to make a start.

WHAT IS SUFFERING?

When applied to ourselves or to other people, we use the word "suffering" as an umbrella term to cover an enormous range of states. We talk about people suffering from thirst, suffering from cold, suffering from a bereavement, suffering from exam nerves as well as suffering from pain or from a facial disfigurement that is not painful. These states are all very different, not just in their physiological manifestations, but also in how people react to them and, above all, in what it is like to consciously experience them. So what makes us apply this one word to such diversity and give it any sort of meaning? The answer is that they are all states that can be described as unpleasant, states that we would rather not be in if we could possibly avoid them, states that we would get out of if we had the means to do so. And the unpleasantness must be either prolonged or severe. We would not count a mild itch as suffering, but an itch that persisted, was so severe that it stopped us doing other things, or both would count as suffering.

The word "suffering" as used in everyday speech about people subtly links together what they are doing (piling on more clothes and huddling over the radiator), their autonomic responses (shivering, white fingers), and what we assume their conscious experiences to be (by using our own experiences of what it is like to be really cold and showing the same symptoms). With other people, this assumption is based on a combination of their anatomical and physiological similarity to ourselves, the fact that they are taking steps to alleviate their situation, and the fact that what they say they are experiencing fits very closely with what we say when we are shivering and huddled over a radiator. When it comes to other species of animals, by following the reasoning from the previous section, we should be careful to consider these different attributes separately. We can observe a rat building a bigger nest and we can record its autonomic responses. We can even be impressed by the fact that the rat learns to press a lever to give itself more heat and is thus taking advantage of the opportunity to change the situation it is in. Thus far, we are still in the realm of the scientifically observable and the objectively measurable. But the conscious experience of the rat—that is still on the other side of the explanatory gap. Strictly speaking, despite similarities of behavior in lever pressing in rats and reported pleasantness of the temperature of different stimuli applied to the skin (Cabanac 1992), it still requires a leap of faith—not a scientific step—to say that the rat consciously experiences cold in the way we do. Even Cabanac's ingenious experiment in which humans and rats had to report the pleasantness or otherwise of different temperatures applied to the skin (the humans verbally, the rats by how much they would press a lever to repeat the stimulus) requires this leap of faith, an untestable assumption of similarity.

Many, if not most, readers of this book may be quite prepared to make this leap of faith, regarding it as a small gesture, indeed, toward the well-being of other species. This is a reasonable and practical decision—one, in fact, that I share—but it should be on record that we go beyond the boundaries of present-day science when we do this and that the very use of the term "suffering" taken from a human to a nonhuman context can be challenged. Because it is in such widespread use, I shall, however, continue to use the word "suffering" for nonhuman animals. For the rest of this chapter, it will be used to describe a range of states indicated by a variety of physiological and behavioral symptoms but having in common that the animals are seen to take steps to change their states in some way, either by following an innate response (such as building a bigger nest) or, even more convincingly, by learning to perform an arbitrary task such as pressing a lever conveniently provided for them by a human to bring about some change in their environments. Major causes of suffering are physical injury, disease, lack of water, lack of food, temperatures that are too low or too high, shortage of space to move around in, lack of stimulation, lack of social companions, and so on. The issue of whether, in addition, the animals with these causes have prolonged or severe unpleasant conscious experiences (pain, thirst, hunger, fear, boredom, frustration, etc.) while they are doing the behavior or showing the physiological symptoms is one which, as I hope I have now explained, is still open.

PHYSICAL HEALTH AND MENTAL HEALTH IN ANIMALS

Good physical health is the foundation of animal welfare. Conversely, disease, injury, and deformity are major sources of suffering. But there is more to good welfare than not dying of disease and injury. A wild animal confined in a cage could be well fed and in apparently good health and yet "suffering" from fear due to the presence of humans or frustration at not being able to run over long distances as it would do in the wild. Equally, an animal that had been injured but was apparently able to behave more or less normally might not be "suffering" from its injury. In each case, we need to take into account not just the animal's physical health but its mental or psychological health as well.

Innumerable attempts have been made over the past 20 years to address this issue of assessing animal psychological health and to define measures of welfare. About the only universally accepted conclusion is that there is no single measure of welfare (Dawkins 1980, Broom 1998, Mason & Mendl 1993). Moreover, there is a distinct lack of agreement about how the various measures that are now available—physiological, biochemical, or behavioral—should be put together to give a picture of whether the animal is suffering. With more and more "measures" of welfare available to us (stress hormones measured from saliva and feces, stereotypies, remotely measured heart rate, changes in skin temperature, vocalizations and so on), the temptation is to draw up longer and longer lists of symptoms in the belief that this gives a more and more accurate picture of whether the animal is suffering. But there are major problems with this approach. Heart rate, respiratory rate, and levels of corticosteroids, for example, rise naturally during coitus, exercise, and in anticipation of food. Many vary naturally with time of day, temperature, or breeding condition (Wingfield et al. 1997). Some stereotypies may be indicative of poor welfare, but others may be an animal's way of calming itself down and coping with its environment (Mason & Latham 2004). Some repeated stereotypic behaviors may even be beneficial enrichments. For example, non-nutritive sucking in calves (repeated sucking on an empty teat that might be interpreted as a sign of "frustration") has beneficial effects on the calves' digestion (de Passille et al. 1993).

The definition of "suffering" given in the previous section, however, suggests that we should not be too concerned by the difficulties posed by these individual measures, but should instead be asking for evidence that animals are in some way taking steps to change the state they are in—either to remove themselves from situations they find aversive or to gain access to something they want. That is the key to whether they are "suffering." Various measures such as heart rate changes or stereotyped behavior do not, in themselves, give us sufficient evidence on this point; an increase in heart rate, for example, could come about because an animal is desperately trying to get away from something it dislikes or because it is happily engaged in a pleasurable activity. The prey animal fleeing from its predator and the predator excitedly chasing it will show very similar autonomic responses (to running fast), but the valence (whether the situation is positive or negative for the animal) could be completely different. The key to identifying animal suffering, then, is to find ways of asking animals how they themselves view the situation. The animals themselves need to tell us whether they want to escape and avoid a situation in the future or whether they have what they want and want to repeat the experience. And, as suffering contains an element of an unpleasant experience that is intense, prolonged, or both, we also need a measure of *how much* an animal wants to escape or repeat the experience so that its negative preferences can be in some way ranked and the worst ones avoided.

The two keys to establishing whether an animal is suffering are thus 1) whether it is physically healthy and 2) whether and how much it wants to change the situation it is in. Good welfare is a situation in which animals are healthy and have what they want. Suffering occurs when they are injured, diseased, deprived of something that is important to them, or desperately trying to escape from something they find aversive—in other words, do not have what they want. Although it may sound simplistic, by asking these two questions—and giving them primacy in all investigations of animal welfare—we can begin to make sense of a whole range of controversial measures of welfare. For example, people have argued both for and against the idea that animals suffer if they are unable to perform the natural behavior patterns shown by wild members of their species. Many behavioral enrichment studies are undertaken on the assumption that the more natural an animal's behavior is, the better its welfare must be. But is this necessarily so? The two key questions can help out here. Does being able to do the behavior improve the animal's health? Does the animal show evidence of wanting to do the behavior, and if so, how much? If the answer to both of these questions is no in a particular instance, then the argument for saying that that particular animal suffers if unable to do that particular natural behavior is weak or non-existent. But if the answers are positive, then the case is much stronger. Similarly, to find out if high levels of corticosteroid hormones or high levels of stereotypic behavior indicate suffering, the same two questions can help to provide the answer.

The two key questions also help us keep our heads when confronted with otherwise apparently intractable questions such as whether broiler (meat) chickens suffer when kept at the high stocking densities that are common in commercial farms. It has been claimed (e.g., Webster, 1994) that at commercial stocking densities, the chickens' welfare is severely compromised and that there should be legislation to compel farmers to give the birds more space. But would this really improve welfare? To find out, we need to know 1) whether it would improve bird health and 2) whether the birds themselves show evidence of wanting more space and of trying to get away from each other if they possibly could. Without this evidence, we flounder in well-meaning but ill-founded speculation about what might or might not reduce bird suffering. With it, we can come to at least some conclusions about how to increase broiler chicken welfare (Dawkins et al. 2004).

Suffering, then, includes both conscious experiences and indications of what animals themselves want. Conscious experiences may remain, strictly speaking, inaccessible to scientific investigation, but as we shall see in the next section, we now have means of establishing what animals want. What is striking about the recent research that has been done in this area is that animals have in many cases told us so accurately and so clearly what they want that it becomes difficult to believe that we have not gained access to what they feel.

MEASURING WHAT ANIMALS WANT

The simplest and most obvious way of establishing what an animal wants is to give it some sort of choice or preference test, such as what sort of flooring it wants to stand on. Although this gives us a first indication of how the animal sees its environment, it has the disadvantage that even plants, which do not have nervous systems, can exhibit preferences and even be said to make choices. Many plants, for example, choose to grow toward light, and the parasitic plant dodder (*Cuscuta europeaea*) finds a new host bush on which to feed by growing rapidly but only "choosing" to insert itself into bushes in a good state of nutrition (Kelly 1992). If the first bush it encounters is poorly nourished, dodder moves (grows) onward to search for something better. Unless we wish to include plants in our discussion of "suffering," we need to find a way of measuring what an animal wants that excludes the vegetable kingdom, which means excluding choice behavior controlled by simple tropisms and taxes.

Tropisms and taxes are innate, fixed responses that enable organisms to approach or avoid different stimuli, such as responses to light by plants or to humidity gradients in woodlice. These fixed responses enable the organism to "choose" the environments that are favorable to them and avoid those that are not, but only in a very simple, preprogrammed way that does not allow much variation or response to novelty. One of the major steps in evolution occurred when organisms evolved the ability to go beyond this simple hard-wiring and learn arbitrary connections between stimuli or learn to do completely arbitrary actions to achieve certain goals (Rolls 1999). If an organism can learn to associate almost any stimulus with, say, a food reward, then natural selection can no longer "build in" the rules for action. If an organism can learn to go away from a red light because it signifies danger and toward a green one because it signals food, but can equally well make the opposite associations, then simple innate rules such as "move toward red" are no longer adequate. Rolls (1999) argues that the learning of arbitrary connections demanded something

new: emotion. Negative emotions such as fear act as negative reinforcers in the sense that the animal learns to avoid or not to repeat a set of arbitrary actions if fear is the consequence of those actions. Positive emotions such as pleasure act as positive reinforcers that lead animals to repeat other arbitrary actions (Broom 1998). Rolls argues that only organisms with the capacity for such arbitrary learning to obtain reinforcers have emotions and therefore, by implication, the capacity for suffering. In this, he differs from Cabanac (1992, 1996), who sees a pleasure-suffering continuum as common to any organism exhibiting choice. Rolls' argument is essentially an evolutionary one. Only organisms with the capacity for building associations using rewards and punishments needed emotions. Before that, there was no need for emotion. All behavior could be hard wired. Rolls' theory provides a justification for distinguishing different types of choice mechanisms. By focusing not so much on choice itself (which would have to include plants) as on what animals find positively and negatively reinforcing, we have an essential tool for assessing emotional states in animals. Let us see how close this can take us to answering the question of whether or not they are suffering.

Broiler chickens have been selected for very fast growth rate, so much so that they reach a slaughter weight of 2–3 kg in only 39–42, or even fewer, days. As a direct result of this abnormal growth, the chickens often become very lame and find it difficult to walk. The exact causes and pathological symptoms of this lameness are quite varied, but whatever the etiology, it constitutes a major welfare issue. Kestin et al. (1992) devised a simple but effective way of scoring the walking ability of large numbers of birds on farms. Each bird is watched and given a score from 0 (walks well) to 5 (extreme difficulty in walking). This 6-point score is widely used on UK farms, and many companies have strict policies of culling birds with scores of 3 or more. The score also correlates well with leg health and biomechanical damage (Corr et al. 1998). There are several ways in which lame birds could potentially suffer, ranging from being physically unable to get to the feeders and drinkers and thus slowly dying of starvation or thirst, to the direct pain caused by deformed or diseased legs. What evidence is there that the birds suffer from being lame?

The most striking evidence is that the birds will learn to associate arbitrary colors with drugs known to have pain-relieving properties in humans (Danbury et al. 2000). Birds with healthy legs and good walking ability (score 0) have no preference for food containing carprofen, which is a non-steroidal anti-inflammatory drug, but birds scored as "lame" (3 or more) learned to choose red or blue food, depending on whether it contained the pain-reliever. Lame birds realized the connection between something arbitrary in their environment (food of different colors) and consequent result (pain reduction). They also started walking better when they had ingested the analgesic. The lame birds were thus meeting all the criteria we have been discussing in relation to suffering, over and above the obvious one of their impaired locomotion. They showed that they wanted to get out of the state they were in by using the only opportunity they had, namely, voluntarily ingesting a pain-relieving drug. Furthermore, their ability to do this extended beyond a simple choice and involved learning an arbitrary association between the color of a food and the long-term consequences of doing so. In the face of such evidence, it becomes very difficult to maintain that lame broiler chickens are simply "going through the motions" without any conscious experience of pain. Of course, it is still possible that they have no accompanying feelings that correspond to what we would call pain, but the explanation of why they choose the analgesic and why their walking improves when they eat it if they do not consciously experience pain becomes quite complex, and the simplest explanation is that they suffer from pain and want to relieve it.

We now have many other examples of animals expressing not only what they want but also how much they want it or want to get away from it. Laboratory rats, for example, do not just choose to be with other rats when given the opportunity; they will also work hard (press a lever many times) to gain access to companion rats—much harder than they will work to gain access to a larger cage or a cage with novel objects (Patterson-Kane et al. 2002). Once again, the animals are showing that they want to change their situation (from being alone to being with other rats), that they can learn to do so by associating an arbitrary and unnatural response (pressing a lever) to achieve their goal, and that the goal is sufficiently important to them that even when it becomes more difficult (the lever does not have the desired effect unless it is pressed a large number of times so that the rat has to expend time and energy to get what it wants). Mink (*Mustela vison*) will learn to push extremely heavy doors to gain access to water where they can swim (Mason et al. 2001), and the rise in urinary cortisol level that occurs when they are locked out of their swimming bath is only slightly lower than that which occurs when they are locked out of the compartment where they are fed. Because being locked out of an empty cage or a cage with an alternative nest site resulted in no change in urinary cortisol level, this suggests that the mink place considerable value on access to water to swim in and could potentially suffer if kept in cages where they had no access to it.

There are, of course, difficulties that can be raised with the interpretation of such experiments (Fraser & Matthews 1997). For example, mink appear to value resources differently depending on whether they can see what they are working for (Mason & Warburton 2003). However, the fact that many factors, including an individual animal's developmental history, the precise choices they are offered, and how they are offered them can all potentially affect what the animal wants and how much it wants it, is no reason for abandoning this approach. For a start, other methods of assessing suffering such as use of cortisol levels, heart rate, or frequency of stereotyped behavior are just, if not more, subject to such factors. Rather, it is a reason for being particularly careful about how and in what circumstances such tests are administered. We need to study animal suffering *in situ*—in the places where there is the greatest concern for their welfare such as commercial farms. Rushen (1986) was concerned about whether sheep suffered from the various things that were done to them in the course of removing their fleeces. By all obvious behavioral criteria such as struggling and running away, sheep find the process of being confined, manhandled, and shorn highly aversive. Rushen used a specific aversion-learning technique to demonstrate which parts of the commercial shearing process were most aversive to commercially kept sheep. He arranged it that the sheep had to run down a race (corridor), at the end of which they were treated in one of three ways: they were allowed to run unhindered back to their flock, they were restrained for a few minutes in a sheep-holding machine, or they were put in the machine and subjected to simulated shearing (clippers were moved backward and forward, but no wool was removed). The sheep were subjected to their respective treatments for a total of seven trials, and on each trial, their speed of running down the race was recorded and used as a measure of how aversive they found the treatment. Sheep that were not caught continued to run down the race at great speed without hesitation and without needing to be pushed. Sheep that were restrained, however, showed increasing reluctance to run, and by the fourth trial, sheep that were both restrained and sheared had to be pushed continuously to make them move at all. Rushen concluded that sheep find both restraint and shearing aversive but find shearing more aversive than restraint alone.

Rushen also investigated whether sheep suffered from being electro-immobilized because manufacturers of commercial electro-immobilization devices claimed that these were an effective but humane way of restraining animals and avoiding stress because the animals didn't struggle. Using the same technique of measuring reluctance to run down a race after repeatedly experiencing either physical or electro-immobilization, Rushen found that electro-immobilization was significantly more aversive and that furthermore, the reluctance of the sheep to keep running down the race was directly proportional to the amount of current applied. Despite the fact that the sheep did not struggle, it was clear that they disliked being electro-immobilized and tried not to repeat the experience.

CONCLUSIONS

Measuring what animals want, particularly by arbitrary operant response or stimulus-response associations, is a powerful tool for assessing one major element of what we mean by suffering—that animals are highly motivated to remove themselves from a situation or to obtain something they have not got. It enables us to be objective about the situations that different animals find aversive or attractive even though this may be very different from our own view of the world; it enables us to rank their preferences or aversions so that we can give them what they most want and remove what is most aversive for them. It requires only a very minimal leap of analogy—that what we experience when we will work hard to avoid or obtain something is not unlike what other animals do when they perform a similar task. Examples such as the self-administration of analgesics makes the leap seem not only minimal but simply the most plausible explanation available. We may not have solved the mystery of consciousness, but for practical purposes of assessing animal welfare and suffering, this may not be necessary.

REFERENCES

Bekoff M (ed). 2000. *The smile of a dolphin: Remarkable accounts of animal emotions.* New York: Discovery Books/Random House.

Berridge KC, Robinson TE. 2003. Parsing reward. *Trends Neurosci* 26:507–513.

Berridge KC, Winkielman P. 2003. What is an unconscious emotion? (The case for unconscious 'liking'.). *Cognition Emotion* 17:181–211.

Broom DM. 1998. Welfare, stress and the evolution of feelings. *Adv Stud Behav* 27:317–403.

Cabanac M. 1992. Pleasure: The common currency. *J Theor Biol* 155:173–200.

Cabanac M. 1996. On the origin of consciousness, a postulation and its corollary. *Neurosci Biobehav R* 20:33–40.

Corr SA, Gentle MJ, McCorquodale CC, *et al.* 1998. The effect of morphology on the musculoskeletal system of the modern broiler. *Anim Welfare* 123:145–147.

Cowey A, Stoerig P. 1995. Blindsight in monkeys. *Nature* 373:247–249.

Damasio AR. 1999. *The feeling of what happens: Body and emotion in the making of consciousness.* London: Heinemann.

Danbury TC, Weeks CA, Chambers JP, *et al.* 2000. Self-selection of the analgesic drug carprofen by lame broiler chickens. *Vet Rec* 146:307–311.

Dawkins MS. 1980. *Animal suffering: The science of animal welfare.* London: Chapman and Hall.

Dawkins MS. 2001. Who needs consciousness? *Anim Welfare* 10:S19–S29.

Dawkins MS, Donnelly CA, Jones TA. 2004. Chicken welfare is more influenced by housing conditions than by stocking density. *Nature* 427:342–344.

Dennett DC. 1996. *Kinds of minds: Toward[the actual title as published is "Towards..."] an understanding of consciousness.* London: Weidenfeld and Nicolson.

de Passille AM, Christopherson R, Rushen J. 1993. Non-nutritive sucking by the calf and posprandial secretion of insulin, CCK and gastrin. *Physiol Behav* 54:1069–1073.

Fischman MW, Foltin RW. 1992. Self-administration of cocaine by humans: A laboratory perspective. In: Bock GR, Whelan J (eds), *Cocaine: Scientific and social dimensions,* Vol. 166. New York, Wiley:165–180.

Fraser D, Matthews LR. 1997. Preference and motivation testing. In: Appleby MC, Hughes BO (eds), *Animal Welfare.* Wallingford, CAB International:159–173.

Griffin DR. 1981. *The question of animal awareness.* New York: Rockefeller University Press.

Griffin DR. 1992. *Animal minds.* Chicago: University of Chicago Press.

Huxley TH. 1866. Lessons in elementary physiology. Reprinted in *Collected essays by T.H. Huxley.* London, Macmillan (1893).

Kelly CK. 1992. Resource choice in *Cuscuta europaea*. *P Natl Acad Sci USA* 889:12194–12197.

Kestin SC, Knowles TG, Tinch AE, *et al.* 1992. Prevalence of leg weakness in broiler chickens and its relation to genotype. *Vet Rec* 131:190–194.

Mason GJ, Cooper J, Clareborough C. 2001. Frustrations of fur-farmed mink. *Nature* 410:389.

Mason GJ, Latham NR. 2004. Can't stop, won't stop: Is stereotypy a reliable animal welfare indicator? *Anim Welfare*: in press.

Mason GJ, Mendl M. 1993. Why is there no simple way of measuring animal welfare? *Anim Welfare* 2:301–319.

Mason GJ, Warburton H. 2003. Is out of sight out of mind? The effects of resource cues on motivation in mink, *Mustela vison*. *Anim Behav* 65:755–763.

Masson J, McCarthy S. 1996. *When elephants weep: The emotional lives of animals*. London: Vintage.

Patterson-Kane EG, Hunt M, Harper D. 2002. Rats demand social contact. *Anim Welfare* 11:327–332.

Rolls ET. 1999. *The brain and emotion*. Oxford: Oxford University Press.

Rushen J. 1986. Aversion of sheep to electro-immobilization and mechanical restraint. *Appl Anim Behav Sci* 15:315–324.

Webster J. 1994. *Animal welfare: A cool eye toward[the actual title as published is "…towards…"] eden*. Oxford: Blackwell Science.

Weiskrantz L. 1997. *Consciousness lost and found: A neuropsychological exploration*. Oxford: Oxford University Press.

Wingfield JC, Hunt K, Breune C, *et al.* 1997. Environmental stress, field endocrinology, and conservation biology. In: Clemmons JR, Buckolz RT (eds), *Behavioral[the actual title as published is "Behavioural…"] approaches to conservation in the wild*. Cambridge, Cambridge University Press:95–131.

Young AW, Block N. 1998. Consciousness. In: Bruce V (ed), *Unsolved mysteries of the mind*. Hove, Psychology Press:149–179.

5

Affective-Social Neuroscience Approaches to Understanding Core Emotional Feelings in Animals

Jaak Panksepp

The study of emotions is undergoing a renaissance in human psychology and brain imaging. Discussion of affective processes is reaching a fever pitch, even though mere words that describe affects hide a deeper mystery that is inaccessible to those who are not willing to probe the brain (Zajonc 1980). Unfortunately, human brain imaging gives some neurogeographic correlates of affective processes, some intriguing relationships among brain areas, but little of the essential neural detail to really know what we are talking about. To understand what affects truly are, one must probe into a neural jungle that seems impenetrable unless we use animal models. And few who work on brain details are willing to grant other animals rich emotional lives.

Except for studies of fear learning (for example, see LeDoux 1996), there is no institutional devotion to the study of emotions in nonhuman animals. Those who support neuroscience research remain hesitant to conceptualize the neuro-mental lives of animals. This is because, for an entire century, we have not had the disciplinary will to move beyond the safe harbor of logical positivism in animal brain research to try to fathom some deeper organizational principles. There is little recognition of the fact that behavioral neuroscience is the only discipline that can profoundly illuminate the nature of affective processes in other animals, and thereby, in humans. I have sought to change this bias in human psychology and animal brain science for the past thirty years. Ultimately, the common scientific denominator for every animal welfare issue is the question: What is the nature of affective experience, and which among the living species have such experiences?

Since the emergence of the Cartesian tradition in psychological science, which definitively split the study of behavior and mind, scientists have deemed it wise to remain paradigmatically skeptical of the position that animals have emotionally experienced mental lives. To this day, those who would deny affective feelings to animals continue to prevail over those who do not. Despite the cognitive revolution starting 40 years ago, this remains true both on the neuroscientific academic landscape and among those who control federal funding policies in the pursuit of behavioral neuroscience research. Attempts to translate work on animal investigations of affective states (through a study of their emotional behaviors) to the human domain are commonly considered misleading and inappropriate. *Anthropomorphism*—the suggestion that human feelings may have substantive parallels in animal brains—remains as much of a sin as ever, despite the emergence of scientific forms of anthropomorphism that are based on the deep functional homologies in mammalian brains that arise from a massively shared genetic heritage (Burghardt 1997; Panksepp 1998a, 2003a).

Too many investigators still believe that human consciousness, affective and otherwise, emerges from higher brain functions that most other mammals do not have. This view often ignores the substantial data-base that suggests that raw affective experiences may reflect an ancient form of consciousness that we share remarkably homologously with many other animals (Panksepp 1998a, 1998b, 2003a, 2003b, 2003c). Having been steeped in British-associationist and American learning-theory traditions, few behavioral neuroscientists are explicitly willing to take a deep evolutionary position and entertain, as did Darwin (1871), the probable existence of human-like emotional feelings in animals.

My own approach has been neuroethological and premised on the data-based assumption that a study of the instinctual emotional circuits in the brains of various other mammals is currently the best strategy to understand affect (Panksepp 1982). This vision is premised on the fact that electrical brain stimulation can evoke several coherent emotional responses with accompanying affective feelings (Panksepp 1998a). The fact that electrical "garbage" applied to specific sites in the brain can yield psychobehavioral coherence indicates that various affect-generating emotional operating systems exist in deep subcortical regions of the brain. Unfortunately, many people wish to envision these systems as psychologically vacuous "output" components. They are probably wrong. This issue was well put by Walter Hess (1957), who received the Nobel Prize for his work on brain stimulation-induced autonomic and behavioral changes in cats from the hypothalamus, including the first descriptions of brain stimulation-induced anger responses. In considering such subcortical conceptual issues, including the rage facilitated by decortication, he noted that "American investigators label this condition 'sham rage.' In our opinion, the behavior that we find manifested here should be interpreted as *true* rage, and its appearance is aided by the suppression of inhibitions that go out from the cortex." This reasonable perspective never became mainstream on the Anglo-American scene, and very little discussion of potential affective states in animals occurs among behavioral neuroscientists.

Silence also prevails about translating animal emotions to the human estate. However, if a profound continuity in the emotions of animals and humans exists, anthropomorphism and zoomorphism may be used as scientific guides to investigate the neural nature of human feelings and the animalian[1] side of our emotionality. This is also the only way we will get credible neuroscientific data about animal emotions and associated feelings. In short, a variety of basic affects arise, most probably, from activities of ancient neural systems that we share with many other animals. As emphasized by pioneers such as Zajonc (1980), affective feelings have an immediacy in consciousness, which leads to rapid preferences that require no cognitive inferences. Less well appreciated is that the scientific analysis of these brain systems cannot proceed effectively without the emergence of new paradigms such as a cross-species *affective neuroscience* (Panksepp 1998a).

NON-NEUROSCIENCE AND RADICAL-NEUROSCIENCE PERSPECTIVES ON AFFECTIVE FEELINGS IN ANIMALS

At present, as has occurred in earlier eras, a growing animal behavior literature exists that vigorously seeks to affirm that other animals have emotional lives (for example, see Bekoff 2000, this volume). At the time of this writing, a most recent offering of this popular genre is Jeffrey Masson's (2003) *The Pig Who Sang to the Moon,* which focuses on the emotional lives of farm animals. Prior to this, Masson had written three other popular books on the emotional lives of domestic dogs and cats and some wild animals. Literature in this vein is largely based on anecdotes, which most experimental scientists would only consider the prelude to rigorous work. Because of ultra-behavioristic biases, LeDoux (2002) has sought to situate my thirty years of work in this genre while ignoring my empirical contributions (for a pointed rebuttal to that approach, see Panksepp 2002). One especially impressive collection of pointedly harvested anecdotes from established scientists makes a compelling case for scientists to open the Pandora's Box of animal feelings once more (*The Smile of a Dolphin,* edited by Bekoff [2000], in which I also shared several observations). Unfortunately, such efforts do not contribute to an understanding of the underlying brain processes but do make a strong statement about what needs to be explained. That type of evidence should coax neuroscientists to openly consider new ontological positions and epistemological strategies to work on problems of ultimate concern that have long been neglected. Hopefully, this is gradually happening, even though long-held scientific beliefs seem as resistant to change as religious beliefs.

Without a "mechanistic" analysis of affect (such as the triangulation method noted above), animal stories must remain forever in the pre-scientific stage of observations, even though their acceptance could lead to a new respect for other creatures and ever better behavioral studies of the true capacities of other animals. One of the aims of the study of animal emotions should be to achieve a point where the evidence for animal feelings is so strong that some type of cultural commitment followed by institutional resources will be available to work out the important underlying principles. There is reason to believe that this type of data will eventually provide a foundation for our understanding of human consciousness.

The ultra-skeptical behavioristic (positivistic) position—still the most common attitude in neuroscience—fails to explicitly acknowledge that the essence of modern science is accurate measurement and productive prediction rather than definitive explanation. It should be quite obvious that coherent causal analysis of affects, as of all dynamic brain functions not clearly evident in behavior, cannot ever be complete and cannot proceed effectively without guiding theory. However, once workable theories have been generated to guide productive predictions (non-circular observations), the main issue that matters is the resulting *weight of evidence.* In my estimation, *the weight* is already massively in favor of the conclusion that many nonhuman animals have various affective experiences that resemble our own, rather than the conclusion that they do not. Most behavioral neuroscientists appear to still be in timid denial about this.

Regrettably, one dimension commonly missing from the non-neuroscience discussion of animal emotions is what type of data should be deemed sufficiently compelling, one way or the other, for agreeing on the general nature of the brain mechanisms by which feelings are generated. This has been one of the great problems in all types of consciousness studies. In the study of the cognitive aspects of consciousness (e.g., sensory awareness), leading thinkers assert that good evidence can be obtained only if one makes levels of consciousness an independent variable in experimental studies (Baars et al. 2003). This can be achieved by concurrently studying stimuli that are presented both unconsciously and supra-liminally (at levels that are clearly perceived by humans) and then determining differences in how the brain processes the two modes of delivery. This, of course, is not a workable strategy when it comes to affective issues. Although emotion-provoking stimuli can certainly be presented subliminally or masked with blocking stimuli, that is not quite the same as having effectively manipulated emotional states. When it comes to affective states of consciousness such as anger or hunger, it is hard to imagine that time-locked delivery of external *information* can be used as a relevant variable. The internal states of the brain-mind must be manipulated by other means. Brain stimulation and pharmacological challenges, at several levels of "dosing," could be envisioned (and this has been done with drugs of abuse, albeit the few published studies are very problematic; for critique, see Panksepp et al. 2004). A bigger dilemma is that we do not have the tools to manipulate many of the relevant neurochemical systems of the brain, for that kind of knowledge necessarily must come from animal brain research (where talk of affect typically continues to be deemed in poor taste).

As noted already, my "triangulation" solution to this problem is as follows. Because most now accept that humans have various emotional feelings, we can utilize animals that seem to exhibit outward indicators of similar experiences as model systems for working out the underlying neuro-details. If we discover seemingly critical variables that appear to control animal emotional experiences, such as certain distinct neurochemical controls, then we can evaluate the quality of the data by doing the converse experiments—predicting and evaluating the types of affective changes that should result in humans. For instance, if we administer the relevant neurochemical agents derived from animal studies to increase or reduce separation distress (as monitored by their vocalizations, *vide infra*), and humans indicate the predicted increases or decreases in affective feelings of sadness, then by the criterion of *weight of evidence*, we are justified in concluding that all the data, taken together, support the conclusion that the animal species tested also *probably* have the corresponding types of emotional experiences. This conclusion would be reinforced if animals exhibit behavioral choices such as conditioned place preferences and aversion, which are congruent with the existence of those types of positive and negative affective states.

The animal behavioral brain research and human mind research could fertilize each other much better than they have for the past half century. An example of this process, proceeding reasonably well with the separation distress system, has recently been summarized (Panksepp 2003a). We originally started to study the separation distress system of animal brains with the theoretical premise that this emotional function (a psychological "pain") evolved from more ancient physical distress systems. As will be detailed toward the end of this chapter, correlative human functional magnetic brain imaging (fMRI) now affirms that the distress of social exclusion does "light-up" some of the pain-mediating areas of the human brain (for example, see Eisenberger et al. 2003). With additional pharmacological studies that are known to modulate separation distress in animal models (e.g., opioids and opioid receptor antagonists), as well as relevant deep brain stimulation studies, if they are medically possible (for example, see Bejjani et al. 1999), we could obtain further triangulation on the critical causal issues. This highlights that the study of affect in animals must eventually go hand in hand with the neuroscientific study of affect in humans. A behavior-only approach in other animals and a psychology-only approach in humans is not a robust enough strategy to understand the deep neuro-evolutionary nature of animal or human feelings.

Also, it is important to remember that the study of animals in the laboratory has a variety of distorting effects on their behavioral capacities. Thus, whatever criticisms one might make about the use of anecdotal data of animal behavior in the "real world," it at least is not subject to the distortions brought about by common laboratory practices. Perhaps the biggest problem during the twentieth century was the widespread use of individual housing, and now we know that these animals should not be deemed the norm. Rather, animals that are socially housed, with abundant opportunities for engagement with complex environments, should always have been the norm if we were going to draw conclusions about the true cognitive and emotional capacities of animals. How investigators could ever have accepted individual housing of animals in sterile environments as the norm from which to contrast behavioral changes is simply perplexing, in retrospect. But even the mere social-housing of animals in restricted laboratory situations should be deemed a questionable practice for deriving estimates of what "normal" animals are like. This is rarely recognized, and before proceeding to a discussion of the core emotional systems of animals, it may be worth dwelling on this typically unrecognized dilemma as well as at least one other spooky type of variable that can easily pollute traditional behavioral experiments.

DISTORTED EMOTIONAL PROCESSES IN "KENNELIZED" ANIMALS

The widespread use of individually housed animals in behavioral research has generally led to the recognition of the possibility that social species tested in this way will not adequately represent the behavior of "normal" animals. As a result, much of the published behavioral work could be deemed to be the study of emotionally abnormal creatures, and because of that (as well as new animal care regulations), test animals are more commonly group housed. Does this solve our problems? Perhaps not.

Animals often seem less intelligent and emotionally flexible than they are because they have been reared for most of their lives in very restricted environments. This is most dramatically the case in *factory farms* where animals are used as mere machines to produce human foodstuffs. In the canine literature, we see a syndrome of emotional inflexibility emerge if animals are kept for most of their early lives in social groups within restricted kennel environments. These kennel-dogs exhibit a behavioral syndrome characterized by extreme and persistent timidity and anxiety, and at times, fear-biting when removed to an unfamiliar environment (Scott et al. 1973). This seems to be a milder form of the syndrome produced by complete isolation housing. Our attempts at providing pharmacologically assisted therapy to such dogs were generally unsuccessful even though opioids such as morphine had some small effect in facilitating obedience training and social rehabilitation (Panksepp et al. 1983). We regret that we could not obtain resources to evaluate the drugs in combination with social therapies, as modern biological psychiatry will need to do in future human studies (Panksepp & Harro 2004).

The "kennel syndrome" raises some important issues for studying emotions in laboratory animals and may help explain why the sophistication of behaviors described in anecdotes (for example, see Bekoff 2000) may be hard to replicate under standardized laboratory conditions. Let us consider whether "simple" laboratory animals such as rats and mice, although reared socially, might become "kennelized" because they are reared in such strictly limited laboratory environments. This possibility emerged recently in a project in which we were following up the fascinating phenomenon of chirping that young rats exhibit during their rough-and-tumble play and that can be markedly amplified by human tickling (Panksepp & Burgdorf 2003). As will be discussed later, there are many reasons to believe that this response reflects a social-joy response. Although adult rats are not as responsive as young animals, they do typically chirp quite a bit if they had been accustomed to such interactions in youth. Females generally remain much more responsive to such social overtures than males; however, in a recent experiment using a large group of five-month-old females who had had little experience with human contact other than routine cleaning, we were in for a surprise. To our initial chagrin, these animals were fearful or unresponsive to our tickling overtures and only with extended experience did some become responsive. As a group, they never became as responsive as animals that had had abundant human contact early in life. Our provisional conclusion is that practically all *adult* rats that have had little social experience outside their typical laboratory "kennel environments" can, in fact, be appropriately deemed "kennel rats." If this is a reasonable interpretation, it is to be expected that their behavior will not represent the behavior of animals that have had rich and diverse early experiences.

The lesson may be simple. To become socially flexible, animals need a variety of early social contacts. A growing literature says that the better the quality of care that mother rats provide to their offspring, the more behaviorally and emotionally robust those offspring will be for the rest of their lives (Meaney 2001). As it turns out, this maternal effect explained decades of earlier research indicating that human handling (or the mere separation of animals from their mothers and littermates for short periods) had a similar effect. Apparently, the main reason this was happening was that mothers were attending to their offspring more intensely when they were returned to their cages. The lesson appears to be clear: If we neglect the emotional and exploratory needs of our animals, they will give us impoverished answers concerning the potential depth of their mental lives. A large environmental and social "enrichment" literature now exists that supports the importance of such factors (for summary and relevant developmental issues, see Panksepp 2001a).

There are many other examples of the contextual effects that may be dramatically influencing our "well" controlled laboratory findings. For instance, rodents are very sensitive to ultrasonic noise that we cannot hear that can be very disturbing to animals. Sales et al. (1988) documented how standard metal cage cleaning practices can be a background stressor that modifies the behavior of laboratory animals. Temple Grandin (this volume) outlines various disturbing stimuli that can exist in the rearing and slaughtering of domestic farm animals. Finally, let us consider the fact that our laboratory rats and mice are dramatically more sensitive to olfactory cues than we are, along with the fact that they have intrinsic olfactory-based fear systems. Thirty years ago, we discovered that some of our pharmacological effects were being biased by the fact that our rat lab was situated close to a cat lab. Once the cat lab was terminated, some of the drug effects we had seen with anxiolytic drugs diminished dramatically. Years later we figured out why—simply returning some cat smell back into the environment was sufficient to resurrect our original findings. We, as many

others, have now evaluated the fear-evoking effects of predatory odors such as those of cats, foxes, and ferrets on rodent behavior, and the effects are striking. Figure 5.1 highlights the effects of a single exposure on the play of rats. The contextual fear effect, in a totally clean cage, long outlasted the short exposure to a small sample of cat hair. This unconditional fear effect was mediated via the vomeronasal systems, as opposed to the main olfactory apparatus (Panksepp & Crepeau 1990).

How many behaviorists have carried predatory odors from their pets to the laboratory, biasing results in indeterminate ways? I know laboratories that to this day keep cats and rats in nearby animal holding rooms, and we must suspect that these background effects may be polluting rigorously controlled results in presently unknown ways. Such mistakes are easy to make if we are not sensitive to the emotional states of our animals. Indeed, even our laboratory rats recognize individual investigators and like some more than others (as could be evaluated by the number of their 50-kHz "happy" chirps as investigators approach their cages, *vide infra*).

Regrettably, the majority of neurobehaviorists remain in denial concerning the likelihood that their animals experience emotions. Let us now examine the major lines of evidence that strongly point toward the existence of various types of affective states in animals.

EVIDENCE FOR INTERNAL AFFECTIVE STATES IN ANIMALS

So what should coax us toward the position that other animals do have affective states? We obviously cannot be certain on such difficult issues, but just as with Pascal's famous wager concerning the existence of a god, we are surely less likely to partake in ethical travesties if we provisionally accept the mind-affirming position that animals do have emotional feelings than by accepting that they do not. But there is also substantial experimental evidence to support this. The existence of affective feelings is premised largely on a behavioral neuroscience evidence 1) that other mammals are attracted to the same drugs of abuse that we humans are; 2) that, as far as we know, our human emotional feelings are dependent on very similar subcortical brain systems situated in deep brain regions where evolutionarily homologous "instinctual" neural systems for emotional responses exist in animals (Panksepp 1998a, Damasio 1999); and 3) that artificial activation of the deep brain systems that can

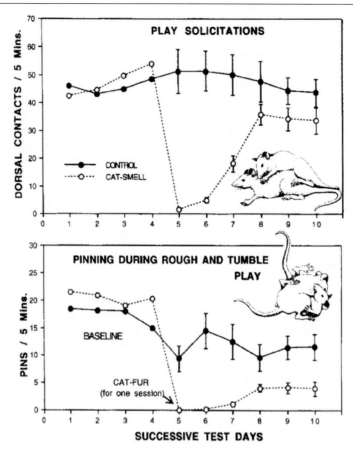

Figure 5.1. A single exposure to a small ~20 mg sample of cat hair on the fifth day of testing inhibited rat rough-and-tumble play completely, and this contextual fear response continued for up to five subsequent test days, at higher levels with the measure of pinning (bottom) and less with the dorsal contact measure of play solicitation (top). Reprinted from Figure 1.1. of *Affective Neuroscience* (Panksepp 1998a) with permission of Oxford University Press.

trigger emotional actions are liked and disliked by animals (as measured by a host of approach and avoidance measures).

1. Perhaps the most robust evidence for affective states in animals comes from the studies of drugs of abuse in humans and animals. Many humans find drugs that activate opiate receptors in the brain, and those that facilitate dopamine activity, to be pleasurable or euphoria-producing. The types of brain changes that correlated with these effects have been documented by Drevets et al. (2001) and Volkow et al. (2002). The fact that animals exhibit strong desires for similar agents and that those approach effects are mediated by similar brain systems is so impressive that skepticism about the existence of

affective states in other animals seems unjustified. Indeed, one can predict drugs that will be addictive in humans quite effectively from animal model studies of this generalized desire system. Animals show anticipatory-positive affective vocalizations (50-kHz "self-reports") in environments where they have received desirable drugs, and negative vocalizations (22-kHz "complaints") when placed in locations where they have received aversive drugs (Burgdorf et al. 2001).

2. The second major line of evidence comes from neurological data suggesting that the major loci of control for affective experiences in both animals and humans is subcortically situated in very similar regions of the brain (Panksepp 1985, Liotti & Panksepp 2004). It is within such deep regions of

the brain where neuroanatomical and neuro-functional homologies abound in all brain functions, to the extent that most neuroscientists feel confident that work conducted on animal models does reveal general principles of function that hold true for the human species. Of course, there is a reticence to accept that a primitive affective form of consciousness exists far below the cerebral mantle, which is substantially independent of neocortical functions, but the evidence is quite consistent (Panksepp 2003a). Even though many fMRI human brain imaging studies of emotion have not yielded clear differentiation of basic emotional systems (Phan et al. 2002, Murphy et al. 2003), the most extensive PET studies have yielded striking differences between sadness, anger, fear, and happiness, with patterns that often match animal data based on localized brain stimulation (Damasio et al. 2000). Although higher cognitive functions add an enormous richness to human emotional life and that of animals as well, the evidence indicates that the "energetic" engines for the Cartesian "Passions of the Soul" find their loci of executive control in homologous cross-species sub-neocortical regions of brains (Panksepp 2000, 2001b, 2001c, 2002, 2003a, 2004a).

3. The third, and perhaps most definitive, line of evidence comes from brain-stimulation studies. The areas that generate behavioral indicators of positive and negative affective states in humans and animals are remarkably similar, and the most powerful effects come from subcortical brain areas where homologies are very striking. The most reasonable conclusion from this is that not only are many affective states related to such deep brain systems but also that the resemblances between animals and humans on such dimensions are truly remarkable. Indeed, localized brain stimulation of specific brain areas, whether electrical or neurochemical, is the most compelling way to try to scientifically dissect what types of emotional systems animals truly have.

In short, the simplest ontological position is a *dual-aspect monism*, which assumes that instinctual emotional behaviors and affective states are pretty much reflections of the global neurodynamics of essentially the same brain systems. This assumption also allows us to develop effective empirical strategies to try to understand human emotional feelings through a careful study of animal brains. I will now briefly summarize some of these universal emotional systems that exist in mammals and many other vertebrates, and then focus on the most inter-esting and subtle of these systems—the ones that mediate social emotions such as separation distress, social bonding, and playfulness. A detailed compendium of the evidence for these and other core emotional systems shared by humans and other animals is available in Panksepp (1998a), so at this juncture, I will provide only a nut-shell listing of the key systems that exist as processes of the affective-emotional apparatus.

SEVEN CROSS-SPECIES CORE EMOTIONAL SYSTEMS AND RELATED MOTIVATIONAL STRUCTURES

Let us briefly consider some of the intrinsic emotional systems that are shared evolutionary "gifts" in all mammals. These systems are important for the emotionally motivated behaviors of both animals and humans. Even though there are bound to be many differences in detail among different species, to the best of our knowledge, the general trajectories and executive neurochemistries are the same. We do not have sufficient room to cover these systems in detail here, so I will merely introduce them with brief evolutionary vignettes. (Interested readers are directed to *Affective Neuroscience* for a more comprehensive coverage [Panksepp 1998a].) After these preliminary introductions, however, three of the systems (1, 6, and 7) will receive a bit more attention. It should also be noted that there are many other affect systems in the brain—e.g., hunger, thirst, disgust, pain, and the various pleasures of sensation—but they are not properly placed in the "emotion" category, where the defining features are intrinsic central nervous system states with strong and complex, instinctually characteristic, action urges such as SEEKING, RAGE, FEAR, LUST, CARE, PANIC, and PLAY.[2]

1. A remarkable system that has emerged from brain research is that which mediates the appetitive desire to find and harvest the fruits of the world. A reasonable label for this general-purpose desire system is the SEEKING system. Animals "love" to self-activate—to self-stimulate—this system in addictive ways. For decades, this system was considered to be a reward-pleasure system, but it is now generally agreed that it is better conceptualized as a basic, positively motivated action system that helps mediate our desires, our foraging, and our positive expectancies about the world rather than the behavioristic concept of *reinforcement*. It courses from the midbrain to the ventro-medial forebrain and is

activated strongly by the meso-limbic dopamine systems (Ikemoto & Panksepp 1999). This system is presently being intensively studied in animals as a general purpose learning system, as it is essential for animals to pursue all the fruits of their environments, including the satisfactions to be had through the emotional systems already discussed, such as the seeking of safety when one is scared or seeking retribution when one is angry (for summary, see Panksepp & Moskal 2004). This system can even energize dreams (Solms 2000). The fact that this system can be used for so many seemingly distinct motivations, operating in both positive and negative emotional situations, has been a difficult finding for psychology to assimilate. However, it is a reasonable way for evolution to have constructed a general-purpose motivational urge that is needed in many situations, helping maintain a fluidity in behavior as well as the operations of the cognitive apparatus (Ikemoto & Panksepp 1999)

2. Where does anger come from? It is commonly aroused by frustration and the inability to behave freely. An easy way to make a baby angry, to arouse its RAGE system, is to restrain its arms to the side of its body. If adults do not get what they want, they are also much more likely to become enraged than they otherwise would be. Of course, adults can modulate their anger in ways that children and animals cannot, because it is often wise to keep this emotional system well regulated. Just like every sub-cortical emotional system, higher cortico-cognitive systems are able to provide inhibition, guidance, and other forms of emotional regulation. We presently have no psychotropic medications that can specifically control pathological anger, but the neuroscientific analysis of RAGE circuitry may eventually yield such tools for emotional self-regulation. Many peptide candidates, most prominently Substance P, have been identified along this amygdala-hypothalamic-midbrain operating system for affective attack, or, as the behavioral neuroscientists prefer, the "defense motivation system."

3. Our world has abundant dangers, many of which we need to learn about, and others which we intrinsically FEAR. Fear is commonly evoked by the anger of other, bigger and stronger, people and animals. Although the stimuli that provoke fearfulness in different species are often different (e.g., darkness in humans and light in rats; we like cats, but rats have an intrinsic fear of cat smells), the core structures of the FEAR system are remarkably similar across all mammalian species. Neuroscientists have unraveled the details of the brain circuitry that mediate some of the fears, but they have tended to focus on information that enters the FEAR system via so-called "high roads" (more cognitive-perceptual inputs to brain areas such as the amygdala), and via the so-called "low road," the more primitive sensory inputs to the same brain regions, from which descends what might be called the "Royal Road"— the evolved FEAR system itself, which governs the instinctual action apparatus that intrinsically helps animals avoid danger (Panksepp 1998a). Several distinct fear systems may exist in the brain, but the FEAR system appears to be the one inhibited by modern anti-anxiety drugs used clinically in humans. These same drugs reduce the affective-motivational impact of fearful stimuli and situations in animals. A host of neuropeptide candidates that could be targets for new drug development exist along this system (Panksepp & Harro 2004).

4. Where would we mammals be if we did not have brain systems to feel LUST for each other? Male and female sexual systems are laid down early in development, while babies are still gestating, but they are not brought fully into action until puberty, when the maturing gonadal hormone systems begin to spawn male and female sexual desires. Because of the way the brain and body get organized, however, female-type desires can exist in male brains, and male-type desires can exist in female brains (see Pfaff 1999). Of course, learning and culture persistently add layers of control and complexity that cannot yet be disentangled by neuroscience; however, I suspect we can work out the mechanisms of social and orgasmic pleasures by studying the neural substrates of rat sexual behaviors. It has long been known that male rats find sexual activity to be a positive reward, but it has only recently been well documented in females, partly because it is harder to establish experimental conditions for females where they can self-pace this activity. It is now known that "only self-paced mating is rewarding in rats of both sexes" (Martinez & Paredes 2001).

5. Where would we mammals be if we did not have brain systems to take CARE of each other? Extinct. The maternal attachment instinct, so rich in every species of mammal (and bird too), allows us to propagate effectively down generations. To have left this to chance or the vagaries of individual learning would have assured the end of our line of ascent. These hormonally governed urges, still present in humans, have produced a sea-change in the way we respond to newborn babies—those squiggly infant lives that carry our hopes and our recombined packages of genes. The changing tides of peripheral

estrogen, progesterone, prolactin, and brain oxytocin figure heavily in the transformation of a virgin female brain into a fully maternal state (see Numan & Insel 2003). Because males and females have such large differences in these brain and body systems, males require more emotional education to become fully motivated, and hence engaged, caretakers.

6. When young children get lost, they are thrown into a PANIC. The young of other mammals and most birds are no different. They cry out for care, and their feelings of sudden aloneness and distress may reflect the ancestral codes on which adult sadness and grief are built. A critical brain system is that which yields separation distress calls (crying) in all mammalian species. Brain chemistries that exacerbate feelings of distress (e.g., corticotropin-releasing factor) and those that powerfully alleviate distress (e.g., brain opioids, oxytocin, and prolactin) are the ones that figure heavily in the genesis of social attachments and probably amelioration of depression (Nelson & Panksepp 1996). These chemistries instigate desires to create inter-subjective spaces with others where both animals and humans can learn the emotional ways of their kind. Many social neurochemistries remain to be found, but when they are, we will eventually have new ways to help those whose social emotional "energies" are more or less than they desire (Panksepp 2003a). This knowledge may also link up with a better understanding of childhood disorders such as autism, because some children with this condition may be socially aloof if they are addicted to their own self-released opioids as opposed to those activated by significant others (Panksepp et al. 1991).

7. Young animals PLAY with each other in order to navigate social possibilities in joyous ways. The urge to play was also not left to chance by evolution, but is built into the instinctual action apparatus of the mammalian brain. We know less about this emotional system than any other, partly because so few are willing to recognize that such gifts could be derived as much from Mother Nature as our kindest nurture. It is even harder to conceive that such systems can even promote a joyous "laughter" in other species (Panksepp & Burgdorf 2003), but these are "experience expectant" systems that bring young animals to the perimeter of their social-knowledge, to psychic places where one must pause to contemplate what one can or cannot do to others. Children who are not allowed safe places to exercise their ludic energies—these urges for rough-and-tumble engagement—may express such ancient urges in situations where they should not. To be too impulsive

within the classroom is to increase the likelihood that one will be labeled as a troublemaker (e.g., with Attention Deficit Hyperactivity Disorder) who "should" be quieted with anti-play drugs, for example, psychostimulants such as Ritalin. Some of us entertain the idea that many of these kids, especially when they are very young, would find better benefits from extra rations of rough-and-tumble activities every day (Panksepp 1998c, Panksepp et al. 2003). It seems likely that this type of social activity can program brain circuits essential for well-modulated social abilities, perhaps partly by activating many genes that promote neuronal growth and health. As Plato said in the *Republic*, "Our children from their earliest years must take part in all the more lawful forms of play, for if they are not surrounded with such an atmosphere they can never grow up to be well conducted and virtuous citizens."

MORE ON THE SEEKING, PANIC, AND PLAY SYSTEMS OF THE BRAIN

Let me now cover three of the above systems in greater detail. These are the ones I have expended most research effort on and that we have rather single-mindedly sought to introduce into neuroscience and psychology, with mixed success. The first system had been well studied under the concepts of brain "reward" and "reinforcement" systems, with some individuals willing to go so far as to postulate that the system was the main source of pleasure. Such views had many paradoxes, leading me to postulate that the system was instead a fundamental substrate of exploration, seeking, and desire. Although most investigators are now heading in that theoretical direction under many seemingly distinct semantic banners (for an overview, see Panksepp & Moskal 2004), let us look at this system in relatively simple conceptual terms.

THE SEEKING SYSTEM

Most of us readily recognize that animals actively do many things "energetically." Animal behavior seems outwardly purposive and with just a little experience with the reward contingencies of the world, it becomes intensely goal-directed in a "magnetized" sort of way. The animals seem to show every indication that they have some level of comprehension of their goals, and if barriers to success are imposed, they persist in quite flexible but insistent ways. If nothing works, they often tend to show frustration and anger, and eventually they give up and "extinguish" (but they do not forget). Although the animals' well-developed behavior patterns seem to make good sense in terms of the apparent cognitive goals, it is the energized nature of their riveted attention to tasks and their focused movement toward things that seem to indicate that they have internal wants and desires. There is every indication that some type of mental process seems to exist in seeking that may reflect rudimentary thought. It is hard to imagine that such goal-seeking patterns could occur in living systems that had no experiences. Although it is much easier for us to think about animals' behaviors in terms of what they are aspiring to find or achieve (the *active* organism perspective) than in terms of what stimuli have impinged on them in the past (passive receivers of information), for ontological reasons, behaviorists have long found the latter option to be the scientifically more-attractive way to view the causes of animal behavior. In any event, the neuroscience evidence indicates that all mammalian brains contain a general purpose SEEKING system that is designed to actively engage the world, and especially its life-sustaining resources, and in this active quest to also integrate a large amount of information about the world for increasing the future efficiency of behavior. Thus, it is easy to see how both views could be easily blended, but until recently there has been little incentive to include the evolutionary perspective that an emotive system for resource acquisition is an intrinsic part of the nervous system and that it has affective feel to it—an invigorated positive feeling of engagement with tasks that can border on euphoria. The affect would be a good way to motivate behavioral richness. Indeed, all the psychostimulants seem to promote such feelings, helping explain not only why certain drugs are addictive but also why goal-directed behaviors have such a wonderful and often obsessive persistence.

THE PANIC SYSTEM

To be a mammal is to be socially dependent and bonded to others. John Bowlby was the first to bring this concept to the psychiatric forefront, and only recently have research programs attempted to clarify the neural underpinnings. I think our own research effort was the first to conceptualize an intrinsic social-emotional system in the mammalian brain. The guiding idea was that severance of social bonds led to painful feelings of separation distress that could be monitored by crying behaviors in young animals separated from their mothers. Endogenous opioids that could regulate feelings of physical pain were hypothesized to inhibit separa-

tion distress. The effects of opioids on the emotional response turned out to be even more robust than on the physical pain, leading to the study of many details (Panksepp et al. 1980b, Panksepp et al. 1985, Panksepp et al. 1988). Along the way, we also discovered other important chemistries that robustly quelled separation distress, such as oxytocin (Panksepp 1988, 1992) and prolactin (Panksepp 1998a). Others beautifully described how oxytocin regulated social dynamics in various species of voles (Carter 2003, Insel 2003). All these findings have now converged on the implicit acceptance of integrated social emotional systems within the brain, although it is hard for most to admit that other animals probably feel the emotional power of these systems in their own lives. Anyone who has seen how persistently both mother and infant, in practically all mammalian species, aspire to achieve reunion when forcibly separated must be rather cold-hearted and wrong not to accept the most likely possible conclusion. The rational point of view is that other animals feel the power of their social needs intensely, even though we can re-symbolize our needs in great literature, music, movies, dance, and other arts. Yes, feelings of loss and loneliness can energize our cortical creative energies, but those higher processes do not create affect on their own.

THE PLAY SYSTEM

Soon after we discovered the locations and cardinal chemistries of separation distress, we sought to consider the opposite side of the social coin, that is, the profound desire of animals to interact with each other in energetic ways, from juvenile play to sexual congress. We decided to focus on rough-and-tumble play as the process that deserved the most attention, not only because it seemed to be the foundational process for the emergence of many other social skills but also because it had largely been neglected in experimental animal behavior and essentially ignored by neuroscientists. We found that play was easy to study in the laboratory, that it was a powerful positive incentive, and we identified many of the attributes, as did a few investigators who joined the search (for summary, see Panksepp 1998a). The underlying brain systems were harder to identify, but we could be confident that they included quite ancient brain systems, because the behavior survived radical decortication. Animals without any neocortex played vigorously (Panksepp et al. 1994).

Although our analysis of sensory systems regulating play highlighted both somatosensory and auditory systems (Siviy & Panksepp 1987), we were especially intrigued by "play sounds" when we listened at ultrasonic levels (Knuston et al. 1998). It took us a few years to consider that those abundant 50-kHz chirps resembled laughter, and we then conducted a great deal of research before we felt confident enough to share that working hypothesis with the scientific community (Panksepp & Burgdorf 1999). Not surprisingly, segments of this community were very unreceptive, as they had been toward our separation distress work (for example, see Blumberg & Sokoloff 2001, LeDoux 2002). We have assembled a critical mass of data for the liberal views we favor that a dozen good reasons exist to believe that all open-minded scientists should entertain the possibility that such sounds reflect a positive affective process which, in its most intense forms, can be emotionally characterized as a playful, social joy (Panksepp & Burgdorf 2003). That such brain functions may exist in other species provides a robust reason to more fully anticipate the existence of other remarkable affective processes in their psychological repertoire. In any event, the evidence strongly suggests that many human emotional feelings are based on these types of ancient brain systems (Panksepp 1985, Heath 1996).

SOCIAL DEPENDENCE, SOCIAL BONDING, SOCIAL PAIN, AND SOCIAL ATTACHMENTS

The fundamental issue is, what are the core neuropsychological dimensions of social attachments that evolution has provided all mammals? Our own work on the topic emerged from the recognition that separation distress, and hence crying circuitry, might be the inroad to this problem (Panksepp 1981, Nelson & Panksepp 1998). As already indicated, the key chemistries discovered were opioids that stimulate *mu* receptors, as well as oxytocin and prolactin sensitivities of the brain. The oxytocin story has received extensive experimental attention because of field mice, such as the prairie voles, that exhibit pair-bonding. Sue Carter (2003) and Tom Insel (2003) have been at the forefront of robust research programs that have highlighted how important oxytocin (and also vasopressin in males) is to the formation of social friendships and allegiances. Others were showing that oxytocin was critical for facilitating mother-infant bonding in sheep, maternal urges in many species, and solidification of social memories in rats (for details, see Panksepp 1998a, or numerous papers by Carter or Insel). Our lab was the first to demonstrate that oxytocin was even more

effective than opioids in reducing separation distress in birds (Panksepp 1988). We proceeded to demonstrate that social bonding from the infant's perspective was also oxytocin-facilitated in rats (Nelson & Panksepp 1996, 1998).

Rather than detail those findings, let me consider the idea that the "painful" experience of social loss, ranging from a perceived lack of social support to the profound internal "ache" resulting from abandonment or death of a loved one, achieves part of its emotional intensity from the brain systems that mediate physical pain (Panksepp 1998a, 2003b). Behavioral brain research on separation distress systems of other animals has long suggested an evolutionary relationship between the sources of social isolation-induced distress and physical pain (Panksepp 1981). Given the dependence of mammalian young on their caregivers, it is easy to understand the strong survival value conferred by neural systems that elaborate both social attachments that may have evolutionary relations and those that mediate the affective qualities of physical pain. If evidence continues to support this relationship, intriguing implications may exist for the clinical management of pain in both humans and other animals.

It has long been common in diverse human cultures for people to talk about the loss of a loved one in terms of painful feelings. This seems to be more than a semantic metaphor. Although we have no time capsule to return to the evolutionary origins of brain emotional systems, close analyses of living brains offer important clues. So far, the strongest evidence for the evolutionary relations between social pain and physical pain systems comes largely from the fact that localized electrical stimulation of subcortical brain areas that have been implicated in the regulation of pain can provoke separation cries, and these responses are regulated by endogenous opioids (Herman & Panksepp 1981, Panksepp et al. 1988). Additional areas of control include the anterior cingulate, the bed-nucleus of the stria terminalis, the ventral septal and dorsal preoptic areas, the dorsomedial thalamus, and the periaqueductal central gray (PAG) of the brain stem (Figure 5.2). Recent human brain imaging has highlighted very similar trajectories of brain activation on humans experiencing intense sadness (Damasio et al. 2000). Some of these areas, especially the last two, are known to control feelings of physical pain. Indeed, the PAG is the brain area from which emotional distress can be most easily evoked in humans and animals with the lowest levels of brain stimulation.

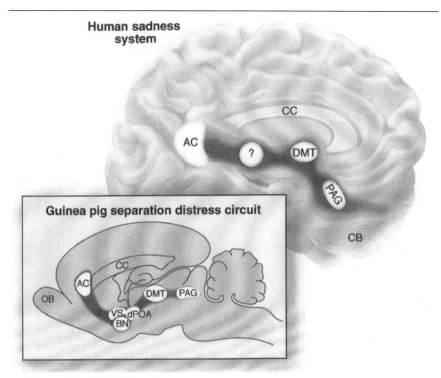

Figure 5.2. Remarkable similarities exist between regions of the guinea pig brain that, when activated, provoke separation distress and areas of the human brain that are activated during feelings of sadness. During separation distress in guinea pigs, the most responsive brain areas are the anterior cingulate (AC), the ventral septal (VS) and dorsal preoptic areas (dPOA), the bed nucleus of the stria terminalis (BN), the dorsomedial thalamus (DMT), and the periaqueductal central gray area of the brain stem (PAG). In humans experiencing sadness, the anterior cingulate is most responsive, but other areas also activated include the DMT, PAG, and insula. The correspondence between the brain regions activated during human sadness and those activated during animal separation distress suggests that human feelings may arise from the instinctual emotional action systems of ancient regions of the mammalian brain. OB, olfactory bulb; CC, corpus callosum; CB, cerebellum. Figure is reprinted from Panksepp (2003b), *Science 302*, p. 238, with the permission of the American Association for the Advancement of Science.

Pursuant to the demonstration that prosocial activites such as play release opioids in the brain (Panksepp & Bishop 1981), human brain imaging has recently highlighted that opioid activity is markedly reduced during the experience of sadness (Zubieta et al. 2003). In sum, it seems likely that certain kinds of psychological pain, especially grief and intense loneliness, have emerged as exaptations from systems that controlled only physical pain at some remote time in our ancestral past.

A growing human psycho-social literature now suggests that the social environment can modulate the affective intensity of pain (for example, see Leary & Springer 2000, Brown et al. 2003). Moreover, results of recent brain imaging studies are consistent with the idea that certain brain areas such as the anterior cingulate cortex (ACC), long implicated in the processing of pain responses (Rainville 2002), also participate in the genesis of distressful social feelings (Eisenberger et al. 2003). Brain research has long indicated that this brain area also helps mediate social processes such as maternal behavior, social bonding, and separation calls (MacLean 1990, Panksepp 1998a).

The Eisenberger et al. (2003) study employed a new behavioral task that allowed feelings of social exclusion/ostracism to be evoked easily in the solitary confines of a modern brain imaging device (Williams et al. 2000). Participants were ostracized during a simulated ball-tossing video game while their cerebral blood oxygenation was monitored via fMRI. Social exclusion distress was experienced by the experimental subjects when the two other "players" (actually computerized stooges) stopped throwing the ball to the subjects. As the subjects were shunned, two brain regions showed substantial arousals. One was the ACC, where the greater the evoked feelings of social distress, the more the ACC was aroused. The other area, in the ventral prefrontal cortex, known to participate in emotional evaluations, showed the opposite pattern. Instead of becoming increasingly aroused with escalating distress, activation diminished as distress increased. The two aroused brain areas were moving in opposite directions with reference to the degree of experienced affect.

These patterns are consistent with the idea that the pain mechanisms of the ACC (Tölle et al. 1999, Price 2000) are important for generating the feelings of distress due to being ostracized, while the prefrontal cortex, a brain region that regulates emotion (for summary see Devinsky et al. 1995), may help counteract the painful feeling of being shunned. Of course, the feelings induced in such laboratory settings are a pale shadow of the real-life feelings that humans and other animals experience during sudden social loss. It will be most interesting when more intense feelings of social loss are studied with a better focus on even deeper regions of the mammalian brain that control separation distress, such as the PAG and ACC (Panksepp et al. 1988), which have also been visualized during intense human sadness (Damasio et al. 2000; Liotti & Panksepp, 2004).

There are, of course, explanations other than direct affect generators in the ACC. The anterior cingulate is aroused in many other attention-grabbing tasks and situations (Paus 2001). The ACC has also long been implicated in re-allocation of attentional resources (Eccleston & Crombez 1999), autonomic nervous system activity, and the mediation of various cognitive functions (Bush et al. 2000, Paus 2001). Recent work has highlighted how heart rate during various cognitive and motor tasks is highly correlated with ACC arousal, leading to the suggestion "that a principal function of the ACC is the regulation of bodily states of arousal to meet concurrent behavioral demand" (Critchley et al. 2003). These are the types of control issues that will

have to be addressed in an attempt to specify affect-mediating brain regions using correlative measures such as fMRI.

Although much work remains to be done before the neural causes of experienced pain are adequately understood, the above findings dovetail well with what we know about the neural substrates of social separation distress in other animals, which first highlighted the potential relationships between the separation distress mechanisms of the brain and the core brain systems for the affective intensity of pain (see Panksepp et al. 1980b, Panksepp 1981 and initial reviews). The obvious fact that crying occurs in response to pain as well as social loss was not our only reason for considering such relationships. Our initial work into the neurochemistry of social attachments a quarter of a century ago was also motivated by the possibility that the loss of a loved one—the painful grief occasioned by sudden loss of social support—could be alleviated by the same brain chemistries that regulate our feelings of physical pain. Opioid alkaloids of plant origin (e.g., morphine), as well as the endogenous opioids of the brain (especially endorphins), proved to be quintessentially effective in alleviating behavioral measures of separation distress (as monitored by the frequency of isolation-cries), in various species including young dogs, guinea pigs, chicks, rats, and primates (Panksepp et al. 1980b, Panksepp et al. 1985). These findings not only affirmed our conjecture that fundamental similarities may exist between the brain dynamics of narcotic dependence and social dependence/bonding but also forged an empirical link between neural mechanisms that regulate feelings of social loss and those that mediate feelings of pain. So far, most of the human studies in this arena, such as that by Eisenberger and colleagues (2003), are correlative in nature.

The relationships between physical pain and social exclusion distress systems of the brain need to be further evaluated with causal studies. Some can be done in humans, for instance, by including pharmacological manipulations such as opiate receptor stimulants and antagonists; however, the animal research leads the way in novel manipulations. Because several other brain chemistries have been identified that powerfully and specifically regulate separation distress, especially oxytocin (Panksepp 1992), a neuropeptide that can also attenuate pain (Lundeberg et al. 1994), additional critical causal tests could be envisioned as soon as clinically useable drugs to modify such neuropeptidergic systems are developed. Many of the needed functional dissections cannot be achieved with human studies, and progress will require investigators to have a new willingness to entertain that psychological processes exist in the minds of other animals. If we are willing to accept that animals experience affective processes, we have a special responsibility to do such studies with a new level of cross-species sensitivity.

Perhaps the biggest stumbling block to future scientific progress in mind sciences interested in fundamental issues of consciousness is the general unwillingness of the scientific community to try to study brain-affect linkages in animal models in which the neural foundations of emotional experiences can be studied in some detail. To the present day, experts claim that most animals do not experience pain. One prominent investigator recently asserted that the anatomical "evidence indicates that they cannot, because the phylogenetically new pathway that conveys primary homeostatic afferent activity direct to thalamocortical levels in primates . . . is either rudimentary or absent in non-primates" (Craig 2003). Although anatomical evidence suggests that many other species do not have the sophisticated forms of reflective *self-awareness* that human do, such views ignore the vast amount of behavioral data concerning the role of many primitive brain systems in the generation of raw emotional experiences (Panksepp 1998a). In fact, the behavioral data is quite compelling that all mammals do experience pain and that, just as in humans, the ACC is involved in the genesis of those experiences (Johansen et al. 2001).

The vigorous social bonding that all infants and mothers in mammalian species show for each other, and the prolonged signs of distress in isolated young animals, are so clearly reflective of a profound affective state that it is hard to imagine that any other position, such as animals having no feelings, could still be accepted as the default position by such a large segment of the neuroscientific community. Clearly, it is both ethically and scientifically wiser to invest in the working hypothesis that other animals do have many affective experiences than to sustain the Cartesian bias that they do not. It is "wise" not only for potential ethical reasons but also because animal models are the only efficient way to work out the underlying causal details.

Now that more and more human investigators recognize that the affective sting of social pain may share evolutionary relations with that of physical pain, many new avenues of understanding and clinically useful interventions may open up. The quality of social environments may contribute much to not only our emotional feelings but also our ability to cope with pain (Gatchel & Turk 2000, McMillan 2002). There has long been evidence that the pain of childbirth is eased with social support (Klaus et al. 1986), and substantial evidence that both cardiac and post-operative pain can be alleviated likewise (Kulik & Mahler 1989, King et al. 1993).

Indeed, the placebo effect could be conceptualized as the cerebral representation of the "healing-touch," which may be partly mediated by opioid release in the brain. Contact-comfort in animals is partly mediated by release of opioids (Panksepp et al. 1980a). Placebos in humans operate partly through opioid release (Petrovic et al. 2002) and can reduce arousal of anterior cingulate regions of the brain that are commonly overactive when people are depressed or in distress (Mayberg et al. 2002). Substantial research has demonstrated placebo effects in animals, and their underlying mechanisms appear to be quite similar to those in humans (for a review, see McMillan 1999a).

The overall message seems obvious. Abundant room still exists to use human empathy and the healing touch in the management of all forms of pain. In humans this can take the form of music, which often quintessentially captures social feelings (Panksepp & Bernatzky 2002); in domestic animals, the mere proximity of friendly and caring others can surely provide substantial relief (for a review, see McMillan 1999b). For instance, animals exhibit diminished vocal indices of emotional pain to nociceptive stimulation when they have abundant social companionship (Panksepp 1980).

SUMMARY AND IMPLICATIONS

The issue of how we should ethically treat animals is integrally linked to the affective quality of their subjective experiences. If it were to turn out that animals had no internal experience of themselves as living creatures, without a variety of emotional and motivational feelings, there might be little reason, other than aesthetic ones, for us to be concerned about how we treat them. However, if the animals' experiences of the world resemble our own, especially in terms of their emotional and motivational feelings, we have profound reasons to reflect on and feel sympathy and responsibility for their life qualities—to respect them for the many ways they contribute to our own quality of life. In the scientific arena, this has become a contentious issue since Descartes brought us the mischief of mind-body dualism, in which animals were granted bodily reflexes but not mental awareness (Rollin 1998). Although those views may bring peace of mind to those who pursue a livelihood through the use of animals (Thomas 1996), it should never have given any solace to those who are scientifically interested in the nature of mind. My goal in this chapter has been to evaluate the evidence, as it currently stands, concerning some of the types of emotional experiences of which the other animals partake.

My position, in a long historical tradition (for example, see Darwin 1871, Hess 1957), is that the weight of evidence indicates that human emotional feelings are critically dependent on primitive neural systems of the mammalian brain that coordinate instinctual actions, and that these systems are comparably represented in the brains of all mammals. There are also reasons to believe that our own capacity for higher levels of conscious experience are based on a solid foundation of affective processes that represent our core biological values as instantiated in brain systems that can be empirically defined. Very little data exist to suggest that the basic affects emerge from the highest regions of the human brain (Liotti & Panksepp 2004), even though few would deny that those regions can parse emotional feelings into a texture of artful living that is uniquely human.

A critical scientific question is how basic affects are instantiated within the complexities of neural tissues. We are on the near-shore of navigating these mysteries empirically; however, I see no evidence to suggest that it requires neocortical areas that are unique to humans. The recent discovery of spindle cells and other specialized cortical cells (Sherwood et al. 2003) in regions such as the anterior cingulate and orbitofrontal cortex that are important for social-emotional strategies and experiences in all mammals (for summary, see Blakeslee 2003) is not a compelling functional correlate for anything *yet*. Although such systems may add a great deal of richness to human emotional life and everyone might agree that emotions profoundly influence how we see the world and process "information," at present, we have no substantive causal evidence that the higher brain areas that contribute uniquely to human mental life are essential for raw emotional experiences. The neurodynamics of extensive subcortical circuits suffice. My philosophical view is that if we assume a dual-aspect monism on such issues—that

certain unconditioned emotional behaviors and their corresponding feelings arise from the same evolutionarily based "instinctual" systems—we will make more progress on understanding the sources of both animal and human emotions than if we continue to work under the assumption that such ancient "energies" need to be "read out" into some type of higher consciousness. The evidence strongly suggests that *affective consciousness* and *cognitive consciousness* are distinct species of mental activities, albeit they interact closely in the regulation of behavior (Panksepp 2003a). Indeed, the natural emotional systems of the brain may be dynamic "attractors" for the higher cognitive-perceptual aspects of mind (Freeman 2003).

To make further scientific progress, we must intensively study such "natural kind" types of psychobehavioral systems in mammalian brains. These core systems help construct long-term cognitive and temperamental structures as they interact with the perceptual processes of higher regions of the brain. The fact that these systems were evolutionarily designed to be centers of gravity for the emotional concerns of animals provides a clear rationale for considering animal welfare issues (Broom 2001). Just as our cultural evolution has aspired to do for human societies, environments for animals should be designed to maximize positive affects and to minimize negative ones (a lesson learned by most zoos). All investigators need to worry about whether "kennelized animals" provide adequate estimates for the questions they are seeking to answer. If one is interested in the breadth and depth of animals' cognitive abilities, there are many such issues to worry about. Although most animals may not have the cognitive ability to dwell deeply on their emotional circumstances the way we humans can, the notion that they have no emotional concerns, no affective inner life, remains a corrupt idea that can promote unethical behaviors toward other sentient species of this world. In experimental psychology and medicine, there have at times been comparable attitudes toward newborn human infants, which have gradually changed as we recognize the emotional sophistication of babies in realms ranging from gustatory (Steiner 1977) to social responsivity (Reddy 2003). However, I still know of several famous developmental psychologists who do not believe that newborn human infants can experience pain.

One belief that prevents many interested investigators from tackling such issues (after all, most modern behaviorists are open to new empirical approaches) is that they realize no institutional commitment exists to support such work. Thus, it is still politically wise to present oneself as soundly behavioristic, if not radically so. At present, the issue of animal feelings is not a mainstream scientific problem. As long as such chilling attitudes prevail, we will make little additional progress on understanding what affective processes really are in either animals or ourselves. And by failing to study such issues, we will continue to deny animals the respect and honor (perhaps even the rights [Wise, 2000]) that they deserve.

The ethical compromises we must make in pursuing neuroscientific research on the mental processes of other animals are difficult ones, but full consideration can only lead to better research (Panksepp 1998a). Of course, some claim that such research should not proceed. That would cut short the possibility of further insight into the nature of our own emotional depths and histories, and it is not a wise option if we want to come to terms with the shared underbelly of the affectively regulated mental apparatus we still share with fellow creatures. There are many societal benefits to be obtained from such knowledge (Panksepp 2004a, 2004b). To pursue that project well, however, research must proceed with a sense of cross-species sensitivity that was not an evident feature of twentieth-century behavioral research.

NOTES

1. The term *animalian,* used by Susan Langer (1951) to describe primitive ancestral psychological forces in the human psyche, is used here to efficiently highlight that same issue. Obviously, humans are also animals, but it is often convenient to reinforce that by also at times using the term "other animals" when referring to nonhuman species.

2. Capitalizations are used for designating emotional systems, as in Panksepp (1998a). This convention serves two purposes: 1) It highlights that the referents are specific neural systems of the brain, all of which are only partly understood; and 2) it hopefully minimizes the likelihood that by using the vernacular, we will be accused of promoting part-whole confusions. Our research aim is to identify the necessary neural components of basic emotions without suggesting that this provides a sufficient explanation for all of the attributes that such emotions connote in the human mind.

ACKNOWLEDGMENTS

I greatly appreciate the editorial comments on this chapter by Frank McMillan and Jeffrey Stewart.

REFERENCES

Baars BJ, Ramsoy TZ, Laureys S. 2003. Brain, conscious experience and the observing self. *Trends Neurosci* 26:671–675.

Bejjani BP, Damier P, Arnulf I, et al. 1999. Transient acute depression induced by high frequency deep-brain stimulation. *New Engl J Med* 340:1476–1480.

Bekoff M (ed). 2000. The smile of a dolphin: Remarkable accounts of animal emotions. New York: Discovery Books.

Blakeslee S. 2003. Humanity? Maybe it's in the wiring. *New York Times* Dec. 9, 2003:D1.

Blumberg MS, Sokoloff G. 2001. Do infant rats cry? *Psychol Rev* 108:83–95.

Broom DM. 2001. *Coping with challenge: Welfare in animals including humans.* Berlin: Dahlem University Press.

Brown JL, Sheffield D, Leary MR, et al. 2003. Social support and experimental pain. *Psychosom Med* 65:276–283.

Burgdorf J, Knutson B, Panksepp J, et al. 2001. Evaluation of rat ultrasonic vocalizations as predictors of the conditioned aversive effects of drugs. *Psychopharmacology* 155:35–42.

Burghardt GM. 1997. Amending Tinbergen: A fifth aim for ethology. In: Mitchell S, Thompson NS, Miles HL (eds), *Anthropomorphism, anecdotes, and animals.* Albany, NY, SUNY Press:254–276.

Bush G, Luu P, Posner MI. 2000. Cognitive and emotional influences in anterior cingulate cortex. *Trends Cogn Sci* 4:215–222.

Carter CS. 2003. Developmental consequences of oxytocin. *Physiol Behav* 79:383–397.

Craig AD. 2003. Interoception: The sense of the physiological condition of the body. *Curr Opin Neurobiol* 13:500–505.

Critchley HD, Mathias CJ, Josephs O, et al. 2003. Human cingulated cortex and autonomic control: Converging neuroimaging and clinical evidence. *Brain* 126:2139–2152.

Damasio AR. 1999. Commentary by Antonio R. Damasio. *Neuro-Psychoanalysis* 1:38–39.

Damasio AR, Grabowski TJ, Bechara A, et al. 2000. Subcortical and cortical brain activity during the feeling of self-generated emotions. *Nat Neurosci* 3:1049–1056.

Darwin C. 1871. *The descent of man, and selection in relation to sex.* Reprinted by Princeton University Press, Princeton, NJ.

Devinsky O, Morrell MJ, Vogt BA. 1995. Contributions of anterior cingulate cortex to behaviour. *Brain* 118:279–306.

Drevets WC, Gautier C, Price JC, et al. 2001. Amphetamine-induced dopamine release in human ventral striatum correlates with euphoria. *Biol Psychiat* 49:81–96.

Eccleston C, Crombez G. 1999. Pain demands attention: A cognitive-affective model of the interruptive function of pain. *Psychol Bull* 125:356–366.

Eisenberger NI, Lieberman MD, Williams KD. 2003. Does rejection hurt? An fMRI study of social exclusion. *Science* 302:290–292.

Freeman WJ. 2003. Neurodynamic models of brain in psychiatry. *Neuropsychopharm* 28,S1:54–63.

Gatchel R, Turk D (eds). 2000. *Psychosocial factors in pain: Critical perspectives.* New York: The Guilford Press.

Heath RG. 1996. *Exploring the mind-brain relationship.* Baton Rough, LA: Moran Printing.

Herman BH, Panksepp J. 1981. Ascending endorphinergic inhibition of distress vocalization. *Science* 211:1060.

Hess WR. 1957. *The functional organization of the diencephalon.* London: Gune & Stratton.

Ikemoto S, Panksepp J. 1999. The role of nucleus accumbens DA in motivated behavior: A unifying interpretation with special reference to reward-seeking. *Brain Res Rev* 31:6–41.

Insel TR. 2003. Is social attachment an addictive disorder? *Physiol Behav* 79:351–357.

Johansen JP, Fields HL, Manning BH. 2001. The affective component of pain in rodents: Direct evidence for a contribution of the anterior cingulate cortex. *P Natl Acad Sci* 98:8077–8082.

King KB, Reis HT, Porter LA, et al. 1993. Social support and long-term recovery from coronary artery surgery: Effects on patients and spouses. *Health Psychol* 12:56–63.

Klaus M, Kennel J, Robertson S, et al. 1986. Effects of social support during parturition on maternal and infant mortality. *Brit Med J* 293:585–597.

Knutson B, Burgdorf J, Panksepp J. 1998. Anticipation of play elicits high-frequency ultrasonic vocalizations in young rats. *J Comp Psychol* 112:65–73.

Kulik JA, Mahler HI. 1989. Social support and recovery from surgery. *Health Psychol* 8:221–238.

Langer S. 1951. *Philosophy in a new key.* New York: Mentor Books.

Leary MR, Springer CA. 2001. Hurt feelings: The neglected emotion. In: Kowalski RM (ed), *Aversive behaviors and interpersonal transgression. Behaving badly: Aversive behaviors in interper-sonal relationships.* Washington DC: American Psychological Association:151–177.

LeDoux JE. 1996. *The emotional brain.* New York: Simon & Schuster.

LeDoux JE. 2002. *The synaptic self: How our brain becomes who we are.* New York: Viking.

Liotti M, Panksepp J. 2004. Imaging human emotions and affective feelings: Implications for biological psychiatry. In: Panksepp J (ed), *Textbook of biological psychiatry.* Hoboken, NJ, Wiley:33–74.

Lundeberg T, Uvnäs-Moberg K, Ågren G, et al. 1994. Anti-nociceptive effects of oxytocin in rats and mice 1994. *Neurosci Lett* 170:153–157.

MacLean PD. 1990. *The triune brain in evolution.* New York: Plenum.

Martinez I, Paredes RG. 2001. Only self-paced mating is rewarding in rats of both sexes. *Horm Behav* 40:510–517.

Masson JM. 2003. *The pig who sang to the moon: The emotional world of farm animals.* New York: Ballantine Books.

Mayberg HS, Silva JA, Brannan SK, et al. 2002. The functional neuroanatomy of the placebo effect. *Am J Psychiat* 159:728–737.

McMillan FD. 1999a. The placebo effect in animals. *J Am Vet Med Assoc* 215:992–999.

McMillan FD. 1999b. Effects of human contact on animal health and well-being. *J Am Vet Med Assoc* 215:1592–1598.

McMillan FD. 2002. Emotional pain management. *Vet Med* Nov:822–832.

Meaney MJ. 2001. Maternal care, gene expression, and the transmission of individual differences in stress reactivity across generations. *Annu Rev Neurosci* 24:1161–1192.

Murphy FC, Nimmo-Smith I, Lawrence AD. 2003. Functional neuroanatomy of emotions: A meta-analysis. *Cognitive, Affective, & Behavioral Neuroscience* 3:207–233.

Nelson E, Panksepp J. 1996. Oxytocin and infant-mother bonding in rats. *Behav Neurosci* 110:583–592.

Nelson EE, Panksepp J. 1998. Brain substrates of infant-mother attachment: Contributions of opioids, oxytocin, and norepinephrine. *Neurosci Biobehav R* 22:437–452.

Numan M, Insel TR. 2003. *The neurobiology of parental behavior.* New York: Springer.

Panksepp J. 1980. Brief social isolation, pain responsivity, and morphine analgesia in young rats. *Psychopharmacology* 72:111–112.

Panksepp J. 1981. Brain opioids: A neurochemical substrate for narcotic and social dependence. In: Cooper S (ed), *Progress in theory in psychopharmacology.* London, Academic Press:149–175.

Panksepp J. 1982. Toward a general psychobiological theory of emotions. *Behav Brain Sci* 5:407–467.

Panksepp J. 1985. Mood changes. In: *Handbook of clinical neurology,* Vol. 1, *Clinical neuropsychology*. Amsterdam, Elsevier Science Publishers:271–285.

Panksepp J. 1988. Posterior pituitary hormones and separation distress in chicks. *Neuroscience Abstracts* 14:287.

Panksepp J. 1992. Oxytocin effects on emotional processes: Separation distress, social bonding, and relationships to psychiatric disorders. *Ann NY Acad Sci* 652:243–252.

Panksepp J. 1998a. *Affective neuroscience: The foundations of human and animal emotions*. London: Oxford University Press.

Panksepp J. 1998b. The periconscious substrates of consciousness: Affective states and the evolutionary origins of the SELF. *J Consciousness Stud* 5:566–582.

Panksepp J. 1998c. Attention deficit disorders, psychostimulants, and intolerance of childhood playfulness: A tragedy in the making? *Curr Dir Psychol Sci* 7:91–98.

Panksepp J. 2000. Affective consciousness and the instinctual motor system: The neural sources of sadness and joy. In: Ellis R, Newton N (eds), *The caldron of consciousness, motivation, affect and self-organization*, Vol. 16, *Advances in consciousness research*. Amsterdam, John Benjamins:27–54.

Panksepp J. 2001a. The long-term psychobiological consequences of infant emotions: Prescriptions for the 21st century. *Inf Mental Hlth J* 22:132–173.

Panksepp J. 2001b. The neuro-evolutionary cusp between emotions and cognitions: Emergence of a unified mind science. *Evolution and Cognition* 7:141–163.

Panksepp J. 2001c. On the subcortical sources of basic human emotions and the primacy of emotional affective action-perception processes in human consciousness. *Evolution and Cognition* 7:134–140.

Panksepp J. 2002. The MacLean legacy and some modern trends in emotion research. In: Cory Jr GA, Gardner Jr R (eds), *The evolutionary neuroethology of Paul MacLean*. Westport, CT, Praeger:ix–xxvii.

Panksepp J. 2003a. At the interface of affective, behavioral and cognitive neurosciences. Decoding the emotional feelings of the brain. *Brain Cognition* 52:4–14.

Panksepp J. 2003b. Feeling the pain of social loss. *Science* 302:237–239.

Panksepp J. 2003c. Can anthropomorphic analyses of separation cries in other animals inform us about the emotional nature of social loss in humans? Comment on Blumberg and Sokoloff, 2001. *Psychol Rev* 110:376–388.

Panksepp J (ed). 2004a. *Textbook of biological psychiatry*. New York: Wiley.

Panksepp J. 2004b. The emerging neuroscience of fear and anxiety: Therapeutic practice and clinical implications. In: Panksepp J (ed), *Textbook of biological psychiatry*. Hoboken, NJ, Wiley:587–519.

Panksepp J, Bean NJ, Bishop P, et al. 1980a. Opioid blockade and social comfort in chicks. *Pharmacol Biochem Be* 13:673–683.

Panksepp J, Bernatzky G. 2002. Emotional sounds and the brain: The neuro-affective foundations of musical appreciation. *Behav Process* 60:133–155.

Panksepp J, Bishop P. 1981. An autoradiographic map of 3H diprenorphine binding in the rat brain: Effects of social interaction. *Brain Res Bull* 7:405–410.

Panksepp J, Burgdorf J. 1999. Laughing rats? Playful tickling arouses high frequency ultrasonic chirping in young rodents. In: Hameroff S, Chalmers D, Kazniak A (eds), *Toward a science of consciousness III*. Cambridge, MA, MIT Press:124–136.

Panksepp J, Burgdorf J. 2003. "Laughing" rats and the evolutionary antecedents of human joy? *Physiol Behav* 79:533–547.

Panksepp J, Burgdorf J, Turner C, et al. 2003. Modeling ADHD-type arousal with unilateral frontal cortex damage in rats and beneficial effects of play therapy. *Brain Cognition* 52:97–105.

Panksepp J, Conner R, Forster PK, et al. 1983. Opioid effects on social behavior of kennel dogs. *Appl Anim Ethol* 10:63–74.

Panksepp J, Crepeau L. 1990. Selective lesions of the dual olfactory system and cat smell-attenuated play fighting among juvenile rats. *Aggressive Behav* 16:130–131.

Panksepp J, Harro J. 2004. The future of neuropeptides in biological psychiatry and emotional psychopharmacology: Goals and strategies. In: Panksepp J (ed), *Textbook of biological psychiatry*. Hoboken, NJ, Wiley:627–659.

Panksepp J, Herman BH, Villberg T, et al. 1980b. Endogenous opioids and social behavior. *Neurosci Biobehav R* 4:473–487.

Panksepp J, Lensing P, Leboyer M, et al. 1991. Naltrexone and other potential new pharmacological treatments of autism. *Brain Dysfunct* 4:281–300.

Panksepp J, Moskal J. 2004. Dopamine, pleasure and appetitive eagerness: An emotional systems overview of the trans-hypothalamic "reward" system in the genesis of addictive urges. In: Barsch S (ed), *The cognitive, behavioral and affective neurosciences in psychiatric disorders*. New York, Oxford University Press: in press.

Panksepp J, Nocjar C, Burgdorf J, et al. 2004. The role of emotional systems in addiction: A neuroethological perspective. In: Bevins RA (ed), *50th Nebraska symposium on motivation: Motivational factors in the etiology of drug abuse*. Lincoln, NE, University of Nebraska Press: in press.

Panksepp J, Normansell LA, Cox JF, et al. 1994. Effects of neonatal decortication on the social play of juvenile rats. *Physiol Behav* 56:429–443.

Panksepp J, Normansell L, Herman B, et al. 1988. Neural and neurochemical control of the separation distress call. In: Newman JD (ed), *The physiological control of mammalian vocalizations*. New York, Plenum Press:263–300.

Panksepp J, Siviy SM, Normansell LA. 1985. Brain opioids and social emotions. In: Reite M, Fields T (eds), *The psychobiology of attachment and separation*. New York, Academic Press:3–49.

Paus T. 2001. Primate anterior cingulate cortex: Where motor control, drive and cognition interface. *Nat Rev Neurosci* 2:417–424.

Petrovic P, Kalso E, Petersson KM, et al. 2002. Placebo and opioid analgesia: Imaging a shared neuronal network. *Science* 295:1737–1740.

Pfaff DW. 1999. *Drive: Neurobiological and molecular mechanisms of sexual motivation*. Cambridge, MA: MIT Press.

Phan KL, Wager T, Taylor SF, et al. 2002. Functional neuroanatomy of emotion: A meta-analysis of emotion activation studies in PET and fMRI. *Neuroimage* 16:331–348.

Price DD. 2000. Psychological and neural mechanisms of the affective dimension of pain. *Science* 288:1769–1772.

Rainville P. 2002. Brain mechanisms of pain affect and pain modulation. *Curr Opin Neurobiol* 12:195–204.

Reddy V. 2003. On being the object of attention: Self-other consciousness. *Trends Cogn Sci* 7:397–402.

Rollin BE. 1998. *The unheeded cry: Animal consciousness, animal pain and science*, 2nd Edition. Ames, Iowa: Iowa State University Press.

Sales GD, Wilson KJ, Spencer KE, et al. 1988. Environmental ultrasound in laboratories and animal houses: A possible cause for concern in the welfare and use of laboratory animals. *Lab Anim* 22:369–375.

Scott JP, Stewart JM, DeGhett VJ. 1973. Separation in infant dogs: Emotional response and motivational consequences. In: Scott JP, Senay EC (eds), *Separation and depression*. Washington, DC, American Association for the Advancement of Science:162–187.

Sherwood CC, Lee PWH, Rivara CB, et al. 2003. Evolution of specialized pyramidal neurons in primate visual and motor cortex. *Brain Behav Evolut* 61:28–44.

Siviy SM, Panksepp J. 1987. Sensory modulation of juvenile play in rats. *Dev Psychobiol* 20:39–55.

Solms M. 2000. Dreaming and REM sleep are controlled by different brain mechanisms. *Behav Brain Sci* 23:843–850

Steiner JE. 1977. Facial expressions of the neonate infant indicating the hedonics of food related chemical stimuli. In: Weiffenbach JE (ed), *Taste and development*. Bethesda, MD, US Dept HEW:173–189.

Thomas K. 1996. *Man and the natural world*. New York: Oxford University Press.

Tölle TR, Kaufmann T, Siessmeier T, et al. 1999. Region-specific encoding of sensory and affective components of pain in the human brain: A positron emission tomography correlation analysis. *Ann Neurol* 45:40–47.

Volkow ND, Fowler JS, Wang GJ. 2002. Role of dopamine in drug reinforcement and addiction in humans: Results from imaging studies. *Behav Pharmacol* 13:355–366.

Williams KD, Cheung CKT, Choi W. 2000. Cyberostracism: Effects of being ignored over the internet. *J Pers Soc Psychol* 79:748–762.

Wise SM. 2000. *Rattling the cage*. Cambridge, MA: Perseus Books.

Zajonc RB. 1980. Feelings and thinking: Preferences need no inferences. *Am Psychol* 116:157–175.

Zubieta JK, Ketter TA, Bueller JA, et al. 2003. Regulation of human affective responses by anterior cingulate and limbic mu-opioid neurotransmission. *Arch Gen Psychiat* 60:1145–1153.

Part II
Emotional Distress, Suffering, and Mental Illness

6

Animal Boredom: Understanding the Tedium of Confined Lives

Françoise Wemelsfelder

INTRODUCTION

Animals play an important role in human industrial society. We keep enormous numbers of animals confined in small enclosed areas for the sake of food production, scientific research, and leisure entertainment and subject these animals to strict procedures of management and control. The animals are housed mostly in functional, standardized environments and are submitted daily to the same feeding and handling routines. Thus, their lives become highly predictable and lack surprising, challenging, or entertaining events. So few opportunities exist for the animal to engage with its surroundings or express preferences that its behavioral repertoire narrows to the functional minimum. The animal has nothing to *do*. The environment might be full of noise, smells, and things to see, but nevertheless, the animal is barred from leading an active, self-motivated life.

For decades, it was assumed that such conditions are not detrimental to animals as long as they reproduce and stay physically healthy; however, recent years have seen such an expansion in our awareness of the intelligence with which animals lead their lives that there is growing recognition that animals can suffer in ways that do not primarily concern physical health (Griffin 2001). It is now acceptable to speak of "psychological" or "mental" well-being in animals and to ask what is required to give them a psychologically wholesome life (McMillan 2002). This in turn has led to a greater willingness to provide animals with various forms of "environmental enrichment." A rapidly growing body of research work reports how the provision of mates, foraging materials, bedding, or toys enlivens animals and reduces abnormal postures and behaviors. Throughout this work, the leading theme of discussion is what constitutes appropriate and manageable enrichment (Shepherdson et al. 1998). Some forms of enrichment are successful in bringing about long-term changes in the way animals behave; others have only a temporary effect. The question is, what does it take to relieve an animal's passivity and re-empower its life (Markowitz & Aday 1998)?

The term "boredom" is a crucial concept in this debate, summing up our sense of what life in confined conditions might be like (Wood-Gush 1973, Wemelsfelder 1990). Boredom is a rich, complex concept that has different layers of meaning and that cannot be measured in a quick, simple way. The purpose of this chapter is to explore that richness and develop a sense of what boredom is about—and to consider how this applies to the welfare of captive animals. The chapter consists of two main sections: The first section takes a closer look at the history and meaning of the term "boredom" and at the circumstances under which boredom may arise. Many more studies have been done on human boredom than on animal boredom, so, inevitably, this discussion relies on human research; however, it goes on to evaluate whether similar circumstances exist that may give rise to boredom in animals. On the basis of this discussion, a working definition of the concept of animal boredom is proposed. The second section of this chapter reviews animal studies providing empirical support for this definition and formulates criteria for recognizing boredom in animals when it occurs. To conclude, the chapter considers what may be effective ways of preventing boredom for animals that are permanently confined.

UNDERSTANDING "BOREDOM" AND HOW IT COMES ABOUT

TRANSIENT BOREDOM: THE DIFFICULTY OF ATTENDING TO REPETITIVE OR MONOTONOUS TASKS

Research on human boredom started to gain momentum early in the twentieth century. It was motivated by the rapidly growing industrialization of workplaces and the concomitant increase of automated, highly repetitive, and/or monotonous labor tasks (Smith 1981). The boredom arising from such tasks was found to be associated with a decrease in alertness and vigilance and an increase in distractibility, restlessness, irritability, fatigue, sleepiness, and daydreaming (Ognianova et al. 1998). This multifaceted syndrome negatively affected the accuracy and efficiency of workers' performances and led to an increased risk of making harmful mistakes (O'Hanlon 1981, Kass et al. 2001a). Most industrial tasks, however, require workers to remain unfailingly vigilant despite their inclination to let their attentions wane. This is experienced as stressful, leading to exhaustion, depression, and complaints about physical health (Thackray 1981). Although in this context the experienced boredom may persist and be severe, it is essentially regarded as transient, that is, as an externally induced state that would correct itself if circumstances would change.

Circumstances exist that also subject animals to repetitive or monotonous tasks. Animals in the entertainment industry (circuses, dolphinaria, film studios), laboratory animals, rescue or police dogs, or guide dogs may all be asked to perform the same task again and again. Few scientific studies have investigated how this affects the animals' welfare. In circuses and dolphinaria, learning to perform routines may bring animals temporary relief from the boredom of their living quarters, especially when training is based on positive interaction and reinforcement (Pryor 1986, Kiley-Worthington 1997). When animals are not sufficiently motivated to perform a task, however, these positive methods may not work. The animals may then have to be forced to sustain vigilance against their will, which may lead to anxiety and boredom (e.g., Anonymous 2003). In laboratories, animals perform repetitive tasks to allow scientists to take certain measurements. The animals do not understand the purpose of such tasks but nevertheless need to stay alert and so may well become fidgety and bored.

CHRONIC BOREDOM: THE DIFFICULTY OF FINDING SOMETHING MEANINGFUL TO DO

The research on automated industrial tasks soon brought to light that not all human individuals respond to these tasks with similar levels of boredom; some people are easily bored, while others are not. This led researchers to see boredom as a more chronic "trait" rather than a transient "state" and to develop a "Boredom Proneness Scale" (Farmer & Sundberg 1986). This scale has provided the starting point for much research on human boredom and the conditions under which it occurs. It became clear that boredom does not arise only in industrial tasks but also in a wider range of social contexts such as family life, school and university education, prisons, and hospitals. Here again, boredom emerges as a complex, multifaceted syndrome. The boredom-prone person is one with a dependency on external excitement and challenge who finds it hard to concentrate and keep him- or herself interested or entertained; has a strong sense of time passing by; and experiences varying degrees of tedium, apathy, restlessness, frustration, anxiety, hostility, loneliness, and depression. He or she perceives day-to-day tasks as requiring effort and often experiences general dissatisfaction with his or her job or life (Vodanovich et al. 1997, Kass et al. 2001b). In sum, the boredom-prone person finds it difficult to experience meaning in the activities with which he or she is engaged (Gemmill & Oakley 1992, Newberry & Duncan 2001).

The question is what causes people to experience such a state—what sort of factors bring on these symptoms of chronic boredom. We tend to assume that people are naturally competent in finding things to do; however, certain circumstances may hinder a person in sustaining personal interests and goals (Csikszentmihalyi 1977, Barbalet 1999). One obvious case is that of enforced confinement such as in prisons, mental health clinics, or even schools. These institutions may provide various forms of exercise and entertainment but crucially, the individual is not free to choose how, where, and when to act. He or she can respond with more or less enthusiasm to proposed activities, but true creative autonomy is not an option. As a consequence, the environment, though offering variable stimulation, may still be experienced as dull and "subjectively monotonous" (Meisenhelder 1985, Perkins & Hill 1985). Indeed, this may happen even if an *overload* of stimulation occurs; if a person is overwhelmed and fails to creatively engage, he or she will still feel bored (Klapp 1986).

Even when not physically confined, people can be constrained in their creative autonomy through various forms of social control. When adolescents are controlled too strongly in their leisure activities by parents or teachers, they typically respond by being bored (Caldwell et al. 1999). To cope with such boredom and "pass the time," they turn their attentions to impulsive, sensation-seeking, disruptive behaviors (e.g., truancy, drug use, casual aggression). Yet stimulating as such behaviors may be, they lack personal meaning and reflect a passive dependency on external excitement. Never truly satisfying, such excitement will set off further cycles of boredom and alienation and, when allowed to develop unchecked, may lead to severe addiction or delinquency (Barbalet 1999, Newberry & Duncan 2001). Thus, "activity" and "sensation" are not in and of themselves meaningful. Dissociated from a person's voluntary, authentic interest, that person's performance becomes incoherent, uncoordinated, and unrewarding. Typically, addicts are disaffected from their compulsive habits; there is no pleasurable engagement, they feel unmotivated to deal with the situation, and they remain hostile and bored.

As with automated industrial tasks, boredom in this context seems a matter of enforced attention and experienced monotony; however, it is no longer transient but has become internalized, disrupting behavioral and psychological organization. Boredom theorists suggest that the chronic impediment of voluntary activity leads to a progressive disintegration of psychological "time" or "flow" (Straus 1966, Csikszentmihalyi 1977, Harris 2000). Typically, our attentive awareness flows in time, connecting past, present, and future and endowing behavior with meaningful coherence. Normally in such flow, we experience alert relaxation, absorbed interest, positive anticipation, personal efficacy, spontaneous creativity, and intrinsic enjoyment. We perceive life as open toward the future and full of potential, and this motivates us to get out and engage with the world. Life is not an effort—it flows (Bargdill 2000).

People for whom this process is somehow blocked, however, lose this experience. In prisons, time is experienced as a burden that must be *made* to flow. Futureless, the passage of time seems maddeningly repetitive and strangely jerky and discontinuous. The alert relaxation of normal life is replaced with a taut, muted awareness; trapped within the past, the prisoner feels dehumanized and depressed (Meisenhelder 1985). Outside the prison environment, people show similar signs of "flow

deprivation" when their expression of voluntary interest is blocked: They become tense, impatient, irritable, and abrupt and feel listless, despondent, grim, and depressed. Life becomes an effort, and psychological atrophy sets in (Harris 2000, Hunter & Csikszentmihalyi 2003). There is growing evidence that such decline also affects a person's physical health, reducing his or her ability to cope with stress and increasing his or her susceptibility to illness (Sommers & Vodanovich 2000). All in all, it is undisputed that this syndrome involves suffering and distress; in suffering boredom, the disintegration of autonomy and identity is resisted and experienced as wrong (Barbalet 1999).

Circumstances that also constrain animals and bar them from expressing voluntary interests are not difficult to find. As indicated in the introduction, virtually all captive animals live in institutionalized conditions. In laboratory and agricultural systems, animals tend to be kept in simple functional environments and are submitted daily to the same feeding and handling routines. Very few opportunities exist for these animals to express individual interests or preferences beyond the bare functional minimum. The cage environment may contain noise, smells, and things to see, and to these, the animal may respond; but this is not to say that the animal can engage creatively and experience attentional flow. For animals, too, it may be true that "activity" and "sensation" do not equal "meaning" and that an animal must be allowed to engage in voluntary activities for this experience to arise (Wemelsfelder 1993).

DEEP BOREDOM: THE DIFFICULTY OF FINDING MEANING IN MODERN SOCIETY

The study of chronic boredom in individual people brought to light the profound effect that social control can have on the fulfillment of their lives. It is therefore not surprising that various thinkers have considered the relationship between boredom and society as a whole, using boredom as a key concept in their critique of the values of the post-modern world (Klapp 1986, Brissett & Snow 1993, Thiele 1997). These values, it is argued, reflect the growing acceleration of tempo of life in the West (Rifkin 1987). Our culture is obsessed with speed, time saving, and efficiency and has an extremely negative attitude toward waiting. Time is a commodity, and we wish our actions to have guaranteed results from beginning to end. Leisure centers offer readily accessible excitement, but the excitement is prescripted, pre-digested, homogenized, and gives the individual little to do. When events are thus stream-lined and made efficient, they lose their edge, their aliveness, subtlety, and uniqueness, and, so it is argued, become shallow and banal (Klapp 1986). A rationalized society offers little to capture our atten-tion; we are pushed along linear time, losing our sense of positive anticipation and flow. Thus, mod-ern society *conquers* time, leaving its inhabitants deeply, helplessly bored (Brissett & Snow 1993, Thiele 1997).

This collective state, often referred to as "deep boredom" or "ennui," has been associated by promi-nent philosophers with a technological, science-dri-ven age (see, for example, Heidegger 1962, Ellul 1967, Fukuyama 1989). The mechanization of our world and its explanation in terms of predictable causal connections may enable us to control that world; however, few people realize that such control *by its very nature* will hamper our propensity for personal interest and engagement. It is thought that slowly but surely, pervasive mechanization will alienate and anesthetize our collective awareness and cause an emptiness that "can find no corrective in the over-production of things" (Thiele 1997). Caught in a cage of our own making, we may suffer the collective breakdown of meaning and joy (Ellul 1967).

It goes too far to ask whether animals may suffer from existential ennui, but this is not to say they could not be caught up in ours. Natural scientists generally insist on regarding animals as complex mechanical systems and often respond with irrita-tion to proposals that animals may also be consid-ered "subjects of a life," capable of suffering in a variety of ways (Regan 1983). There has long been a tendency in animal science to not necessarily regard expressions of emotional distress (e.g., fear) as signs of suffering. Commendably objective as this may sound, however, when facing or holding a screaming animal, this stance is hard to maintain (Arluke & Sanders 1996). One may ask whether the distrust toward empathy felt by many scientists might not be a manifestation of the collective anaes-thesia that "deep boredom" supposedly brings about (Thiele 1997). For example, on the one hand, scien-tists are content to use animals as models for human depression, but on the other hand, many resist the idea that when kept under oppressive conditions, animals may actually suffer from depression them-selves. Thus, animals may well be subjected to "deep boredom" as passive recipients. If such a thing as collective emptiness exists, it engulfs them too.

ANIMAL BOREDOM: A WORKING DEFINITION

The discussion above indicates that human boredom is generally understood as the experience of impaired voluntary attention, leading to listlessness, irritability, and other expressions of disrupted atten-tional "flow." Much of human boredom research is based on verbal reports and questionnaires, so it is therefore perhaps not surprising that few, if any, authors in this field discuss the applicability of their findings to animal lives. Social scientists tend to conceive of boredom within the complex network of socio-cultural relationships that constitute human society (e.g., Gemmill & Oakley 1992, Brissett & Snow 1993). Animals are not considered part of this society; as Eric Fromm in his book *The Sane Society* (1955) bluntly states, "Man is the only ani-mal that can be bored."

The justification of de-personalizing animals and excluding them from social society, however, is increasingly questioned in a variety of academic fields (Midgley 1983, Arluke & Sanders 1996, Wolch & Emel 1998, Bekoff & Goodall 2002). It does not seem a matter of evidence or well-substan-tiated thought that animals are disqualified from experiencing meaning; rather, it seems to reflect a conviction that we ought to explain animal behavior purely in functional terms. An animal's actions, even when intelligent, are presumed to have mean-ing primarily in that they are adaptive and geared toward survival and reproduction; one is not very likely to hear scientists suggest that animals do things because they *like* doing them (but see Sjölander 2000). Thus, a difficulty arises in apply-ing the sort of language that human boredom researchers use to animals. If we are uncertain whether animals can have voluntary interests, it may be difficult for us to see how, when safe and well-fed, they could suffer from "having nothing to do."

But why should animals, in addition to the need to survive, not have such interests and enjoy what they do for the activity's sake? Being curious, trying out new skills, cavorting with their mates? Whether or not animals engage in voluntary activity is, in the first instance, an empirical question that should be addressed through the skilled observation of animal behavior. The question then arises whether and how captive conditions affect the expression of voluntary attention—whether any evidence exists of listless-ness, irritability, and other signs of disrupted atten-tional flow. Again, this is an empirical question requiring empirical research. Thus, the broad definition for human boredom given above may serve as a working definition for animal boredom as well.

RECOGNIZING ANIMAL BOREDOM: SIGNS OF DISRUPTED ATTENTIONAL FLOW

ANIMAL EXPRESSIONS OF VOLUNTARY ATTENTION

Ample evidence indicates that the propensity of animals to attend to their environments does not depend on external circumstances (Archer & Birke 1983, Wemelsfelder & Birke 1997). Certainly, unexpected or novel events will immediately attract an animal's attention; however, animals continuously orient themselves toward their surroundings, regardless of whether something novel has occurred. They move their bodies, heads, and sensory organs in different directions, often accompanied by synchronous rhythmic vibrations of nostrils, antennae, whiskers, or other sensors (Welker 1964). Scientists in the early twentieth century showed considerable interest in this stream of attention and found that it enables animals to efficiently familiarize themselves with an environment, memorize its features, solve current problems, and anticipate future tasks (Krechevsky 1932, Tolman 1948, Goss & Wischner 1956). This led the scientists to interpret "attentiveness" as a process of actively structuring and organizing one's response, bringing anticipated consequences of behavior into the psychological present, and adjusting behavior accordingly—a capacity they referred to as "means-end-readiness," "hypothesis-testing," or "volition" (Tolman 1932, Mowrer 1960). In a similar vein, Thelen (1981) links the rhythmic synchronous movements that human babies make with their arms, legs, and whole bodies to the emergence of "voluntary control."

Recently, the interest in attentiveness seems to have waned. This is perhaps not surprising, given how scientists, as indicated above, prefer to discuss behavior in functional terms. And of course, attentive behavior does fulfill an important function—that of acquiring information and reducing an animal's uncertainty about the environment (Inglis 1983, Inglis et al. 2001). The persistence and versatility with which animals attend to their surroundings, however, appears to go beyond any functional endpoint. Animals *experiment* with their environments and deliberately create opportunities for trying out and perceiving novel things. Most of the

time that animals are forcibly confined to experimental tests, they are not often left free to enter these tests and explore their contents in whatever way and for however long they like, but when given this chance in studies of "inquisitive exploration," animals sustain interest much longer than under forced conditions and show a preference for objects that can be manipulated and keep them occupied (Harlow 1950; Welker 1956, 1957; Wood-Gush & Vestergaard 1991, 1993; Markowitz & Aday 1998; Newberry 1999). Equally, animals in the wild can spend long periods creatively exploring aspects of their environments, together or alone. Common ravens, for example, will fly upside down, slide down snowy slopes on their backs, play tug-of-war, or play pass-the-stick in midair (Heinrich & Smolker 1998).

The boundary between such explorative activities and play is very thin. Manipulations of other animals or objects are often interspersed with loose running, jumping, or flying movements, and the relaxed, free-flowing character of such interactions leads researchers to generally refer to them as "play" (Bekoff & Byers 1998). Play occurs in a wide variety of species, but particularly birds and mammals are known to develop inventive rituals and games (Kummer & Goodall 1985, McDonnell & Poulin 2002). Whether play has an identifiable function has long been the subject of debate; it has recently been proposed, for example, that in mammals, play helps animals to cope with unexpected events and the sudden loss of control (Spinka et al. 2001). This may well be true; however, for the purpose of this chapter, it is beside the point. The point is that through attentiveness, exploration, and play, animals engage with the environment for the sake of interaction in its own right. They behave in a way that is open-ended, versatile, innovative, and that allows animals to experience "doing things" as an end in itself (White 1959, Fagen 1982, Wemelsfelder & Birke 1997). Whether it has a function or not, the activity appears spontaneous, "in the moment," and relaxing, and it is hard to avoid the impression that playing animals, like children, are having fun (Fagen 1992, Sjölander 2000, Spinka et al. 2001).

Given such evidence, then, it seems to me justifiable to accept that animals can engage in voluntary attention and are capable of experiencing attentional flow. The form and style in which this occurs may vary throughout the animal kingdom; however, expressions of voluntary attention have been observed right down the phylogenetic scale (see, for example, Best 1963), and so it seems justified to not exclude any particular species from this approach. Like the early twentieth-century theorists, I am of the view that voluntary attention reflects a general principle of behavioral organization. Through attentiveness, animals organize their own activity and are engaged and absorbed in its meaning. Like humans, they are not automata but *experience* what they do (Wemelsfelder 1997, Wemelsfelder et al. 2001).

THE EFFECT OF CLOSE CONFINEMENT ON ANIMAL ATTENTIVENESS

The overriding characteristic of the enclosures in which most farm and laboratory animals are kept is the severe restriction of horizontal and vertical space. The cages of these animals do not allow them to make much more than a small series of steps, hops, or jumps, or they may even prevent normal movement altogether (see, for example, Gunn & Morton 1995). In this respect, those cages truly resemble prison conditions. The space restrictions, in turn, do not allow for more than the most basic provisions to be placed in the cage: a food-dispenser, a drinker, and perhaps some bedding, nesting material, or small objects for exploration. Sometimes, particularly with larger species, not even the space for a social companion or family group exists, so the animal is kept in isolation. The sparseness of such cages certainly makes them easy to clean and makes it easy to inspect or capture animals; however, it also severely narrows the range of behaviors in which animals can engage.

A primary effect of this restriction, not surprisingly, is that animals simply cease to be active. They spend a large proportion of their time lying down, sleeping, or dozing (Gunn & Morton 1995, Zanella et al. 1996). They may also go through extended periods of motionless sitting or standing, often with drooping heads and ears, half-closed eyes, abnormally bent limbs, and pressing themselves against a wall or stall division. Such passive postures have been characterized as drowsy, listless, apathetic, helpless, or depressed (Buchenauer 1981, Wood-Gush & Vestergaard 1991, Wemelsfelder 2000, Martin 2002). How inactive animals are in small barren pens comes to light most clearly in comparison with their behavior in more-enriched pens or enclosures. Many studies, for a range of species, report that enriched conditions significantly reduce the time animals spend lying, sitting, or standing in favor of various types of activity (Schapiro et al. 1997, Beattie et al. 2000, Kells et al. 2001, Morrison et al. 2003, Celli et al. 2003). Thus, it appears that

for substantial amounts of time, confined animals withdraw attention from their surroundings.

As animals stay longer in their cages, they begin to direct their attention to inadequate substrates. They may lick, suck, or chew the floors and bars of their cages or start pecking, sucking, or chewing their cage mates' bodies (Huber-Eicher & Wechsler 1998, Day et al. 2002, Waters et al. 2002, Margerison et al. 2003). They appear tense, restless, and agitated and respond aggressively to other animals around them (Beattie et al. 2000, Hansen & Berthelsen 2000, Van Loo et al. 2002). They may also respond to their own bodies in this way, forcefully plucking fur or feathers or chewing their own limbs, genitals, or tail; they may also eat their own excrement or regurgitate and reingest previous meals (Baker & Easley 1996, Wielebnowski et al. 2002). In addition, animals may perform behaviors that appear to have no substrate at all, such as air-chewing, tongue-rolling, wind-sucking, or sham dust-bathing (Buchenauer 1981, Zanella et al. 1996, Lindberg & Nicol 1997, Marsden 2002). All of these behaviors are likely to develop into compulsive habits that are difficult, if not impossible, to break. This may lead to self-mutilation or infliction of physical damage on other animals, sometimes so severe as to cause their deaths (Lutz et al. 2003). As a rule, such behaviors are not observed in natural or semi-natural conditions and are sometimes addressed as a confinement "vice," as if it were the animal's fault. But like human addicts, the animal does not perform such behavior out of choice. Rather, its behavior appears relentlessly driven, not providing much reward other than perhaps calming the animal (Marsden 2002).

As abnormal activities develop, the animal's behavior loses its open-ended versatility and narrows down through a process of behavioral fixation (Dantzer 1986, Golani et al. 1999). The usual diversity of behavior is reduced, and fewer elements of behavior begin to dominate the animal's repertoire (Haskell et al. 1996). This is particularly evident when the animal is presented with novel objects or testing conditions. The animal may explore the situation but is less likely to show the bold agility and playful inquisitiveness that enriched animals do. It will be more anxious to approach and will restrict its attention to fewer, less complex stimulus-aspects of the situation (Renner 1987, Wemelsfelder et al. 2000, Meehan & Mench 2002). Thus, the animal's repertoire closes in and often starts to include strikingly repetitive, stereotyped patterns of movement (Lawrence & Rushen 1993).

Stereotyped behavior patterns occur in a wide range of captive species, in many shapes and forms. Research indicates that these patterns tend to emerge when the animal cannot engage in behavior it is highly motivated to perform, such as searching or hunting for food, seeking social interaction, or just trying to escape (Spoolder et al. 1995, Wurbel & Stauffacher 1997, Martin 2002, Bashaw et al. 2003). This association is often taken to suggest that stereotypies reflect the frustration of specific functional drives, and this may well be the case (Carlstead 1998). However, there is more to stereotypies than that; their repetitive, rigid character also signals a more general deterioration of behavioral flexibility and control (Wemelsfelder 1993, Garner & Mason 2002). Stereotypies affect how efficiently animals organize their behavior and how well they learn and adapt to new tasks (Garner & Mason 2002, Garner et al. 2003). In sum, it appears that the process of behavioral fixation observed in confined animals may, in addition to specific traumas, also reflect a malfunctioning of their attentive capacities and ability for voluntary control.

Thus, ample evidence seems to exist indicating that captive animals endure a chronic disruption of attentional flow. This is not to say that animals completely cease to pay attention to what goes on in and around their cage. They may be physically mobile and respond to perceived stimuli; what matters is whether their interest in these responses is actively, voluntarily engaged. Do they interact resourcefully and playfully with their environment and are they busy and absorbed in organizing their lives? The passive, abrupt, unvaried, and rigid nature of the behavior of many captive animals suggests that this is not the case. They are prevented from sustaining activities that they are motivated to perform, and as a result, their voluntary engagement with the environment deteriorates. There are things to do, but not many things they'd *like* to do, and so the versatility and flow of their behavior dries up.

Does this mean that animals, like humans, are bored? By and large, the signs of chronic boredom identified in humans have been reported in animals as well: apathy, listlessness, compulsive habits, frustration, restlessness, hostility, and the disappearance of inquisitive play. The complex, multifaceted character of these symptoms makes it unlikely that the diagnosis of animal boredom could be supported with unambivalent "proof." However, if we can accept that through attentional flow, animals experience meaning and enjoyment in what they do, no reason seems to exist why the chronic disruption of

that flow should not be experienced as debilitating and profoundly dull. With very little to absorb the animals' interest, time ticks by and animals can either try to fill that time or wait for it to pass. But filling time is not the same as having fun, so animals that appear to be active could still be very bored. This is not to suggest that animals intellectually contemplate their situations but rather that they emotionally resist those situations. Boredom in animals seems best conceived not as a cognitive event but as a psychological response (Wemelsfelder 2001).

CRITERIA FOR RECOGNIZING ANIMAL BOREDOM

How, then, can we recognize boredom in captive animals when it occurs? Again, the complex, multifaceted character of boredom means that one or two criteria are unlikely to provide sufficient clarity by themselves. Each of the symptoms discussed above is open to other explanations; heightened aggression, for example, may be a sign of social disruption, territorial strife, or the result of genetic selection, and so it cannot be regarded as a reliable indicator of boredom *per se*. However, "attentional flow" is very much a dynamic notion, which suggests that rather than consider symptoms in isolation, we may be more effective conceiving them as interrelated aspects of an animal's overall behavioral style.

Over time the animal appears to become both more lethargic and more irritably reactive; there is a tense, uneasy responsiveness allowing the animal neither to truly relax nor to positively express itself. The animal may wander around, sniffing or nibbling different substrates but never staying with any for long. Unsure of what it is doing, it is easily provoked or spooked. Or the animal might sit uncomfortably crouched on its legs, looking around as if waiting for something to happen. In all this, the animal appears rather forlorn, never fully absorbed in what it is doing. It is listless, tense, restless, anxious, and hostile, all at the same time—all fluctuating signs of a chronic absence of meaning, which, in their totality, suggest that the animal is bored. By the time the animal begins to develop a fixation on inadequate substrates, the situation has become severe. It is well established in human beings that symptoms of chronic boredom and depression are closely related (see, for example, Sommers & Vodanovich 2000), and the same may be true with animals. Eventually, chronically bored animals may give up looking for things to do; they stop resisting monotony, give in to lethargy, and become helpless and depressed (Wemelsfelder 1993).

To be able to recognize such shifts in an animal's behavioral style requires patience, good knowledge of individual animals, and, above all, well-honed observational skills. The precise form of the process of "flow deterioration" is likely to differ between species, depending on their physical shapes and motor and sensory skills. Some animals swim and float rather than walk or sit; others may rely on sensors other than their eyes. Given that attentiveness is a general animal trait, however, it seems safe to assume that each species can show symptoms of lethargy and irritability in its own species-typical way. When looking for those symptoms, it is important that we know an animal's biological background and understand how it prefers to spend its time under more natural conditions. This gives an idea of the animal's priorities and needs and suggests where we might look for signs that those needs are not met. Nothing exists like a stark contrast to open one's eyes: We may not be struck at first by an animal's lethargy, but when we see the animal come to life in enriched conditions, we may realize how "not its normal self" it previously was.

The question remains whether and how we may scientifically describe and record symptoms of animal boredom. Most quantitative scientific methods break the stream of behavior into separate elements and measure these independently. This approach, of course, has its usefulness, but it leaves the flow of behavior untouched (Wemelsfelder 1997, 2001). Addressing attentional flow requires a more qualitative approach that evaluates the behavior of animals as a dynamic, coherent whole. Qualitative assessments of behavioral style play a prominent role in studies of animal temperament and personality, describing animals as friendly, hostile, anxious, or relaxed (Gosling 2001), for example. However, making such assessments in the context of animal welfare and taking seriously their implications for understanding an animal's emotional state is more controversial and still relatively rare (see, for example, Grandin 1993, Kessler & Turner 1997, Cambridge et al. 2000). Scientists traditionally fear that qualitative assessments are subjective, anthropomorphic judgments that fall outside the scientific domain (Caporael & Heyes 1997). This is a preconception, however; there is no *a priori* reason why addressing the animal as a whole rather than in fragmented parts should be less valid or real.

Research based on a recently developed method for "whole animal" assessment supports this contention. It shows that observers from different backgrounds can qualitatively evaluate the behavioral style of pigs (e.g., as tense, playful, restless, or calm) in a highly reliable and repeatable way (Wemelsfelder et al. 2001). Furthermore, such qualitative assessments correlate well to quantitative measures of behavior obtained through a conventional ethogram (Wemelsfelder et al. 2003). This research has now been extended to other farm animal species, and its aim is to develop a practical tool for assessing animal welfare in "the field," whether that is a farm, zoo, or lab (Wemelsfelder & Lawrence 2001). The point of this and other researchers' qualitative work is that it puts our highly sophisticated human observational skills to good scientific and practical use. Those who work with animals daily (e.g., farmers, veterinarians, animal trainers, laboratory technicians) depend on this skill to read their animals' "body language" and to determine whether the animals are ill, languishing, or doing well. Animals may not provide us with verbal reports, but that does not mean they do not express themselves in an intelligible way (Hearne 1986). This chapter hopes to stimulate and support our sensitivity to these expressions so that we recognize boredom if and when it arises in the animals for whom we care.

CONCLUSION

The research reviewed in this chapter suggests that the effects of boredom on captive animals and the organization of their behavior may be severe. Boredom is not a luxury problem; it disrupts an animal's attentiveness and with that, its ability for voluntary control. There are indications that such loss of control physically affects the brain and as a consequence, compromises the validity of laboratory animal research (Garner et al. 2003; Markowitz & Timmel, this volume). It also seems likely that as with humans, loss of voluntary control may affect an animal's resistance to stress and increase its chance of becoming physically ill (for a review, see McMillan 1999). Such effects would further confound the validity of laboratory animal research and would increase the effort and cost of keeping farm and zoo animals healthy and alive. The level of antibiotics present in farm animals has become a hazard for human health, and so awareness is slowly growing that perhaps keeping animals in highly restrictive-intensive systems creates more problems than it solves (Fox 1996).

A fast-growing body of research indicates that, although severe, the damaging effects of close confinement on animals can be counteracted. Many studies report that providing animals with various forms of environmental and social enrichment appears to revive interest in their surroundings and restore the versatility with which they respond (see, for example, Brent et al. 1991). Passive and abnormal behaviors are reduced, and appropriate appetitive behaviors (e.g., foraging) re-appear; moreover, a creative engagement with the wider environment may return. Various studies report that giving animals the opportunity to search for food not only stimulates them to forage but also causes them to explore their pens, manipulate objects, scamper around, peer at visitors, or play with their mates (Kastelein & Wiepkema 1989, Carlstead 1998, Bashaw et al. 2003). Thus it appears that functional behavior and voluntary attention are two sides of the same coin and that, as previously argued, it is not useful to distinguish functionally motivated behavior from what animals "like to do." Feeding, to the animal, is a *meaningful* goal; it activates the animal's interest and creativity and, in contrast to compulsive habits, appears to be something the animal enjoys. With social enrichment, the same is true. The building of a social group (which may include human handlers) evokes not only specific functional interactions but also a stream of attentiveness that affectionately and playfully maintains social bonds. Clearly, this is a most meaningful way of engaging an animal's interest and time.

What, then, does all this tell us about how chronic boredom in captive animals may be prevented? It should be clear from the material presented in this chapter that the principal purpose of enrichment should be to enhance the animal's active, creative role in organizing its own life. Providing the means for sensory stimulation, physical movement, or both (e.g., television screens, brightly colored objects, exercise wheels, or arenas) is not enough. This is better than nothing and may engage the animal's attention for a while but will not lead to the sustained, versatile sort of interaction that prevents boredom and enhances the animal's behavioral and cognitive skills (Ferchmin & Eterovic 1977, Rosenzweig & Bennet 1996). This seems true for all forms of enrichment that are too artificial and too far removed from the animal's natural environment; they do not activate the animal's senses as organic materials do and will not keep the animal occupied in the long run (Hutchins et al. 1984).

To be able to create a meaningful life, the animal must be provided with materials that are biologically salient and enable it to fulfill its primary needs

in an inventive, varying, and flexibly adaptive way (Newberry 1995, Van de Weerd et al. 2003). If this works, the animal will become lively, energetic, inquisitive, and eager to play, and it should be given the means to express such outgoing exuberant moods. In addition, places should exist where the animal can hide or withdraw from others or can rest or sleep. Inevitably in such environments, animals will endure a certain amount of stress through aggressive conflicts, competition for food, or greater vulnerability to physical illness and harm (Baer 1998). It is becoming increasingly clear that a great deal can be done to alleviate such stress through appropriate environmental design (Van de Weerd et al. 1998). The solution invariably is to give animals more choice in how to deal with challenges—not to take those challenges away. The occasional exposure to alarming or threatening events does not necessarily cause long-lasting distress (Chamove & Moody 1990). Animals are perfectly capable of dealing with difficulties; it is all part of a competent, invigorating life.

ACKNOWLEDGEMENTS

Many thanks to Marianne Farish, Emily Patterson-Kane, and Emma Baxter for their help with and comments on earlier versions of this chapter. The financial support of the Scottish Executive Environment and Rural Affairs Department and The Department for Environment, Food and Rural Affairs, is gratefully acknowledged.

REFERENCES

Anonymous. 2003. Serving a life sentence for your viewing pleasure: The case for ending the use of great apes in film and television. Report by The Chimpanzee Collaboratory. Retrieved 1/30/04. at http://www.chimpcollaboratory.org/projects.

Archer J, Birke LIA (eds). 1983. *Exploration in animals and humans*. London: Van Nostrand Reinhold.

Arluke A, Sanders CR. 1996. *Regarding animals*. Philadelphia: Temple University Press.

Baer JF. 1998. A veterinary perspective on potential risk factors in environmental enrichment. In: Shepherdson DJ, Mellen JD, Hutchins M (eds), *Second nature: Environmental enrichment for captive animals*. Washington, DC, Smithsonian Institution Press:277–302.

Baker KC, Easley SP. 1996. An analysis of regurgitation and reingestion in captive chimpanzees. *Appl Anim Behav Sci* 49:403–415.

Barbalet JM. 1999. Boredom and social meaning. *Brit J Sociol* 50:631–646.

Bargdill RW. 2000. The study of life boredom. *J Phenomenol Psychol* 31:188–219.

Bashaw MJ, Bloomsmith MA, Marr MJ, et al. 2003. To hunt or not to hunt? A feeding enrichment experiment with captive large felids. *Zoo Biol* 22:189–198.

Beattie VE, O'Connell NE, Kilpatrick DJ, et al. 2000. Influence of environmental enrichment on welfare-related behavioural and physiological parameters in growing pigs. *Anim Sci* 70:443–450.

Bekoff M, Byers JA. 1998. *Animal play: Evolutionary, comparative, and ecological perspectives*. Cambridge: Cambridge University Press.

Bekoff M, Goodall J. 2002. *The ten trusts: What we must do to care for the animals we love*. San Francisco: HarperSanFrancisco.

Best JB. 1963. Protopsychology. *Sci Am* 208:55–62.

Brent L, Lee DR, Eichberg JW. 1991. Evaluation of a chimpanzee enclosure. *J Med Primatol* 20:29–34.

Brissett D, Snow RP. 1993. Boredom: Where the future isn't. *Symb Interact* 16:237–256.

Buchenauer D. 1981. Parameters for assessing welfare, ethological criteria. In: Sybesma W (ed), *The welfare of pigs*. The Hague, Martinus Nijhoff:75–95.

Caldwell LL, Darling N, Payne LL, et al. 1999. "Why are you bored?": An examination of psychological and social control causes of boredom among adolescents. *J Leisure Res* 31:103–121.

Cambridge AJ, Tobias KM, Newberry RC, et al. 2000. Subjective and objective measurements of postoperative pain in cats. *J Am Vet Med Assoc* 217:685–690.

Caporael LR, Heyes CM. 1997. Why anthropomorphize? Folk psychology and other stories. In: Mitchell RW, Thompson NS, Miles HL (eds), *Anthropomorphism, anecdotes and animals*. Albany, State University of New York Press:59–73.

Carlstead K. 1998. Determining the causes of stereotypic behaviors in zoo carnivores: Toward appropriate enrichment strategies. In: Shepherdson DJ, Mellen JD, Hutchins M (eds), *Second nature: Environmental enrichment for captive animals*. Washington, DC, Smithsonian Institution Press:172–184.

Celli ML, Tomonaga M, Udono T, et al. 2003. Tool use task as environmental enrichment for captive chimpanzees. *Appl Anim Behav Sci* 81:171–182.

Chamove AS, Moody EM. 1990. Are alarming events good for captive monkeys. *Appl Anim Behav Sci* 27:169–176.

Csikszentmihalyi M. 1977. *Beyond boredom and anxiety*. San Francisco: Jossey-Bass.

Dantzer R. 1986. Behavioral, physiological and functional aspects of stereotyped behaviour: A review and a re-interpretation. *J Anim Sci* 62:1776–1786.

Day JEL, Burfoot A, Docking CM, et al. 2002. The effects of prior experience of straw and the level of straw provision on the behaviour of growing pigs. *Appl Anim Behav Sci* 6:189–202.

Ellul J. 1967. *The technological society*. New York: Vintage Books.

Fagen R. 1982. Evolutionary issues in the development of behavioural flexibility. In: Bateson PPG, Klopfer PH (eds), *Perspectives in ethology*, Vol. 5. New York: Plenum Press:365-383.

Fagen R. 1992. Play, fun, and communication of well-being. *Play Culture* 5:40–58.

Farmer R, Sundberg ND. 1986. Boredom proneness—The development and correlates of a new scale. *J Pers Assess* 50:4–17.

Ferchmin PA, Eterovic VA. 1977. Brain plasticity and environmental complexity: Role of motor skills. *Physiol Behav* 18:455–461.

Fox MW. 1996. *Agricide: The hidden farm and food crisis that affects us all*. Melbourne: Krieger Publishing Co.

Fromm E. 1955. *The sane society*. New York: Rhinehart.

Fukuyama F. 1989. The end of history? *The National Interest* (Summer) 3:18.

Garner JP, Mason GJ. 2002. Evidence for a relationship between cage stereotypies and behavioural disinhibition in laboratory rodents. *Behav Brain Res* 136:83–92.

Garner JP, Mason GJ, Smith R. 2003. Stereotypic route-tracing in experimentally caged songbirds correlates with general behavioural disinhibition. *Anim Behav* 66:711–727.

Gemmill G, Oakley J. 1992. The meaning of boredom in organizational life. *Group Organ Manage* 17:358–369.

Golani I, Kafkafi N, Drai D. 1999. Phenotyping sterotypic behaviour: Collective variables, range of variation and predictability. *Appl Anim Behav Sci* 65:191–220.

Gosling SD. 2001. From mice to men: What can we learn about personality from animal research? *Psychol Bull* 127:45–86.

Goss AE, Wischner GJ. 1956. Vicarious trial and error and related behaviour. *Psychol Bull* 53:35–54.

Grandin T. 1993. Behavioural agitation during handling of cattle is persistent over time. *Appl Anim Behav Sci* 36:1–9.

Griffin DR. 2001. *Animal minds: Beyond cognition to consciousness*. Chicago: The University of Chicago Press.

Gunn D, Morton DB.1995. Inventory of the behaviour of New Zealand Whiterabbits in laboratory cages. *Appl Anim Behav Sci* 45:277–292.

Hansen LT, Berthelsen H. 2000. The effect of environmental enrichment on the behaviour of caged rabbits (*Oryctolagus cuniculus*). *Appl Anim Behav Sci* 68:163–178.

Harlow HF. 1950. Learning and satiation of response in intrinsically motivated complex puzzle performance by monkeys. *J Comp Physiol Psych* 43:289–294.

Harris MB. 2000. Correlates and characteristics of boredom proneness and boredom. *J Appl Soc Psychol* 30:576–598.

Haskell M, Wemelsfelder F, Mendl M, et al. 1996. The effect of substrate-enriched and substrate-impoverished housing environments on the diversity of behaviour in pigs. *Behaviour* 133:741–761.

Hearne V. 1986. *Adam's task: Calling animals by name*. London: Heinemann.

Heidegger M. 1962. *Being and time*. Oxford: Blackwell.

Heinrich B, Smolker R. 1998. Play in common ravens. In: Bekoff M, Byers JA (eds), *Animal play: Evolutionary, comparative, and ecological perspectives*. Cambridge, Cambridge University Press:27–45.

Huber-Eicher B, Wechsler B. 1998. The effect of quality and availability of foraging materials on feather pecking in laying hen chicks. *Anim Behav* 55:861–873.

Hunter JP, Csikszentmihalyi M. 2003. The positive psychology of interested adolescents. *J Youth Adolescence* 32:27–35.

Hutchins M, Hancocks D, Crockett C. 1984. Naturalistic solutions to the behavioral problems of captive animals. *Zoologische Garten* 54:28–42.

Inglis IR. 1983. Towards a cognitive theory of exploratory behaviour. In: Archer J, Birke LIA (eds), *Exploration in animals and humans*. London, Van Nostrand Reinhold:72–117.

Inglis IR, Langton S, Forkman B, et al. 2001. An information primacy model of exploratory and foraging behaviour. *Anim Behav* 62:543-557.

Kass SJ, Vodanovich SJ, Callender A. 2001. State-trait boredom: Relationship to absenteeism, tenure, and job satisfaction. *J Bus Psychol* 16:317–327.

Kass SJ, Vodanovich SJ, Stanny CJ, et al. 2001. Watching the clock: Boredom and vigilance performance. *Percept Motor Skill* 92:969–976.

Kastelein RA, Wiepkema PR. 1989. A digging trough as occupational therapy for Pacific Walrusses (*Odobenus rosmarus divergens*) in human care. *Aquatic Mammals* 15:9–17.

Kells A, Dawkins MS, Borja MC. 2001. The effect of a "freedom food" enrichment on the behaviour of broilers on commercial farms. *Anim Welfare* 10:347–356.

Kessler MR, Turner DC. 1997. Stress and adaptation of cats (*Felis silvestris catus*) housed singly, in pairs and in groups in boarding catteries. *Anim Welfare* 6:243–254.

Kiley-Worthington M. 1997. *Animals in circuses and zoos: Chiron's world?* Harlow: Little Eco-Farms Publishing.

Klapp OE. 1986. *Overload and boredom: Essays on the quality of life in the information society*. New York: Greenwood Press.

Krechevsky I. 1932. "Hypothesis" versus "chance" in the pre-solution period in sensory discrimination learning. Reprinted in: Levine M (ed). 1985. *A cognitive theory of learning*. Hillsdale: Lawrence Erlbaum.

Kummer H, Goodall, J. 1985. Conditions of innovative behaviour in primates. *Philos T Roy Soc B* B308:203–214.

Lawrence AB, Rushen J. 1993. *Stereotypic animal behaviour: Fundamentals and applications to welfare*. Wallingford: CAB International.

Lindberg AC, Nicol CJ. 1997. Dustbathing in modified battery cages: Is sham dustbathing an adequate substitute? *Appl Anim Behav Sci* 55:113–128.

Lutz C, Well A, Novak M. 2003. Stereotypic and self-injurious behavior in rhesus macaques: A survey and retrospective analysis of environment and early experience. *Am J Primatol* 60:1–15.

Margerison JK, Preston TR, Berry N, et al. 2003. Cross-sucking and other oral behaviours in calves, and their relation to cow suckling and food provision. *Appl Anim Behav Sci* 80:277–286.

Markowitz H, Aday C. 1998. Power for captive animals: Contingencies and nature. In: Shepherdson DJ, Mellen JD, Hutchins M (eds), *Second nature: Environmental enrichment for captive animals*. Washington, DC, Smithsonian Institution Press:47–59.

Marsden D. 2002. A new perspective on stereotypic behaviour problems in horses. *In Practice* November/December:558–569.

Martin JE. 2002. Early life experiences: Activity levels and abnormal behaviours in resocialised chimpanzees. *Anim Welfare* 11:419–436.

McDonnell SM, Poulin A. 2002. Equid play ethogram. *Appl Anim Behav Sci* 78:263–290.

McMillan FD. 1999. Influence of mental states on somatic health in animals. *J Am Vet Med Assoc* 214:1221–1225.

McMillan FD. 2002. Development of a mental wellness program for animals. *J Am Vet Med Assoc* 220:965–972.

Meehan CL, Mench JA. 2002. Environmental enrichment affects the fear and exploratory responses to novelty of young Amazon parrots. *Appl Anim Behav Sci* 79:75–88.

Meisenhelder T. 1985. An essay on time and the phenomenology of imprisonment. *Deviant Behav* 6:39–56.

Midgley M. 1983. *Animals and why they matter*. Athens: The University of Georgia Press.

Morrison RS, Hemsworth PH, Cronin GM, et al. 2003. The social and feeding behaviour of growing pigs in deep-litter, large group housing systems. *Appl Anim Behav Sci* 82:173–188.

Mowrer OH. 1960. *Learning theory and the symbolic processes*. New York: Wiley.

Newberry AL, Duncan RD. 2001. Roles of boredom and life goals in juvenile delinquency. *J Appl Soc Psychol* 31:527–541.

Newberry RC. 1995. Environmental enrichment—increasing the biological relevance of captive environments. *Appl Anim Behav Sci* 44:229–243.

Newberry RC. 1999. Exploratory behaviour of young domestic fowl. *Appl Anim Behav Sci* 63:311–321.

Ognianova VM, Dalbokova DL, Stanchev V. 1998. Stress states, alertness and individual differences under 12-hour shiftwork. *Int J Ind Ergonom* 21:283–291.

O'Hanlon JF. 1981. Boredom: Practical consequences and a theory. *Acta Psychologica* 49:53–82.

Perkins RE, Hill AB. 1985. Cognitive and affective aspects of boredom. *Brit J Psychol* 76:221–234.

Pryor KW. 1986. Reinforcement training as interspecies communication. In: Schusterman RJ, Thomas JA, Wood FG (eds), *Dolphin cognition and behavior: A comparative approach*. Hillsdale, NJ, Lawrence Erlbaum:253-266.

Regan T. 1983. *The case for animal rights*. Berkeley: University of California Press.

Renner MJ. 1987. Experience-dependent changes in exploratory behavior in the adult rat (*Rattus norvegicus*): Overall activity level and interactions with objects. *J Comp Psychol* 101:94–100.

Rifkin J. 1987. *Time wars*. New York: Henry Holt.

Rosenzweig MR, Bennett EL. 1996. Psychobiology of plasticity: Effects of training and experience on brain and behavior. *Behav Brain Res* 78:57–65.

Schapiro SJ, Bloomsmith MA, Suarez SA, et al. 1997. A comparison of the effects of simple versus complex environmental enrichment on the behaviour of group-housed, subadult rhesus macaques. *Anim Welfare* 6:17–28.

Shepherdson DJ, Mellen JD, Hutchins M, (eds). 1998. *Second nature: Environmental enrichment for captive animals*. Washington, DC: Smithsonian Institution Press.

Sjölander S. 2000. Singing birds, playing cats, and babbling babies: Why do they do it? *Phonetica* 57:197–204.

Smith RP. 1981. Boredom: A review. *Hum Factors* 23:329–340.

Sommers J, Vodanovich SJ. 2000. Boredom proneness: Its relationship to psychological—and physical—health symptoms. *J Clin Psychol* 56:149–155.

Spinka M, Newberry RC, Bekoff M, 2001. Mammalian play: Training for the unexpected. *Q Rev Biol* 76:141–168.

Spoolder HAM, Burbidge JA, Edwards SA, et al. 1995. Provision of straw as a foraging substrate reduces the development of excessive chain and bar manipulation in food restricted sows. *Appl Anim Behav Sci* 43:249–262.

Straus EW. 1966. Disorders of personal time. *Phenomenological psychology: The selected papers of Erwin W. Straus*. London: Tavistock.

Thackray RI. 1981. The stress of boredom and monotony: A consideration of the evidence. *Psychosom Med* 43:165–176.

Thelen E. 1981. Rhythmical behavior in infancy: An ethological perspective. *Dev Psychol* 17:237–257.

Thiele LP. 1997. Postmodernity and the routinization of novelty: Heidegger on boredom and technology. *Polity* 29:489–517.

Tolman EC 1932. *Purposive behavior in animals and man*. New York: Appleton Century Crofts.

Tolman EC. 1948. Cognitive maps in rats and men. *Psychol Rev* 55:189–208.

Van de Weerd HA, Docking CM, Day JEL, et al. 2003. A systematic approach towards developing environmental enrichment for pigs. *Appl Anim Behav Sci* 84:101–118.

Van de Weerd HA, Van Loo PLP, Van Zutphen LFM, et al. 1998. Preferences for nest boxes as environmental enrichment for laboratory mice. *Anim Welfare* 7:11–25.

Van Loo PLP, Kruitwagen CJJ, Koolhaas JM, et al. 2002. Influence of cage enrichment on aggressive behavior and physiological parameters in male mice. *Appl Anim Behav Sci* 76:65–81.

Vodanovich SJ, Weddle C, Piotrowski C. 1997. The relationship between boredom proneness and internal and external work values. *Soc Behav Personal* 25:259–264.

Waters AJ, Nicol CJ, French NP. 2002. Factors influencing the development of stereotypic and redirected behaviours in young horses: Findings of a four year prospective epidemiological study. *Equine Vet J* 34:572–579.

Welker WI. 1956. Some determinants of play and exploration in Chimpanzees. *J Comp Physiol Psych* 49:84–89.

Welker WI. 1957. "Free" versus "forced" exploration of a novel situation by rats. *Psychol Rep* 3:95–108.

Welker WI. 1964. Analysis of sniffing of the albino rat. *Behaviour* 22:223–244.

Wemelsfelder F. 1990. Boredom and laboratory animal welfare. In: Rollin BE, Kesel ML (eds), *The *experimental animal in biomedical research.* Boca Raton, FL, CRC Press:243–272.

Wemelsfelder F. 1993. The concept of animal boredom and its relationship to stereotyped behaviour. In: Lawrence AB, Rushen J (eds), *Stereotypic animal behaviour: Fundamentals and applications to animal welfare.* Wallingford, CAB-International:65–95.

Wemelsfelder F. 1997. The scientific validity of subjective concepts in models of animal welfare. *Appl Anim Behav Sci* 53:75–88.

Wemelsfelder F. 2000. Lives of quiet desperation. In: Bekoff M (ed), *The smile of a dolphin: Remarkable accounts of animal emotions.* New York, Discovery Books:132–134.

Wemelsfelder F. 2001. The inside and outside aspects of consciousness: Complementary approaches to the study of animal emotion. *Anim Welfare* 10:S129–S139.

Wemelsfelder F, Batchelor C, Jarvis S, et al. 2003. The relationship between qualitative and quantitative assessments of pig behavior. Proceedings of the 37th International Congress of the International Society for Applied Ethology:42.

Wemelsfelder F, Birke LIA. 1997. Environmental challenge. In: Appleby MC, Hughes BO (eds), *Animal welfare.* Wallingford, CAB International:35–47.

Wemelsfelder F, Haskell M, Mendl M, et al. 2000. Diversity of behaviour during novel object tests is reduced in pigs housed in substrate-impoverished conditions. *Anim Behav* 60:385–394.

Wemelsfelder F, Hunter EA, Mendl MT, et al. 2001. Assessing the "whole animal": A Free-Choice-Profiling approach. *Anim Behav* 62:209–220.

Wemelsfelder F, Lawrence AB. 2001. Qualitative assessment of animal behaviour as an on-farm welfare monitoring tool. *Acta Agriculturae Scandinavica* S30:21–25.

White RW. 1959. Motivation reconsidered: The concept of competence. *Psychol Rev* 66:297–333.

Wielebnowski NC, Fletchall N, Carlstead K, et al. 2002. Noninvasive assessment of adrenal activity associated with husbandry and behavioral factors in the North American clouded leopard population. *Zoo Biol* 21:77–98.

Wolch J, Emel J. 1998. *Animal geographies: Place, politics, and identity in the nature-culture borderlands.* London: Verso.

Wood-Gush DGM. 1973. Animal welfare in modern agriculture. *Brit Vet J* 129:167–174.

Wood-Gush DGM, Vestergaard K. 1991. The seeking of novelty and its relation to play. *Anim Behav* 42:599–606.

Wood-Gush DGM, Vestergaard K. 1993. Inquisitive exploration in pigs. *Anim Behav* 45:185–187.

Wurbel H, Stauffacher M. 1997. Age and weight at weaning affect corticosterone level and development of stereotypies in ICR-mice. *Anim Behav* 53:891–900.

Zanella AJ, Broom DM, Hunter JC, et al. 1996. Brain opioid receptors in relation to stereotypies, inactivity, and housing in sows. *Physiol Behav* 59:769–775.

7

Stress, Distress, and Emotion: Distinctions and Implications for Mental Well-Being

Franklin D. McMillan

Despite intensive research and analysis spanning a majority of the twentieth century, stress remains a confusing and controversial concept. Remarkable advances in the understanding of the physiological, psychological, and pathological correlates of the stress response have yet to lead to a unified, integrative framework for stress, and no consensus on a definition or methods for measurement has been reached (Burchfield 1979). Stress is currently a widely and very loosely used term for describing complex and incompletely understood somatic, emotional, and cognitive responses to novel, challenging, and threatening stimuli, as well as many other energy-demanding events (Riley 1981). Unfortunately, stress has now come to serve as an over-simplified catch-all term used to refer to virtually any aversive physical or psychological condition (Clark et al. 1997a).

Much of the confusion surrounding the definition of stress is due to the fact that in the extensive body of stress literature, the term is used to encompass several different ideas and processes (Rose 1980, Clark et al. 1997a). Stress has been used to describe an aversive *stimulus* (often termed a *stressor*), the physiologic *effect* within the animal (referred to as "the stress response"), the *conscious mental experience* of the animal (often termed *distress*), and any combination or interaction of these. Lax usage of the term is commonplace, leaving the reader to guess whether "stress" in such ubiquitous phrases as "being stressed," "reduce stress," or "controlling stress" refers to an aversive stimulus, a physiologic response, an unpleasant emotional experience, or some combination thereof.

In veterinary medicine and animal care in general, stress is a frequently used term to describe a wide variety of physical and psychological states, environmental stimuli, and welfare conditions.

Animals are said to experience "emotional stress," "psychological stress," "psychosocial stress," and "mental stress." When the author attempts greater precision, the animal is said to experience "crowding stress," "hospitalization stress," "isolation stress," "noise stress," and so on. Stress is sometimes used to describe the stimulus, such that a family's move, a change of food, a new baby in the house, a dominant "bully" animal companion, cage confinement, or loud construction next door are each stress for, on, or to the animal. Moreover, the previous examples are also frequently labeled "stressful," thereby, in essence, equating "stress" and "stressful." Animals are frequently said to "encounter stress," "experience stress," "be stressed," "be under stress," "endure stress," "suffer stress," "exhibit signs of stress," "go through stress," "have times of stress," "resist stress," "avoid stress," and "cope with stress," yet such language is of little heuristic value.

EMOTION AND STRESS: FRAMING THE PROBLEM

Stress and emotion are deeply intertwined concepts. Each is mutually dependent on the other; they coexist in many, and possibly all, situations in which stress mechanisms are activated (Lazarus 1999). The ambiguity over the relationship between stress and emotion is reflected in the terminology used, which routinely blends and frequently equates the two concepts. In the scientific literature, "stress" and "unpleasant emotion" (e.g., fear, anxiety, etc.) are often treated as one and the same and are regularly used interchangeably. For example, two recent treatises on the association of stress and emotion (LeDoux 1996, Lazarus 1999) use the terms as virtual equivalents throughout the texts, making no meaningful effort to differentiate the two. Typical examples from scientific journal reports include "Anxiety, as well as other emotional or psychosocial stresses in experimental animals, produces . . . " (Riley 1981), "Animal conditioning . . . can minimize the level of stress, anxiety, and fear in animals" (Martini et al. 2000), and "Anxiety or stress caused by the many examinations to which the dogs were subjected . . . " (Pedersen et al. 1999). Some authors address the problem by switching back and forth between an emotion (such as anxiety) and stress throughout their reports (for example see, Kallet et al. 1997) or by using a combined term such as "stress/emotion" (for example see, Leventhal & Patrick-Miller 2000).

Another method of circumventing the issue of differentiation is through the use of vague labels such as "psychosocial stress" (Riley 1981), "psychological stress" (Carlstead et al. 1993a) "emotional stress" (Riley 1981), or the like. Consider, for instance, two scientific reports in which the researchers induced what they termed "emotional stress" in animal subjects. In one study with rats, the emotional stress was induced by bringing about an experience of social defeat in which one rat is defeated in an aggressive encounter with an experienced fighter (Engelmann et al 1999). In the other (Kuzmin et al. 1996), in which mice were forced to witness another mouse being subjected to electric shocks, the authors concluded that the changes measured in the nonshocked mice "confirmed that they experienced emotional stress." However, while a reasonable list of active emotions in these studies would include fear, anxiety, anger, frustration, conflict, and helplessness, no mention is made by the authors as to which emotion or emotions the "emotional stress" may be referring.

All of these strategies allow the writer to sidestep the formidable task of distinguishing stress and emotion, but in so doing, propagate the confusion and impede progress in the understanding of both concepts. However, another major problem becomes readily apparent when comparing the emotion literature and the stress literature. It is common for authors in each area to describe the same thing but give it a different name. For example, discussions of neuroendocrine and physiological reactions (e.g., activation of the autonomic nervous system [ANS] and hypothalamic-pituitary adrenal [HPA] axis) can be identical in two reports, yet in one, the author is writing about emotion (for example see, Plutchik 1984, Zajonc 1984, Damasio 1999), and in the other, the author is writing about stress (for example see, Rose 1980, McNaughton 1989, LeDoux 1996, Panksepp 1998, Sapolsky 1999).

That is, what some authors call stress responses, others call emotional reactions. The same is true regarding function (e.g., homeostasis regulation, approach-avoidance, and fight-or-flight responses) (Plutchik 1984). Consider Damasio's (1999) discussion of emotion: "[a] biological function of emotion is the regulation of the internal state of the organism such that it can be prepared for the specific action. For example, providing increased blood flow to arteries in the legs so that muscles receive extra oxygen and glucose, in the case of a flight reaction, or changing heart and breathing rhythms, in the case of freezing on the spot." Whereas Damasio is writing here of emotion, essentially identical descriptions are commonly used by other authors to describe stress. For example, Sapolsky (1999) describes what stress in nature looks like: "A wildebeest, seeing a lion charging toward it, may immediately mobilize the stress response—increasing its heart rate and blood pressure, diverting energy to its muscles— even though it has not yet been torn asunder."

To frame the problem inherent in the relationship between stress and emotion, we can look at two key goals in animal care: (1) minimize unpleasant emotions and (2) minimize stress. Are the two goals, and the methods of achieving them, the same? If not, how do they differ? Do aversive events, such as separation from a bonded social companion, elicit stress, emotion, or both? Or do aversive events elicit an emotion, which elicits stress, or stress, which elicits emotion? Is the process in Sapolsky's wildebeest above stress, fear, or both? When a dog with severe separation anxiety is left at home and destroys furniture and frantically claws the door to escape, is the dog experiencing stress, anxiety, fear, or something altogether different? Or is the dog experiencing *dis*tress, and is that different from stress or emotion? This confusion permeates the scientific literature, a prime example being a report of emotional stress in rats (Buwalda et al. 1991) that includes the statement, "Cardiac monitoring during the conditioned *emotional stress of* fear of inescapable electric footshock showed that only the high dose of AVP attenuates the bradycardiac stress response" (italics added). That this sentence has the identical meaning when the italicized words are removed demonstrates that the concept of stress is at best ambiguous, and at worst meaningless, when the accompanying emotion is specified.

The confusing treatment of stress and emotion is further muddled by the careless and interchangeable use of the terms *stress* and *distress*. A typical example is found in a report on emotional stress in mice, in which a switch from stress to distress occurs from one sentence to the next without explanation: "The C57BL/6 mice, which initially failed to demonstrate stable self-administration, started to self-administer morphine after emotional but not physical stress. Emotional distress may increase the individual sensitivity to the rewarding effects of morphine. . . . " (Kuzmin et al. 1996). In other articles, distress is routinely substituted for stress, sometimes to infer a more severe type of aversive situation, other times with no distinction (for example see, Hastings et al. 1992, McEwen & Wingfield 2003).

Other problems in conceptualizing stress include the routine failure to identify and distinguish the conscious and unconscious components of stress. From the animal's point of view, the conscious affect (feelings[1]) is the only aspect of stress that appears to *matter* to the animal and thereby have an influence on its mental well-being and quality of life (Rollin 1989, McMillan 2000). Furthermore, when bodily health becomes harmed by persistent activation of the stress response (discussed in a later section), it is the unpleasant affect associated with the subsequent effects that matters to the individual. That affect is the main, and possibly sole, aspect of stress that matters to the individual is supported by studies in humans, in which it has been demonstrated that of the three main methods used clinically for the diagnosis of stress—personal interviews (or questionnaires), biochemical measures, and physiological measures—the face-to-face medical interview appears to be the best way to diagnose stress (Noble 2002). Because affect is the element that people are self-reporting—i.e., how they are *feeling*—this suggests that the best measure of stress is the experienced affect. Therefore, an understanding of the conscious feelings of stress is essential for us to devise the most effective strategies to minimize the unpleasantness accompanying stress mechanisms and to promote optimal mental well-being. The goal of this chapter is to attempt to disentangle the indiscriminately intermixed aspects of stress—namely, physiologic stress responses, emotion, affect, and the conscious experience of stress.

MAINTAINING HOMEOSTASIS

Despite the lack of consensus on the definition of stress, most researchers agree that central to the concept of stress is the preservation of homeostasis. Homeostasis refers to a dynamic state of psychological and physiologic equilibrium or balance in which vital physiological parameters such as body temperature, acidity, blood glucose level, and so on, are all maintained in a range, often narrow, that is optimally supportive of well-being and survival (Lazarus 1999, Sapolsky 1999, McEwen 2000, Charmandari et al. 2003). Most definitions of stress are framed in terms of homeostasis—specifically, an organism's response to a deviation—actual or threatened—from a state of homeostasis. For instance, stress has been defined as "a threat, real or implied, to homeostasis," (McEwen 2000, McEwen & Wingfield 2003) "the reaction of an organism to a perturbation in homeostasis," (Salmon & Gray 1985) and "the effect of physical, physiologic, or emotional factors (stressors) that induce an alteration in the animal's homeostasis or adaptive states" (Kitchen et al. 1987).

Animals have evolved to be adapted to their environments (more precisely, their ancestors' environments [Tooby & Cosmides 1990]), which is equivalent to saying that the environment in which an animal's ancestors successfully survived and reproduced is the environment in which that animal is best equipped to maintain homeostasis. If an environment—internal as well as external—were unchanging, homeostasis would never be threatened, and the animal organism would have no need to act or react. However, no environment is static; all environments pose virtually constant challenges to homeostasis. Aversive, noxious, and threatening stimuli are a part of life for all animal organisms. Consequently, a state of complete harmony with the environment or perpetual homeostasis is not attainable (or necessarily desirable) for animals, and maintaining homeostasis is a constant endeavor in animal life (Clark et al. 1997a, Charmandari et al. 2003). The entire collection of homeostasis-maintaining processes (termed "allostasis" by some researchers [McEwen 2000]) governs life moment-by-moment in every cell of the animal body (Panksepp 1998). Deviations from homeostasis represent a threat to and reduced chances for fitness; hence, animals have evolved effective mechanisms for detecting and correcting such deviations (Panksepp 1998). The CNS assesses the importance of stimuli to homeostasis and, for those stimuli representing a meaningful threat, organizes and initiates the responses necessary to maintain or restore biological equilibrium (Panksepp 1998). In fact, it has been said that the present day mammalian brain is constructed to seek homeostasis (Panksepp 1998).

Living organisms are highly ordered and complex biological organizations whose interactions with the environment require ordered and "logical" responses to aversive and threatening stimuli (Hinkle 1974). To preserve the integrity of the organism, responses to threats cannot be random or generalized; to the contrary, responses must be highly specific to the stimulus or situation that elicits them (Rolls 2000). The vast array of threats to homeostasis requires an equally vast array of defensive responses; such threats include oxygen deprivation, burned skin, a full urinary bladder, presence of a predator, noxious fumes, a nearby cliff edge, inadequate drinking water, cold or hot temperatures, unsteady surface underfoot, hemorrhage, virus infection, diminished vision, confinement, nasal foreign body, being alone, being exposed and uncovered in the middle of an open field, and a torn ligament, to name just a small fraction.

Somatic, or physiologic, responses operate primarily outside of consciousness to maintain homeostasis and protect the organism. These responses include a wide range of major and minor responses the animal body is making all the time, including increased tear production in response to a corneal irritant, breakdown of body fat for energy in response to a deficient intake of calories, shivering to generate body heat in response to exposure to a cold environment, antibody production in response to a bacterial invasion, an increased heart rate in response to a drop in blood pressure, vomiting in response to ingestion of a toxic substance, a sneeze or cough in response to inhaling an irritant, the righting reflex in cats when falling, pupillary constriction in response to bright light, blister formation as a response to friction against the skin, as well as the innumerable and constant physiologic responses of vasopressin, calcitonin, insulin, glucagon, gastrin, serotonin, renin, and myriad others to maintain chemical and cellular balances. The specificity of the response is essential; an animal whose body responded to a respiratory obstruction by increasing insulin secretion or to a deep laceration of the leg by increasing sperm production would not survive very long (Hinkle 1974).

Emotional responses, like somatic responses, function to preserve, protect, or otherwise maintain homeostasis. The neural organization of emotional systems is very similar across vertebrate species (LeDoux 1996), and substantial evidence supports the view that emotions evolved as specific conscious and unconscious brain mechanisms constructed to generate those behavioral responses that optimally enhance reproductive fitness and survival (Tooby & Cosmides 1990, LeDoux 1996, Panksepp 1998, Rolls 2000). Examples of the specificity of

emotions include fear when approaching a cliff edge, loneliness (or other feelings of isolation and separation) when social animals are separated from companions, and frustration when unable to achieve a desired goal (Rolls 2000). As is the case for somatic defense responses, the specificity of emotional and behavioral responses is imperative; a chipmunk that responds to the rapid approach of a hawk by looking around for food will soon *become* food. The chimpanzees that respond to an intrusion by a group of outsider chimps by self-grooming will soon find themselves without resources, without their territory, and possibly without their lives. In contrast, the chimps whose brains respond to the outsiders by generating anger will be strongly motivated—and physiologically equipped—to chase off the intruders.

In considering all affects—pleasant and unpleasant, physical or emotional—a highly structured and goal-oriented system appears to have evolved in all mammals, and probably birds and reptiles (Cabanac, this volume). In this evolutionary development, pleasant affective states have arisen in association with states beneficial to homeostasis (corresponding to natural selection goals of survival and reproduction), and unpleasant affective states have evolved in association with states threatening homeostasis (Panksepp 1998). It is believed that affective states serve as motivational guides to promote behavior beneficial to overall well-being and to discourage behavior contrary to these goals, through the internally generated reward and punishment of pleasant and unpleasant feelings (Bindra 1978, Panksepp 1998).

In all, a fundamental development of evolved defense mechanisms is the ability to recognize and respond in a non-random, goal-oriented, and specific fashion to threats to the individual's homeostasis. On encountering a stimulus that is perceived by the animal as endangering homeostasis, the animal activates a highly specific homeostasis-preserving response. I will refer to this highly specific response as the *primary mechanism*.

Although specificity appears to be the most important requirement for homeostasis-preserving mechanisms, another important feature is urgency. The primary homeostasis-preserving mechanism—physical or emotional—is activated with an urgency corresponding to the degree of threat to homeostasis. Low-grade threats require low-level responses; high-grade threats (emergency situations) require rapid and intense responses. If the urgency is low, such as a predator spotted far off in the distance, the emotional response will generally function at a low level, eliciting, for example, an increase in alertness and vigilance. However, if a predator is spotted in very close proximity and rapidly approaching, the intensity of the emotional response will function at a high level of urgency. Some threats are of such critical urgency that the homeostasis-preserving response draws on every resource possible, often utilizing both physical and emotional processes. For example, one vitally important threat to homeostasis—and life—is inadequate oxygen intake. When this occurs at a low level, such as being at a higher altitude than one is accustomed to, the body will respond with changes such as an increased respiratory rate (for acute situations) and increased red blood cell production (for longer-term situations) to maintain or restore homeostasis. These responses are elicited unconsciously. Because oxygen deprivation is a survival threat of the highest urgency, however, the homeostasis-restoration process is not limited to a purely physical response, but also utilizes very strong emotions such as panic and terror (Panksepp 1998). This is why humans—and by all evidence, animals—that may be trapped underwater and running out of breath are infused with extremely intense fear and panic, which compels immediate and powerful corrective action. This response is observed frequently in animals, such as in the cat with severe pleural effusion when positioned on its back for radiographs. In the face of compromised oxygen intake, the cat will take the most forceful and aggressive action to restore homeostasis. If the degree of urgency of homeostasis-restoration mechanisms did not match the severity of the threat, the animal's responses would be inadequate and would almost certainly, sooner or later, result in severe harm or death.

PHYSIOLOGY AND FUNCTION OF THE STRESS RESPONSE

The process referred to as "the stress response" is traditionally viewed as comprising a set of neuroendocrine responses to aversive stimuli. Stress research has focused largely on the autonomic, or sympathoadrenal (SA), and HPA systems. The SA response involves the sympathetic nervous system (SNS), adrenal medulla, and catechalamine release. The HPA response involves the hypothalamus, anterior pituitary gland, adrenal cortex, and glucocorticoid release (Clark et al. 1997a). In addition to these two major neuroendocrine components of the stress response—which are present to some degree in most, but not all, stress responses—numerous other

hormones are secreted (e.g., prolactin, vasopressin, endorphins, enkephalins, vasoactive intestinal peptide, substance P, serotonin, glucagon, and renin) (Mason 1975, Mason et al. 1976, Moberg 1987). While the hormonal and neural events comprising the stress response are relatively stereotyped among vertebrates (Sapolsky 1999), research has shown that Selye's (1950) original proposal that a variety of stimuli elicit a common nonspecific stress response is now known to be incorrect and that the physiologic patterns of responses to aversive stimuli vary depending upon the type, duration, and intensity of the stimulus. It is now well accepted that there is no single invariant metabolic stress response and that "the stress response" actually refers to a relatively diverse array of different patterns of physiologic changes observed when organisms encounter different types of aversive or threatening stimuli (Mason 1975, Mason et al. 1976, Moberg 1987). Much current stress research focuses on determining whether each neuroendocrine pattern—termed "hormonal signature"—is distinct and specific for the different eliciting stimuli, homeostatic alterations, and emotions. It is important to note that because there is no *single* invariant stress response, mentions in this and other sources to "the stress response" are usually referring collectively to the variety of responses elicited by different threats to homeostasis. (Although a thorough discussion of this key point is beyond the scope of this chapter, it is no small matter that these individual neuroendocrine patterns are another source of confusion in the differentiation of emotion and stress. Consider a passage by Nicolaidis [2002]: "When a *stressor* elicits behavior directed toward preserving self . . . , there is arousal of the limbic system followed by one of several possible patterns of neuroendocrine response, each of which is peculiar to the *emotion* involved" [italics added]. Are these distinct emotion patterns the same or different than the stress patterns occurring at the same time? The answer is not at all clear.)

On presentation of a sufficiently threatening aversive stimulus, the sympathoadrenal response is activated (Dunn & Berridge 1990). The SNS exerts efferent neural control over a number of diverse mechanisms that contribute to homeostasis restoration (Clark et al. 1997a). The SNS is the primary component of the *fight-or-flight* response (which, to be accurate, should be termed the *fight-or-flight-or-freeze* response) in emergency situations (Moberg 1987, Clark et al. 1997a). The secretion of the catecholamines epinephrine and norepinephrine causes numerous changes supportive of the need for emergency action. Physiologic changes include increased heart rate and contractility, vasoconstriction in nonvital organs, and enhanced gluconeogenic activity of glucocorticoids (Bond & Johnson 1985). Cognitive mental changes include heightened arousal and vigilance (Sapolsky 1994). The HPA response is activated concurrently with the SNS response, but its effects manifest more slowly (Clark et al. 1997a). The aversive stimuli shown to initiate HPA responses include a wide array of physical (e.g., heat, cold, electric shock, sleep deprivation, disease, and injury) and psychological (e.g., uncertainty, unpredictability, anxiety, fear, conflict, social conflict, and lack of control) factors (Clark et al. 1997a, Miller & O'Callaghan 2002). Of the two, psychological factors have been demonstrated to be the most potent stimuli for HPA activation (Clark et al. 1997a).

For their diversity, the complex physiologic changes of the stress response appear to compose a remarkably logical and cohesive functional picture. Taken as a whole, the stress response can be seen as a well-organized set of reactions, all apparently oriented toward a common goal of readying and equipping the animal organism for a prompt response to a threat (or, in some cases, to beneficial opportunities such as mating and playing) (Mason 1968, 1975). Stress responses appear to have evolved because they conferred an adaptive advantage in natural selection by providing means to anticipate and react rapidly to threats to survival or well-being through rapid and short-term adjustments in activities of several physiologic and psychological systems (Clark et al. 1997a, Miller & O'Callaghan 2002). The adaptive value of the stress response is most evident from observations of individuals incapable of generating the appropriate neuroendocrine responses. Due in part to an insufficient secretion of corticosteroids, individuals with hypoadrenocorticism often experience a rapid deterioration of health when encountering challenges to which a healthy individual can successfully respond, such as trauma, infection, surgery, or an aversive emotional event (Reusch 2000). Similarly, the Lewis rat—a strain of rats genetically unable to mount an adequate HPA response when encountering a stressor—has an increased susceptibility to infectious, inflammatory, and immunologic disorders (Sternberg et al. 1989).

THE HARM OF STRESS

The harm of stress comes from the stressful experience and the stress response itself. Although the literature is vast and spans nearly 100 years on the effects of the stress response—the long-term effects of a prolonged activation of the stress response leading to adverse health effects—very little attention has been paid to the short-term effects—the conscious affective experience. Many reasons account for this, not the least of which is that the short-term harm required the concession that animals experience the conscious mental states of emotion and suffering, and scientists did not want to risk being accused of anthropomorphism (Rollin 1989). It is, however, the short-term harm of stressful experiences that animal caregivers are working the hardest to minimize.

SHORT-TERM HARMFUL EFFECTS

The harm to the animal during the acute stressful event appears to be the same as for people: the unpleasant affect that is experienced. When someone is "stressed," he or she is likely to be enduring unpleasant feelings. These feelings may be associated with emotions, such as fear or grief, or physical factors, such as extreme heat or a full urinary bladder. Regardless of the source of unpleasant affect, the individual is *hurting*—emotionally, physically, or both—during the stressful experience. The source of unpleasant feelings during stress will be discussed in a later section, but here we can regard the immediate and short-term harm of stress—the aspect that the animal would presumably most desire to be rid of—is the experienced unpleasant *feelings*. Short-term harm can also occur in the form of adverse health effects ranging from mild somatic disturbances up to and including death (Riley 1981). Health effects, however, appear to be of much greater importance in the chronic stress states.

LONG-TERM HARMFUL EFFECTS

The protective function of the stress response—energy mobilization, suppression of noncritical bodily functions, mental arousal and vigilance—is adaptive in the short run but not suited for and very costly in the long run. In an animal's natural environment, threats rarely persist for more than a few minutes, which would appear to be the most likely reason that stress mechanisms have evolved to be beneficial only for the short term. When the stress response remains activated for prolonged periods—in situations rarely occurring in the natural environment, such as confinement, deficient stimulation, and chronic or extreme overcrowding—the harm becomes manifest in the form of somatic and mental pathology. This makes the effectiveness of turning off of the stress response as critical to well-being as its turning on. Virtually no aspect of the animal organism escapes harm, including a wide array of disorders of the immunologic, hemolymphatic, gastrointestinal, cardiovascular, musculoskeletal, nervous, urinary, and reproductive systems (Riley 1981, McEwen 2002, Schulkin 2003).

THE STRESS RESPONSE AS AN ASSIST MECHANISM

Stress responses appear to have evolved as a specialized part of the body's defense system, activated in some, but not all, aversive conditions (Moberg 1985, 1987; Kitchen et al. 1987; LeDoux 1996; Clark et al. 1997a). As the magnitude of the threat—and the degree of aversiveness—increases, a mechanism to arouse, alert, and prepare the organism (physically and psychologically) to respond rapidly would be of immense adaptive value—not to *replace* primary homeostasis-preserving mechanisms, but to *assist* them by mobilizing energy substrates and inhibiting non-emergency bodily functions. Minor alterations in homeostasis are constantly occurring in the animal body and eliciting corrective responses without the involvement of stress mechanisms. Many examples exist of mildly aversive stimuli and the responses they elicit, and include a physical insult such as chronic friction against skin eliciting the activation of mechanisms to form a callus, a single somatic cell that undergoes neoplastic transformation eliciting an immune response, exposure to sunlight eliciting increased melanin deposition in the skin, ingestion of an irritating substance eliciting vomiting, a high blood glucose level eliciting insulin secretion, sitting in one position for a length of time eliciting discomfort in the areas bearing the greatest pressure of the body's weight and motivating the individual to shift to a new position, absorption of toxic substances eliciting detoxifying actions in the liver, bright light eliciting a squint, a small itch eliciting a scratch, and nasal cavity irritation eliciting a sneeze. In these cases, minor aversive stimuli evoke physical and behavioral responses to restore homeostasis and comfort. These responses may involve only the CNS and involuntary muscle activity, and there may be little or no measurable physiologic changes of the neuroendocrine systems, that is, no detectable stress response (Moberg 1985). As one moves along the gradient toward an increasing degree of aversiveness, threats may no longer be alleviated by specific but minor physiologic and behavioral

responses. When stimuli are threatening and aversive enough to necessitate urgent, rapid, or forceful responses, then additional physiologic, biochemical, and cognitive resources may be required. In these circumstances, the primary homeostasis-preserving mechanisms (e.g., the behavioral responses and the emotional states that motivate them) appear to benefit by a prioritizing and preparatory assist mechanism that mobilizes energy substrates and deactivates non-emergency bodily functions. I suggest that these additional physiologic reactions—a *part* of the total defensive response— constitute the stress response. This would mean that when stimuli are aversive or otherwise threatening enough to activate a stress response, primary defense mechanisms are assisted by, *but not replaced by*, a stress response. An illustration: A toenail cut slightly short and oozing a single drop of blood would elicit platelet activity at the site, whereas an acute and massive hemorrhage would elicit the blood's coagulation mechanisms *and* a stress response. Likewise, the inhalation of a few small particles of matter would stimulate the respiratory cilia to remove the particles from the airways, whereas inhalation of a large foreign body would elicit the most forceful respiratory clearance mechanisms *and* a stress response. Emotional stimuli and responses function similarly. For example, observations suggest that in social animals, low-intensity isolation or separation feelings motivate the individual to seek the proximity of conspecifics (e.g., a sheep looks up from its grazing to see that the flock has started to move away, which prompts a scurrying to rejoin the flock), but prolonged isolation or acute separation of bonded companions (often referred to in the literature as "isolation stress" and "separation distress" [Panksepp 1998]) are accompanied by a physiologic stress response (Hatch et al. 1965).

The distinction between the primary homeostasis-preserving mechanisms and the stress response has been vividly elucidated by Mason and colleagues in studies with monkeys (Mason 1968, Mason et al. 1976) and humans (Mason 1975, Mason et al. 1976). They designed a method whereby an aversive stimulus would be presented to the subjects in such a way that it was not consciously perceived by the subjects as a threat. Using a variety of physically challenging stimuli such as heat exposure and food deprivation, the investigators were able to eliminate the psychological component of the aversive stimulus, for example, by very gradually increasing the degree of heat intensity such that change was not recognizable or by gradually substituting a placebo noncaloric food for real food. The results showed that if the animal could not readily detect the threat to homeostasis, a stress response—as measured by elevated corticosteroid levels—was not activated. In this way, the experimenters had effectively uncoupled the primary homeostasis-preserving mechanism from the stress response. When the animal is presented with challenging stimuli dissociated from their psychological components, the physiological (i.e., primary homeostasis-preserving) response specific to each stimulus remains operational (Burchfield 1979), but the HPA-mediated stress response is absent. For example, when the exposure to gradually increasing heat was unrecognizable by the animals and absent a corticosteroid elevation, the homeostasis-restoration response to the increased heat continued to protect the integrity of the organism without an HPA-mediated stress response.

Similar findings were revealed in an older study by Symington et al. (1955), in which the investigators were able to show that in human patients, unconsciousness eliminated the adrenocortical responses to intense physical stressors such as fatal injury or illness. For patients who remained unconscious while they were dying of injury or disease, corticosteroid concentrations (assessed during autopsy) were not elevated above normal. In contrast, those who were conscious during the dying process showed elevated adrenal cortical concentrations.

These studies suggest that in situations where the primary homeostasis-preserving mechanism is uncoupled from the stress response (by preventing the conscious assessment during a challenge to homeostasis), the primary mechanism remains necessary and operational but may function independently of a stress response.

Further support for the distinction of primary homeostasis-preserving mechanisms and the stress response comes from studies demonstrating that activation of the stress response in animals and humans is not limited to aversive and unpleasant events but also occurs in association with pleasant affect, such as ecstasy, play, sexual excitement and mating, and triumph (Rose 1980). For example, Colborn et al. (1991) found that stallions secreted similar amounts of glucocorticoids whether they were restrained, exercised, or sexually stimulated. It appears that a stress response is elicited when an animal deviates substantially from homeostatic balance in any direction. As Sapolsky (1994) has pointed out, diametrically opposite emotions can

have surprisingly similar physiological underpinnings. The increase in catecholamines observed in intensely pleasurable situations has been suggested to be associated with the arousal or vigilance aspects of the pleasurable stimuli (Rose 1980), not unlike the cortical arousal and attention-focusing functions of the stress response in threatening situations. This would suggest a general "alert and prepare" function to the stress mechanisms accompanying emotional responses. In pleasurable as well as unpleasurable situations, therefore, an assist-preparation mechanism appears to have important functional similarities. The stress reactions are distinguished from the primary homeostasis-preserving mechanisms, the latter being, in emotional situations, the emotions themselves. It is the affect of the emotions that appear to motivate behaviors that promote return to homeostasis. Such a system suggests that because homeostasis can be altered in ways associated with the entire spectrum of emotions ranging from pleasant to unpleasant, it is reasonable to propose that stress-related responses do not *direct* the restoration of homeostasis but rather *provide the means and resources to assist* the primary mechanism in correcting homeostatic alterations.

The evidence supports the thesis that the primary homeostasis-preserving mechanism is integrated with—but differs from—the accompanying and integrated stress response, the latter functioning, through arousal and preparation, as an *assist mechanism for the primary mechanism*. The physiological and psychological effects of the stress response enable and equip the body with the added resources to respond fully, rapidly, and effectively to threatening stimuli.

In my view, this account of the role of stress mechanisms in homeostasis preservation is analogous to another type of defense system—our country's national defense. In response to a meaningful threat to national security, the Joint Operation Planning and Execution System, headed in the Pentagon by the Joint Chiefs of Staff, initiates an immediate analysis of the events and executes a defense strategy (US Department of Defense 1999). A system of progressive alert postures—the defense readiness condition system, or DEFCON for short—is activated to match the degree of threat severity. Commensurate with the degree of threat is a mobilization of defense forces, which includes assembling and organizing personnel, supplies, and weaponry and an activation of reserve components of the armed forces. This organizational, alerting, and preparatory mechanism is not activated for minor threats such as a single soldier being attacked at a guarded border by a lone gunman.

The key pertinence of the analogy is that specific defense responses for specific kinds of threats exist for the nation's defense system. Threats such as a land invasion elicit responses very different than a nuclear missile attack or terrorist attack with biological weapons. All responses are ready for activation at all times. However, the additional mechanism activated by the more serious threats—the DEFCON system—serves to heighten alert status, organize and prioritize responses, and reinforce and deploy defense resources rapidly to the areas with urgent needs and away from areas less in need. In addition, by mobilizing reserve forces, the defense response is fortified by manpower not normally called into action. Without this system, our defenses would still operate but would be slow to respond, lack rapid mobilization and appropriate distribution of resources, and risk failure to mount a response commensurate with the degree of threat. Importantly, the specific defense response for a specific threat continues to function but is assisted by the additional mechanism that alerts, prepares, and fortifies the standard specific response. This organizational mechanism, in cases of major threats, becomes *part of* the defensive response. Minor threats do not require the organizational and preparatory assist. This additional defense mechanism is analogous to the animal body's stress response, whereby primary defense responses to serious threats remain intact and operational but receive a rapid organizational and preparatory assist in the overall defense response.

DISTINGUISHING EMOTION AND STRESS

Stress responses are intimately associated with emotional states. When emotional states coexist with a stress response, the nature of the association is not always clear. The emotional state and its associated affect may be the cause or effect of the stress response or may be elicited by a common stimulus as for the stress response (LeDoux 1996, Lazarus 1999). This complex interrelationship of emotion and stress is a primary reason why in stress discussions in scientific literature, the two concepts are not typically differentiated and are commonly used interchangeably as synonyms.

A major source of the problem in distinguishing stress and emotional states stems from the fact that physiologically, behaviorally, and functionally, certain emotional states overlap extensively with stress mechanisms. The limits of current methodology do not permit us to draw a clear line between any emotion and the associated stress response when both are activated. In humans, self-reports make identification of the predominant emotion of the stress experience relatively straightforward. Of the emotions in people known to be associated with a stress response—fear, anxiety, anger, boredom, guilt, shame, jealousy, and sadness—all are typically recognizable by the person experiencing them (Lazarus 1999). Lacking the investigative tool of self-report evaluations in animals, specific emotional states are inferred primarily by interpretation of behavior and environmental circumstances (Panksepp 1998). For example, when animals in situations of sensory deprivation demonstrate a rise in plasma cortisol concentrations, we can reasonably conclude that insufficient stimulation elicits the emotion of boredom, which is accompanied by a stress response (Wemelsfelder 1984).

As stated, when emotions and stress responses coexist, many emotions appear to be recognizable as the primary component of the stress experience. However, in all animals—human and nonhuman—the emotions of fear and anxiety appear to be special cases, differing from the other emotions in their exceptionally close resemblance to stress mechanisms and experiences. Extensive functional and physiological overlap exists among anxiety, fear, and the stress response (LeDoux 1996). The emotion of fear is believed to be the most primitive mental defense mechanism, having evolved as a system that detects danger and produces behavioral responses that maximize the probability of surviving a dangerous situation in the most beneficial way (LeDoux 1996). This is, of course, also a function commonly ascribed to stress mechanisms. Anatomically, fear, anxiety, and stress mechanisms share common neural pathways, encompassing the thalamic tracts, amygdala, and hypothalamus (LeDoux 1996). The neural pathways of fear and stress mechanisms are so closely related that they are inseparable, and in some ways indistinguishable. Functionally, all three processes increase cortical arousal and alertness, prepare the body for rapid defensive responses, and are, or may be, high-energy demand states (Kitchen et al. 1987, LeDoux 1996). For activation of both fear and the stress response, aversive stimuli are perceived and transmitted by thalamic pathways to the amygdala. The amygdala in turn activates many bodily systems, including the ANS, and, through the hypothalamus, stimulates release of corticotropin releasing factor

(CRF), which ultimately causes corticosterone release from the adrenal cortex (LeDoux 1996). Studies have demonstrated that destruction of the amygdala impairs expression of fear-motivated behaviors and that stimulation of the amygdala produces changes in autonomic, neuroendocrine, and behavioral responses that strongly resemble those seen in a variety of stress paradigms (Van de Kar et al. 1991, LeDoux 1996). The pathways for stress mechanisms and anxiety also overlap extensively. Once released from the hypothalamus, CRF elicits a number of responses normally regarded as associated with both anxiety and stress (Dunn & Berridge 1990). Experimental administration of CRF intracerebrally has resulted in activation of the SNS (Brown et al. 1985), the entire spectrum of responses observed in stress (Koob & Bloom 1985), and an anxiogenic effect (Dunn & File 1987, Britton et al. 1988). Furthermore, CRF antagonists are able to attenuate or reverse the effects of various stress-inducing stimuli (Britton et al. 1988), indicating that CRF appears to be a mediator of stress responses (Dunn & Berridge 1990). Finally, the methods of measurement of fear, anxiety, and stress responses also overlap extensively and include such criteria as changes in heart rate and blood pressure, behavioral signs (e.g., freezing), analgesia, autonomic responses, and increased levels of stress hormones (LeDoux 1996).

In all, we do not have the ability to definitively distinguish fear and anxiety from stress responses in animals (Riley 1981, Dunn & Berridge 1990). Because of this, it is difficult to view stress distinct from the associated emotional states when those states are fear or anxiety. This may be the reason that in everyday discourse, the connotation of stress is most readily equated to anxiety-type emotional states. "Feeling stressed," "being under stress," and "easing one's stress level" all commonly convey the general sense that the experience of stress is that of nervous tension, nervous pressure, or nervous strain (Lazarus 1999).

If we are correct in assuming that the stress response is an adaptive response that occurs in anticipation of and in the service of energy expenditure, it is important to note that many emotional states are high-energy need states (LeDoux 1996). Therefore, in situations involving strong emotional responses, it is not surprising that the stress response is also activated. For all of their shared characteristics, however, emotions and stress are not the same. This is true for all emotions, including the one that seems to most closely resemble stress: fear. Fear is not stress, and stress is not fear. Experimental studies have failed to demonstrate, for example, that the peripheral arousal of sympathetic activation (a predominant component of the stress response) is a necessary condition for an emotional state (Reisenzein 1983); hence, emotions in general appear capable of functioning independently of at least some stress mechanisms (with the possible exception of fear and anxiety). In addition, individuals who are unable to mount effective stress responses (e.g., individuals with hypoadrenocorticism) still experience fear and other emotions. Moreover, emotions have important attributes that distinguish them from stress, most notably specific motivational properties. By necessity, emotional states are activated by specific stimuli and elicit specific responses. Anger, boredom, loneliness, grief, and fear are associated with motivations for specific behaviors designed to respond to the specific challenges eliciting the emotion. The stress response, in contrast to emotion, appears to have little if any specific motivational function; rather, it functions primarily as an arousal and preparatory mechanism. Finally, studies by Diener et al. (1991) have shown that when people were beeped at random moments throughout the day, they reported some emotion virtually all of the time, leading the researchers to conclude that emotion gives either a pleasant or an unpleasant quality to virtually all of one's waking moments. If emotion and stress were the same process, then these studies would suggest that at all times, one would, to some degree, report feeling "stressed."

Taken as a whole, on the basis of the experimental evidence, we can conclude that stress mechanisms are neither fully distinct from the associated emotional state nor the same as the emotional state. The stress response is actually a component part of the emotion it is associated with (LeDoux 1996, Lazarus 1999). In my view, the principal distinguishing feature is that the emotion is the primary homeostasis-preserving mechanism and the stress response functions as an enhancing, assist mechanism to the emotion processes when such an assist—by intensity or urgency—is required for optimal preservation of homeostasis.

THE FEELING OF STRESS

The paramount factor that appears to ultimately matter most to the animal is the affective states associated with stress. This includes the affect at the time of the stressful experience and the affect associated with any adverse health effects to which stress mechanisms may lead.

Because a large portion of emotional processing occurs unconsciously (LeDoux 1996), distinguishing emotion and stress still does not address another important distinction—that between the conscious and unconscious components of stress. This distinction is of critical importance because it recognizes and addresses the mental experience of stress-related events—in the form of pleasant and unpleasant subjective feelings—rather than viewing stress in broad, nonspecific, physiologic-mechanical terms. In general, the scientific literature presents stress in terms of stimulus and response, revealing little about the mental states of animals and essentially nothing about how the animal *feels*. Despite the value of viewing stress mechanisms as a whole, it is, ultimately, how the animal feels about events, perceives what is happening, and experiences the complex interaction between itself and aversive stimuli that determine its mental well-being.

As I have already mentioned, there is an intuitive sense that stress is primarily associated with the feeling of emotional pressure or tension. However, this is clearly not the case for all situations in which "feeling stressed" is used. For example, in people, extreme guilt can be a source of great stress, as can loneliness and boredom. Therefore, to start, we can say that, at least in humans, there is no one feeling of stress. It seems highly probable that the same holds true for nonhuman animals.

To understand the nature of the feeling of stress, we must first consider the contribution of the primary emotion associated with the stressful state. The primary emotion (such as fear, anxiety, anger, or loneliness), which remains operational during activation of the stress response, will account for some portion of the feeling of the stress experience. The question is, how much? All? Some? If only some, what accounts for the other portion? Several studies in humans and animals help provide answers to these questions.

Determining the origin of the feeling of stress requires that we separate the stress response from the primary emotional state. To accomplish this, researchers have utilized two methods: (1) block the physiologic stress mechanisms and (2) reproduce a physiological stress response independent of an emotional state. The change in affect following such experimental or naturally occurring events can then help determine the contribution of stress mechanisms to the overall affect of a stressful experience.

A blocking of the autonomic response has been reported in clinical and experimental conditions. Disconnection of the peripheral autonomic response (as a result of damage to the spinal cord or the sympathetic and vagus autonomic nerves) does not abolish emotional feelings (Hohmann 1966). In addition, the feelings of emotions persist in the presence of pharmacologic blockade of the peripheral autonomic system. Several studies have investigated the effects of beta-adrenergic blockade on the emotions of anxiety and anger in human subjects (Gottschalk et al. 1974, Tyrer 1976, Erdmann & van Lindern 1980). In all of these studies, no reduction in the feelings of the emotions were reported, suggesting little or no contribution of the sympathetic component of the stress response to the experienced affect. Pharmacologic studies must be interpreted with a degree of caution, however, because numerous pathways of autonomic feedback remain unaffected by beta-blocking agents (Reisenzein 1983).

For us to study the subjective feelings associated with physiologic stress responses, our closest approximation of the stress-related changes has been achieved by the exogenous administration of drugs that mimic the physiologic mechanisms activated in the stress response. To achieve this, researchers have used sympathomimetic drugs to simulate the SNS discharge, and have experimentally simulated HPA pathway activation by administering glucocorticoids or ACTH.

The HPA response, when activated by the administration of ACTH or glucocorticoids, does not appear to be associated with meaningful affect in most subjects in most studies. Data compiled from several reports (The Boston Collaborative Drug Surveillance Program 1972, Ling et al. 1981, Lewis & Smith 1983, Minden et al. 1988), showed that 82 to 97 percent of people receiving these compounds reported no specific feelings, and the type of feeling was inconsistent between individuals who reported feelings.

Epinephrine induces effects that are generally believed to be a near-perfect mimicry of the sympathetic portion of the stress responses (for a contrasting view, see McNaughton 1989). Several studies (Maranon 1924, Cantril & Hunt 1932, Landis & Hunt 1932, Schachter & Singer 1962) have demonstrated that subjects to whom epinephrine was administered by injection showed numerous physiologic changes consistent with SNS activation, but the large majority of subjects reported no feelings, pleasant or unpleasant. Cantril and Hunt (1932) concluded in their study that, in general, the injection of epinephrine was not sufficient to produce an emotion.

Animal studies have provided evidence that the same effects are seen in nonhuman species. Singer

(1963) investigated the effects of epinephrine on fear behavior in rats exposed to emotional stimuli. Results demonstrated that in the fear-induced group, rats injected with epinephrine were significantly more frightened (as measured by fear behavior such as activity, defecation, urination, face-washing, and trembling) than placebo-injected rats. The rats not exposed to fear-inducing stimuli showed no differences between the epinephrine and placebo-treated groups, neither group showing any fear behavior. Thus, animals that undergo sympathetic arousal by exogenous epinephrine in emotionally neutral situations display no more fear than a control animal, whereas animals given epinephrine in fear-induced conditions show markedly more fear than a placebo-injected animal. These results have been replicated in various forms, most recently by Haroutunian and Riccio (1977). The findings demonstrate that sympathetic activation by itself does not *produce* fear responses, but when fear is present, sympathetic activation *enhances* fear responses.

Some studies have reported that pharmacologic simulation of the SNS elicits unpleasant affect (Marshall & Zimbardo 1979, Maslach 1979, Cassel 1982). As mentioned earlier, the stress response shares pathways and physiologic mechanisms with anxiety, and the physiology and affect of anxiety may be a part of the stress response. If there is any affect attributable to the stress response, it appears to be generalized anxiety (Maslach 1979).

Notwithstanding the few conflicting studies, the preponderance of experimental evidence substantiates a conclusion reached in a 1932 report that stated, "the theories which base unpleasantness upon activation of the sympathetic division of the ANS are palpably unfounded" (Cantril & Hunt 1932). Current evidence supports the thesis that, in humans and animals, sympathetic activation and arousal is not the primary source of the affect experienced during stressful events but does act to heighten or enhance an existing affect. These studies suggest that activation of the HPA axis is generally not associated with a specific affective state and thus does not likely contribute meaningful affect to the feeling of stress experiences. Hence, taking all of the evidence into account, it appears that the predominant feeling of stress comes not from stress mechanisms, but rather from the primary emotional state(s) elicited by the aversive event. The stress response appears to modulate the intensity of affect. Such a system would make evolutionary sense. The specific emotional state would serve as the primary homeostasis-preserving mechanism, and the physi-

ologic stress response, by enhancing the prevailing emotion and thereby amplifying motivation, would elicit a more rapid and forceful response to the threatening stimulus. This conscious affective component of motivation-enhancement would coincide logically and functionally with the previously discussed physiological "alert and prepare" boost function.

On the basis of the current research findings, we can reasonably propose that the overall feeling during stress is a combined affect—that of the primary affective state(s) (e.g., fear, pain, hunger, disease) and the affect intensity modulation and potential anxiety contributed by the stress response. Just as the stress response becomes part of the emotional response physiologically, so too does the conscious component of affect. The unpleasantness of the feeling during stress is predominantly attributable to the primary emotion, but the stress response appears to contribute to the quality of the unpleasantness.

WHAT IS DISTRESS?

The affect of stress is profoundly linked to, and takes on its greatest significance for well-being in, the concept of *distress*. To the individual experiencing it, distress is the most important conscious component of stress. In contrast to stress, which involves both conscious and unconscious elements, distress appears to be exclusively a conscious, unpleasant affective state (DeGrazia 1996). Distress cannot occur below consciousness; the idea of "unconscious distress" is nonsensical. However, nothing close to a consensus on the definition of distress exists, and discussions of the concept often ambiguously blend unconscious (physiologic) processes and conscious aspects of stress.

In the stress literature, distress has been conceptualized in numerous ways but is generally classifiable into three basic interpretations: (1) the state that results from the inability to cope with or adapt to an aversive condition or event (Kitchen et al. 1987, Kopin et al. 1988, Clark et al. 1997a), (2) the state that exists when pathologic changes or maladaptive behaviors occur in response to aversive stimuli (Kopin et al. 1988, Clark et al. 1997a), and (3) the unpleasant affect elicited by an aversive situation or stimulus (DeGrazia 1996). These three conceptualizations are not mutually exclusive, and some writers use a combination of them when discussing the subject (for example see, Wolfle 2000).

My view is that distress is an affect that resembles, or is, that of anguish, experienced when the individual is unable to adapt to, cope with, or otherwise lessen the intensity of an unpleasant affect in a timely manner. For example, as an unpleasant affect such as loneliness, nausea, fear, or ambient heat increases in intensity, at some level, a mental state of distress—an anguish-like feeling—that compounds the unpleasantness of the original affect will arise. Whether distress represents an affect separate and distinct from the underlying unpleasant affect is unclear.

The extensive literature on *control*, with special reference to studies of escapable versus inescapable shock (Visintainer et al. 1982, Seligman 1975), leads me to propose that it is the degree of perceived control over the intensity of the primary affect that is the main, and possibly sole, factor that raises or lowers the threshold level at which point an unpleasant primary affect elicits distress. In what may be a direct correlation, as the degree of control rises, the threshold of distress elicitation rises. This is saying that as the animal (or person) perceives more control over the unpleasant affect—that is, that he or she has the power to turn down or turn off the unpleasantness at any time—the level of intensity of that unpleasant affect at which distress is elicited becomes higher. Studies of hospitalized human patients with pain have shown that the patients who are given the ability to self-administer morphine (patient-controlled analgesia, or PCA) end up using significantly less of the drug than patients who receive morphine by continuous infusion (CI), for the same degree of pain control (Mackie et al. 1991). In a review of 32 trials comparing PCA with CI, researchers found that when the total drug intake was equal between the groups, the PCA group reported less pain intensity and greater relief than did the CI group (Walder et al. 2001). In these studies, having control in some way appears to lessen the potential for distress when experiencing the unpleasant affect of pain. Anecdotal observations of a wide array of aversive situations in humans, from holding an appendage in icy water to withstanding a rising ambient temperature to holding one's urine, also strongly suggest that the discomfort is tolerated to a substantially higher degree when the individual perceives that he or she has the control to end the discomfort at any time. Whether the effect of control is an actual lessening of the experienced intensity of the unpleasant affect, a change in the brain/mind's tolerance of the same degree of affect intensity, or a combination of both is unknown.

Modifying earlier definitions and establishing affect as the primary focus, I propose the following

definition: *Distress may be conceived as the unpleasant affective state, akin to or the same as anguish, resulting from an inability to control or otherwise cope with or adapt to the unpleasant affect generated by altered or threatened homeostasis.* For example, insufficient mental stimulation leads to the emotion and affect of boredom, which, when exceeding the animal's coping ability, leads to the unpleasant affective state of distress. Likewise for physical pain, thirst, hunger, nausea, loneliness, fear, and, in humans, guilt, shame, and embarrassment. In this sense, distress is a function of how an animal copes with the unpleasant affect elicited by aversive events rather than the quantity of aversive stimulation it actually encounters (Novak & Suomi 1988).

Distress shares many attributes with *suffering*, in that both are unpleasant affective mental states attributable to an underlying unpleasant affect. In my view, it is not at all clear that distress and suffering are different concepts, and I make no attempt to differentiate them. In this interpretation of distress and suffering, I am claiming that neither exists on its own; an underlying unpleasant affect of physical or emotional origin always exists. Accordingly, a person cannot say he is simply in distress or suffering—he has to be in distress or suffering *from* something—and that something can be labeled, or at least described, as a specific unpleasant affect.[2]

STRESS: A WORKING ANALYSIS

In situations where homeostasis is threatened or disturbed, one or more homeostasis-preserving mechanisms are activated. In addition to these mechanisms, a stress response may be activated. Stress is not an independent process; it coexists with and augments a primary homeostasis-preserving mechanism. Stress is not separate from the primary homeostasis-preserving mechanism; rather, it is superimposed on and functions in an assist capacity as part of the primary mechanism. Evidence suggests that stress mechanisms make several contributions to the effort to protect homeostasis, including cognitive arousal and heightened alertness, establishing a sense of urgency and mental focus and preparing the body for the necessary physiologic and behavioral responses.

Psychological stress in all cases coexists with emotions. When the primary homeostasis-preserving mechanism is an emotion, stress is not the emotion. However, it serves, functionally and affectively, as *part of* the emotional response through arousal enhancement, optimal preparation, and affect amplification of the emotional state.

The conscious aspect of stress is the experienced affect. Substantial evidence supports the contention that the affect of stressful experiences derives predominantly from the primary emotion and may contain some contribution of negative affect from stress mechanisms. Anxiety, physiologically and affectively, may be a part of the experience of stress. The unpleasant feeling of stress ("being stressed") may therefore be seen as a combination of the affect of the primary emotion (the predominant affect), the stress response, and potentially, anxiety.

Now let us revisit Sapolsky's wildebeest fleeing the lion. The question at the time was whether the process in the animal is fear, stress, or both. It is both. Fear, the primary emotion, motivates the animal to flee. Stress mechanisms equip the animal to react and flee *faster*.

IMPLICATIONS FOR MENTAL WELL-BEING

The importance of understanding the distinctions among stress, distress, and emotion can be summarized in one word: harm. Harm in all its forms—emotional and physical—is what the animal's defense systems, of which stress mechanisms are a part, are designed to prevent. From the animal's point of view, the unpleasant feelings associated with the emotional and physical harm are what *hurt*; hence, minimizing these feelings assumes the priority in animal care. An understanding of the feelings associated with stressful experiences and the stress response is essential for us to devise the most effective strategies to promote optimal mental well-being. Most important to this goal is to understand the source of the unpleasant feelings, and, more specifically, because the source of unpleasant affect is something other than the stress mechanisms, then a focus on the stress process is not the approach that will bring the animal maximal relief, comfort, and mental well-being.

We can now re-examine some of the problems discussed in the first part of this chapter and consider some frequently used passages from one of many books on the care of pet animals (all italics are added): (1) "A cat that has lived most or all of her life outdoors and is converted to an indoor cat may *show more stress-related behavior* than a cat that has never seen the outdoors"; (2) the cat "may begin to *exhibit signs of stress* . . . "; and (3) "One of the best *stress reducers* . . . for your cats . . . is play" (Church 1998). It should now be clear just how imprecise and unhelpful these statements are. For example, if play is a stress-reducer, what happens if the stress is due to extreme fear of humans? Or due to illness or injury? In such instances, play, rather than reducing stress, could actually increase the degree of emotional or physical harm to the animal. Clearly, to give the cat the proper care and relief from its unpleasantness, we must know that the cat is experiencing the emotion of fear or is afflicted with an illness rather than rely on the catch-all label of "stress." This terminology is also frequently made about animals kept in confinement, such as, "The way to reduce stress in zoo elephants is through environmental enrichment." But, again, what if the elephant's stress is associated with profound depression induced by the recent shipment of her companion of 20 years to another zoo?

Another area in which it is important that we distinguish stress and emotion is pharmacotherapy. Specific drugs are effective for specific emotions but not others, and it is therefore essential to attempt to identify the primary emotion that is active in the stressful experience rather than try to treat "stress." For example, certain pharmacologic agents, such as anxiolytics, are effective in some conditions labeled as "stressful" (e.g., anxiety, fear, anger), but not in others (e.g., boredom, loneliness). The same is true for antidepressant drugs.

The central problem, and the basis for harm, of chronic stress is the failure of the stress response to shut off (Sapolsky 1999). The pathologic consequences of a chronic activation of the stress response have been shown to be attributable to the sustained neurochemical alterations, specifically the elevation of corticosteroids. It has been proposed that a good strategy for short-circuiting the deleterious effects of chronic stress would be to directly alter the activity of the HPA axis by inhibiting the activity of corticotrophin releasing factor (CRH) (Miller & O'Callaghan 2002). Recent work has shown the promise of such pharmacologic agents as antalarmin, a CRH blocker, which helped to reverse the protracted release of glucocorticoids but did not impair the ability to respond fully to a new challenge or threat (Wong et al. 1999, Miller & O'Callaghan 2002).

The need for distinguishing emotion and stress also comes into play in the measurement of stress. It has been proposed that "measuring stress" will provide an assessment for animal well-being (Moberg 1987). The allure of focusing on stress rather than emotional states is that this approach offers at least *something objective* to measure (i.e., "stress hormones"). In contrast, obtaining objective and accurate measurement of emotions, and especially the affective component of each emotion, is currently not possible. However, focusing on stress is misleading and potentially harmful, as stress indices and emotional feeling states are not well correlated. Current measurements of stress may not be sensitive to all forms of discomfort and suffering (Yuwiler 1971), and not all emotional states that can cause suffering have a measurable physiologic stress component (Wemelsfelder 1984), making the absence of a stress response no assurance of positive mental well-being. The presence of a stress response does not necessarily indicate a poor well-being, as the stress response is part of a healthy defense system and may represent a successful response to a threat (Moberg 1987). Finally, glucocorticoid concentrations are not an accurate indicator of long-term aversive stimulation; for example, serum concentrations may remain in the normal range during prolonged illness (Clark et al. 1997b). Problems of correlation are further elucidated in a study comparing the effects of restraint in hand-reared deer and free-range deer (Hastings et al. 1992). Although measurement of stress-related hormones showed that the physiologic response to restraint was lower in the hand-reared animals, the latter struggled just as violently against restraint as the free-range deer, suggesting that the magnitude of change in stress hormones does not correlate with the intensity of emotional affect (in this case, fear). In humans, phobic patients confronted with the object of their phobia reported very large increases in feelings of anxiety despite normal plasma cortisol levels (Curtis et al. 1976). When infant squirrel monkeys were separated from their mothers, their distress vocalizations decreased over time, yet their cortisol levels remained elevated, suggesting that emotional behavior and physiological arousal responses can change independently of one another (Coe et al. 1983). It has been demonstrated in human patients that the degree of perceived burden from a given symptom and the physiological change from a given disease do not perfectly correlate (Stewart et al. 1999). In all, no physiologic parameter of the stress response has been shown to reliably correlate with the intensity or quality of the unpleasant subjective experience in human or nonhuman species (Moberg 1987). As a whole, research has repeatedly demonstrated a poor correlation between measurements of stress and those of mental well-being. Because the wide array of unpleasant emotions in which stress

responses play a role is commonly labeled collectively as "stress," the effectiveness of treatments based on measurements of "stress hormones" is highly unreliable. Together, these findings argue strongly for the need to focus on emotion rather than stress when striving to maximize mental well-being.

Further evidence demonstrating the error of focusing on and trying to prevent stress rather than unpleasant affect is, as mentioned earlier, the finding that a physiologic stress response may occur in association with pleasant as well as unpleasant situations (Moberg 1987, Manser 1992). In these instances, identifying a physiologic stress response and instituting some method of stress management in an effort to eliminate the eliciting stressful stimulus could actually result in a *diminished* mental well-being.

Frequently in animal welfare discussions, it is implied that stress is a bad thing and should be eliminated (Moberg 2000). However, because some stress (i.e., an event that leads to activation of the stress response) in life is known to be beneficial and desirable, the goal of animal care should not be to eliminate all stress but to minimize the *harm* of stressful events. For short-term (acute) stress, our foremost objective is to minimize the unpleasant affect of the primary emotion—the emotional pain (McMillan 2002). We want to reduce the unpleasantness to a level that the animal can successfully cope with, or give the animal the resources to cope with the negative affect. In other words, our goal is to *eliminate distress* (as defined in this chapter). Whereas there is good stress, there is no good distress. Protecting the animal from distress thereby minimizes the harm of acute stressful experiences without eliminating stress entirely. The most potent method for raising the threshold for unpleasant affect to elicit distress appears to be the perception of control over the unpleasantness; hence, the single best tool for equipping an animal to prevent or lessen distress would seem to be control, real or perceived (see Markowitz & Eckert, this volume). To achieve this objective, we must identify the emotional component(s) that contribute the unpleasant affect. Declaring that the dog in the kennel is "stressed" provides little if any useful information for providing control over the prevailing unpleasant affect; the stress could be due to fear, anxiety, separation distress, isolation/loneliness, boredom, frustration, helplessness, pain, hunger, constipation, or other unpleasant emotional or physical states.

Stress management for long-term stress also involves the prevention of distress through reduction of unpleasant feelings. An additional objective in sustained stressful conditions is the prevention of the pathologic health consequences. As for acute stress, we want to give animals the resources (e.g., control) to cope with the aversive situation. This approach was demonstrated by Carlstead et al. (1993a) in a study of leopards. When the cats were housed in a barren enclosure with other large feline species such as lions, tigers, and pumas, which are predators of the smaller cats in the wild, the leopards showed much pacing behavior and high levels of corticosteroids, suggesting high activity of the stress response. When the researchers placed hollow logs, boxes, branches, and platforms in the enclosure, the leopards were then able to hide from the predator cats, and their pacing and hormone levels decreased dramatically. Having hiding places apparently gave the cats control over the degree of unpleasantness (they could lessen their fear by hiding), thereby allowing the animals to cope with the situation. A study in domestic cats (Carlstead et al. 1993b) showed similar effects. Overall, given the vital role of the stress response in animal defense systems, the ideal goal of stress management programs would be to lessen the intensity and/or mental impact of the unpleasant affect and protect against pathologic somatic and mental effects while ensuring that the body's ability to mount an effective defensive response to a new challenge or threat remains intact (Miller & O'Callaghan 2002).

Developing effective strategies to maximize mental well-being in animals necessitates an understanding of the relationship and distinctions between stress, emotion, and distress. Therapeutic and preventive approaches—e.g., environmental, behavioral, medicinal, and nutritional—can never achieve precision and maximal efficacy if the mental and physiological processes for which they are intended remain a nebulous conglomeration of ambiguous concepts. In optimizing mental well-being of animals, it appears that focusing on stress may be addressing the wrong target. Distinguishing stress and emotion, and then focusing on the emotion and its accompanying feeling, appears to be the most direct and effective means for alleviating distress and suffering and maximizing the animals' mental well-being.

NOTES

1. Disagreement exists among researchers as to the definition of "affect." In this chapter it is used to indicate any feeling, emotional or physical in origin. Examples would include fear, pain, anger, full urinary bladder, pruritus, warming of the skin by the sun, nausea, hunger, sadness, dizziness, and so on.

2. Because I am saying that the underlying unpleasant affect elicits the distress, it is irrelevant whether the underlying affect is itself about something (i.e., has an object). For example, humans experience at least two affective states that often have no object—free-floating anxiety and clinical (biochemical) depression. These states can have no known eliciting event; hence, they are apparently not *about something*. When I claim that distress is about something, I am suggesting that the underlying unpleasant affect itself is the object, whether that affect itself has an object or not. In other words, the source of distress in free-floating anxiety or clinical depression is the unpleasant affect—anxiety or depression—itself. My view of distress (and suffering) is that these are unique types of affect, arising when the intensity of other unpleasant affects rise to a certain level. Pain is just pain until it increases in intensity, at which point the individual begins to experience distress. Mild embarrassment is a slight unpleasantry, but when it becomes intense, it elicits distress. All of this, of course, is much more complex than simply a matter of affect intensity, as other factors, especially control, strongly influence when or if a particular unpleasant affect will elicit distress. The reason I claim that distress and suffering (which may be the same thing) are unique types of unpleasant affects is that to me, they, unlike all other unpleasant affects, do not elicit distress and suffering.

ACKNOWLEDGMENTS

I am grateful to Robert Sapolsky for his helpful comments on this chapter.

REFERENCES

Bindra D. 1978. How adaptive behavior is produced: A perceptual-motivational alternative to response-reinforcement. *Behav Brain Sci* 1:41–91.

Bond RF, Johnson G. 1985. Vascular adrenergic interactions during hemorrhagic shock. *Fed Proc* 44:281–289.

The Boston Collaborative Drug Surveillance Program. 1972. Acute adverse reactions to prednisone in relation to dosage. *Clin Pharmacol Ther* 13:694–698.

Britton KT, Lee G, Koob GF. 1988. Corticotropin releasing factor and amphetamine exaggerate partial agonistic properties of benzodiazepine antogonist Ro 15-1788 in the conflict test. *Psychopharmacology* 94:306–311.

Brown MR, Fisher LA, Webb V, et al. 1985. Corticotropin-releasing factor: A physiologic regulator of adrenal epinephrine secretion. *Brain Res* 328:355–357.

Burchfield SR. 1979. The stress response: A new perspective. *Psychosom Med* 41:661–672.

Buwalda B, Nyakas C, Koolhaas JM, et al. 1991. Effects of neonatal administration of vasopressin on cardiac and behavioral responses to emotional stress in adult rats. *Physiol Behav* 50:929–932.

Cantril H, Hunt WA. 1932. Emotional effects produced by the injection of adrenalin. *Am J Psychol* 44:300–307.

Carlstead KJ, Brown J, Seidensticker J. 1993a. Behavioral and adrenocortical responses to environmental changes in leopard cats (*Felis bengalensis*). *Zoo Biol* 12:1–11.

Carlstead K, Brown JL, Strawn W. 1993b. Behavioral and physiological correlates of stress in laboratory cats. *Appl Anim Behav Sci* 38:143–158.

Cassel EJ. 1982. The nature of suffering and the goals of medicine. *New Engl J Med* 306:639–645.

Charmandari E, Kino T, Souvatzoglou E, et al. 2003. Pediatric stress: Hormonal mediators and human development. *Horm Res* 59:161–179.

Church C. 1998. *Housecat*. New York: Howell Book House.

Clark JD, Rager DR, Calpin JP. 1997a. Animal well-being II. Stress and distress. *Lab Anim Sci* 47:571–579.

Clark JD, Rager DR, Calpin JP. 1997b. Animal well-being IV. Specific assessment criteria. *Lab Anim Sci* 47:586–597.

Coe CL, Glass JC, Wiener SG, et al. 1983. Behavioral, but not physiological, adaptation to repeated separation in mother and infant primates. *Psychoneuroendocrino* 8:401–409.

Colborn DR, Thompson DL, Roth TL, et al. 1991. Responses of cortisol and prolactin to sexual excitement and stress in stallions and geldings. *J Anim Sci* 69:2556–2562.

Curtis G, Buxton M, Lippman D, et al. 1976. "Flooding in vivo" during the circadian phase of minimal cortisol secretion: Anxiety and therapeutic success without adrenal cortical activation. *Biol Psychiat* 11:101–107.

Damasio AR. 1999. *The feeling of what happens: Body and emotion in the making of consciousness*. New York: Harcourt Brace.

DeGrazia D. 1996. *Taking animals seriously*. Cambridge: Cambridge University Press.

Diener E, Sandvik E, Pavot W. 1991. Happiness is the frequency, not the intensity, of positive versus negative affect. In: Strack F, Argyle M, Schwarz N (eds), *Subjective well-being: An interdisciplinary perspective*. Elmsford, NY, Pergamon Press:119–139.

Dunn AJ, Berridge CW. 1990. Physiological and behavioral responses to corticotropin-releasing factor administration: Is CRF a mediator of anxiety or stress responses? *Brain Res Rev* 15:71–100.

Dunn AJ, File SE. 1987. Corticotropin-releasing factor has an anxiogenic action in the social interaction test. *Horm Behav* 21:193–202.

Engelmann M, Ebner K, Landgraf R, et al. 1999. Emotional stress triggers intrahypothalamic but not peripheral release of oxytocin in male rats. *J Neuroendocrinol* 11:867–872.

Erdmann G, van Lindern B. 1980. The effects of beta-adrenergic stimulation and beta-adrenergic blockade on emotional reactions. *Psychophysiology* 17:332–338.

Gottschalk LA, Stone WN, Gleser GC. 1974. Peripheral versus central mechanisms accounting for antianxiety effects of propranolol. *Psychosom Med* 36:47–56.

Haroutunian V, Riccio DC. 1977. Effect of arousal conditions during reinstatement treatment upon learned fear in young rats. *Dev Psychobiol* 10:25–32.

Hastings BE, Abbott DE, George LM. 1992. Stress factors influencing plasma cortisol levels and adrenal weights in Chinese water deer (*Hydropotes inermis*). *Res Vet Sci* 53:375–380.

Hatch AM, Wiberg GS, Zawidzka Z, et al. 1965. Long-term isolation in rats. *Toxicol Appl Pharm* 7:737–745.

Hinkle LE. 1974. The concept of "stress" in the biological and social sciences. *Int J Psychiat Med* 5:335–357.

Hohmann GW. 1966. Some effects of spinal cord lesions on experienced emotional feelings. *Psychophysiology* 3:143–156.

Kallet AJ, Cowgill LD, Kass PH. 1997. Comparison of blood pressure measurements obtained in dogs by use of indirect oscillometry in a veterinary clinic versus at home. *J Am Vet Med Assoc* 210:651–654.

Kitchen H, Aronson AL, Bittel JL, et al. 1987. Panel report on the colloquium on recognition and alleviation of animal pain and distress. *J Am Vet Med Assoc* 191:1186–1191.

Koob GF, Bloom FE. 1985. Corticotropin-releasing factor and behavior. *Fed Proc* 44:259–263.

Kopin IJ, Eisenhofer G, Goldstein D. 1988. Sympathoadrenal medullary system and stress. In:

Chrousos GP, Loriaux DL, Gold PW (eds), *Mechanisms of physical and emotional stress*. New York, Plenum Press:11–24.

Kuzmin A, Semenova S, Zvartau EE, et al. 1996. Enhancement of morphine self-administration in drug naïve, inbred strains of mice by acute emotional stress. *Eur Neuropsychopharm* 6:63–68.

Landis C, Hunt WA. 1932. Adrenalin and emotion. *Psychol Rev* 39:467–485.

Lazarus RS. 1999. *Stress and emotion*. New York: Springer.

LeDoux J. 1996. *The emotional brain*. New York: Simon & Schuster.

Leventhal H, Patrick-Miller L. 2000. Emotions and physical illness: Causes and indicators of vulnerability. In: Lewis M, Haviland-Jones JM (eds), *Handbook of emotions*. 2nd edition. New York, The Guilford Press:523–537.

Lewis DA, Smith RE. 1983. Steroid-induced psychiatric syndromes. *J Affect Disorders* 5:319–332.

Ling MHM, Perry PJ, Ming TT. 1981. Side effects of corticosteroid therapy. *Arch Gen Psychiat* 38:471–477.

Mackie AM, Coda BC, Hill HF. 1991. Adolescents use patient-controlled analgesia effectively for relief from prolonged oropharyngeal mucositis pain. *Pain* 46:265–269.

Manser C. 1992. *The assessment of stress in laboratory animals*. Causeway, Horsham, West Sussex, UK: Royal Society for the Prevention of Cruelty to Animals.

Maranon G. 1924. Contribution a l'etude de l'action emotive de l'adrenaline. *Rev Francaise Endocrin* 2:301–325.

Marshall GD, Zimbardo PG. 1979. Affective consequences of inadequately explained physiological arousal. *J Pers Soc Psychol* 37:970–988.

Martini L, Lorenzini RN, Cinotti S, et al. 2000. Evaluation of pain and stress levels of animals used in experimental research. *J Surg Res* 88:114–119.

Maslach C. 1979. The emotional consequences of arousal without reason. In: Izard CE (ed), *Emotion in personality and psychopathology*. New York, Plenum Press:565–590.

Mason JW. 1968. Organization of the multiple endocrine responses to avoidance in the monkey. *Psychosom Med* 30:774–790.

Mason JW. 1975. Emotion as reflected in patterns of endocrine integration. In: Levi L (ed), *Emotions: Their parameters and measurement*. New York, Raven Press:143–181.

Mason JW, Maher JT, Hartley LH, et al. 1976. Selectivity of corticosteroid and catecholamine responses to various natural stimuli. In: Serban G (ed), *Psychopathology of human adaptation*. New York, Plenum Press:147–171.

McEwen BS. 2000. The neurobiology of stress: From serendipity to clinical relevance. *Brain Res* 886:172–189.

McEwen BS. 2002. Protective and damaging effects of stress mediators: The good and bad sides of the response to stress. *Metabolis* 51 Suppl 1:2–4.

McEwen BS, Wingfield JC. 2003. The concept of allostasis on biology and biomedicine. *Horm Behav* 43:2–15.

McMillan FD. 2000. Quality of life in animals. *J Am Vet Med Assoc* 216:1904–1910.

McMillan FD. 2002. Emotional pain management. *Vet Med* 97:822–834.

McNaughton N. 1989. *Biology and emotion*. Cambridge: Cambridge University Press.

Miller DB, O'Callaghan JP. 2002. Neuroendocrine aspects of the response to stress. *Metabolis* 51 Suppl 1:5–10.

Minden SL, Orav J, Schildkraut JJ. 1988. Hypomanic reactions to ACTH and prednisone treatment for multiple sclerosis. *Neurology* 38:1631–1634.

Moberg GP. 1985. Biological responses to stress: Key to assessment of animal well-being. In: Moberg GP (ed), 2000. *Animal stress*. Bethesda, MD, American Physiological Society:28–49.

Moberg GP. 1987. Problems defining stress and distress in animals. *J Am Vet Med Assoc* 191:1207–1211.

Moberg G. 2000. Biological response to stress: Implications for animal welfare. In: Moberg G, Mench JA (eds), *The biology of animal stress: Basic principles and implications for animal welfare*. Wallingford, CABI Publishing:1–22.

Nicolaidis S. 2002. A hormone-based characterization and taxonomy of stress: Possible usefulness in management. *Metabolis* 51 Suppl 1:31–36.

Noble RE. 2002. Diagnosis of stress. *Metabolis* 51 Suppl 1:37–39.

Novak MA, Suomi SJ. 1988. Psychological well-being of primates in captivity. *Am Psychol* 43:765–773.

Panksepp J. 1998. *Affective neuroscience: The foundations of human and animal emotions*. New York: Oxford University Press.

Pedersen HD, Haggstrom J, Falk T, et al. 1999. Auscultation in mild mitral regurgitation in dogs: Observer variation, effects of physical maneuvers, and agreement with color doppler echocardiography and phonocardiography. *J Vet Intern Med* 13:56–64.

Plutchik R. 1984. Emotions: A general psychoevolutionary theory. In: Scherer KR, Ekman P (eds), *Approaches to emotions*. Hillsdale, NJ, Lawrence Erlbaum Associates:197–219.

Reisenzein R. 1983. The Schachter theory of emotions: Two decades later. *Psychol Bull* 94:239–264.

Reusch CE. 2000. Hypoadrenocorticism. In: Ettinger SJ, Feldman EC (eds), *Textbook of veterinary internal medicine: Diseases of the dog and cat*, 5th ed. Philadelphia, W.B. Saunders:1488–1499.

Riley V. 1981. Psychoneuroendocrine influences on immunocompetence and neoplasia. *Science* 212:1100–1109.

Rollin BE. 1989. *The unheeded cry: Animal consciousness, animal pain and science*. Oxford: Oxford University Press.

Rolls ET. 2000. Precis of *The brain and emotion*. *Behav Brain Sci* 23:177–234.

Rose RM. 1980. Endocrine responses to stressful psychological events. *Psychiat Clin N Am* 3:251–276.

Salmon P, Gray JA. 1985. Opposing acute and chronic behavioural effects of a beta-blocker, propranolol, in the rat. *Psychopharmacology* 86:480–486.

Sapolsky RM. 1994. *Why zebras don't get ulcers: A guide to stress, stress-related diseases, and coping*. New York: W.H. Freeman.

Sapolsky RM. 1999. The physiology and pathophysiology of unhappiness. In: Kahneman D, Diener E, Schwarz N (eds), *Well-being: The foundations of hedonic psychology*. New York, Russell Sage Foundation:453–469.

Schachter S, Singer JE. 1962. Cognitive, social, and physiological determinants of emotional state. *Psychol Rev* 69:379–399.

Schulkin J. 2003. Allostasis: A neural behavioral perspective. *Horm Behav* 43:21–27.

Seligman ME. 1975. *Helplessness: On depression, development, and death*. San Francisco: W.H. Freeman.

Selye H. 1950. *The physiology and pathology of exposure to stress*. Montreal: Acta.

Singer J. 1963. Sympathetic activation, drugs, and fear. *J Comp Physiol Psych* 56:612–615.

Sternberg EM, Young WS, Bernardini R, et al. 1989. A central nervous system defect in biosynthesis of corticotrophin-releasing hormone is associated with susceptibility to streptococcal cell wall-induced arthritis in Lewis rats. *P Natl Acad Sci* 86:4771–4775.

Stewart AL, Teno J, Patrick DL, et al. 1999. The concept of quality of life of dying persons in the context of health care. *J Pain Symptom Manag* 17:93–108.

Symington T, Currie AR, Curran RC, et al. 1955. The reaction of the adrenal cortex in conditions of stress. In: *Ciba Foundation Colloquia on Endocrinology. The human adrenal cortex*, Vol. 8. Boston, Little and Brown:70–91.

Tooby J, Cosmides L. 1990. The past explains the present: Emotional adaptations and the structure of ancestral environments. *Ethol Sociobiol* 11:375–424.

Tyrer P. 1976. *The role of bodily feelings in anxiety*. (Institute of Psychiatry Maudsley Monographs, No 23). Oxford: Oxford University Press.

US Department of Defense. 1999. *Dictionary of military terms*. London: Greenhill Books.

Van de Kar LD, Piechowski RA, Rittenhouse PA, et al. 1991. Amygdaloid lesions: Differential effect on conditioned stress and immobilization-induced increases in corticosterone and renin secretion. *Neuroendocrinology* 54:89–95.

Visintainer MA, Volpicelli JR, Seligman MEP. 1982. Tumor rejection in rats after inescapable or escapable shock. *Science* 216:437–439.

Walder B, Schafer M, Henzi I, et al. 2001. Efficacy and safety of patient-controlled opioid analgesia for acute postoperative pain. A quantitative systematic review. *Acta Anaesth Scand* 45:795–804.

Wemelsfelder F. 1984. Animal boredom: Is a scientific study of the subjective experiences of animals possible? In: Fox MW, Mickley LD (eds), *Advances in animal welfare science 1984/85*. Washington, DC, The Humane Society of the United States:115–154.

Wolfle TL. 2000. Understanding the role of stress in animal welfare: Practical considerations. In: Moberg G, Mench JA (eds), *The biology of animal stress: Basic principles and implications for animal welfare*. Wallingford, CABI Publishing:355–368.

Wong ML, Webster EL, Spokes H, et al. 1999. Chronic administration of the non-peptide CRH type 1 receptor antagonist antalarmin does not blunt hypothalamic-pituitary-adrenal axis responses to acute immobilization stress. *Life Sci* 65:PL53–PL58.

Yuwiler A. 1971. Stress. In: Lajtha A (ed), *Handbook of neurochemistry*, Vol. 6. New York, Plenum Press:103–171.

Zajonc RB. 1984. On primacy of affect. In: Scherer KR, Ekman P (eds), *Approaches to emotions*. Hillsdale, NJ, Lawrence Erlbaum:259–270.

8

Interrelationships Between Mental and Physical Health: The Mind-Body Connection

Michael W. Fox

Conventional Western human and veterinary medicine still bear the legacy of French philosopher René Descartes (1970), who promoted the false dualism of the mind being separate from the body, and of the belief that animals were unfeeling machines. Such mechanomorphization of nonhuman animals became the scientific consensus that condemned the belief and empirical evidence of emotional states in animals as sentimentally misguided anthropomorphism. In spite of Charles Darwin's work (notably his book *The Expression of Emotions in Man and Animals* [Darwin 1920]) and other scientists' and philosophers' opposition to Cartesian dualism and mechanistic reductionism, the resistance to accepting that animals have minds and emotions endured for more than three hundred years after Descartes. This was especially true in scientific, biomedical, and related circles of animal use and abuse, in part because of even deeper religious and cultural attitudes toward nonhuman life (Fox 1996). As late as the 1960s, skepticism was expressed by some veterinarians over empirical evidence that dogs will feign injury to a limb to seek attention (Fox 1962). Some members of the profession scoffed at such evidence, contending that they would be called on to be pet shrinks or behavioral therapists, while others acknowledged the need for more expertise and research in normal and abnormal behavior in animals.

The mind-body psyche-soma dichotomization greatly limited progress in human, veterinary, and comparative medicine and contributed to much animal cruelty and suffering. This was compounded by specialization that led to the "fragmentation" of seeing and treating the animal and human patient as a whole being, and of the conceptualization of health and disease processes. Another product of dualism and reductionism was the dichotomization of the essential organism-environment unity that tended to preclude the consideration and recognition of social and environmental influences on mind and body (i.e., on the animals' emotional and physical well-being).

ETHOS, ECOS, AND *TELOS*

Animal health depends on animal well-being, the bioethical and scientific parameters and indices of which include provision of an environment (the *ecos*) that is optimal for animals' basic physical, behavioral, and psychological requirements (their *ethos*, or spirits), and which maximizes animals' *telos*, their natural, ecological purpose and biological values and roles (Fox 2001). Human-imposed and -directed influences on animals' *ecos* include housing and husbandry conditions and standards of care and environmental quality; on animals' *telos* include economic, cultural, and other human values and interests; and on animals' *ethos*, as affected by selective breeding, genetic engineering as well as early handling and socialization, or lack thereof (Figure 8.1).

These three spheres of animal life—*ethos, ecos* and *telos*—translate into the mind-body-organism-environment interfaces that provide a more holistic paradigm for addressing animal health and welfare concerns (Fox 1997).

Because the mind is in the body, the body is in the mind. Likewise, because the elephant is in the forest and the forest is in the elephant, how can we put elephants in chains and force them to help people destroy the last of their forests, or put them in circuses and zoos and expect them to be healthy and reproductive and not go berserk? Elephants and other animals, wild and domesticated, under our

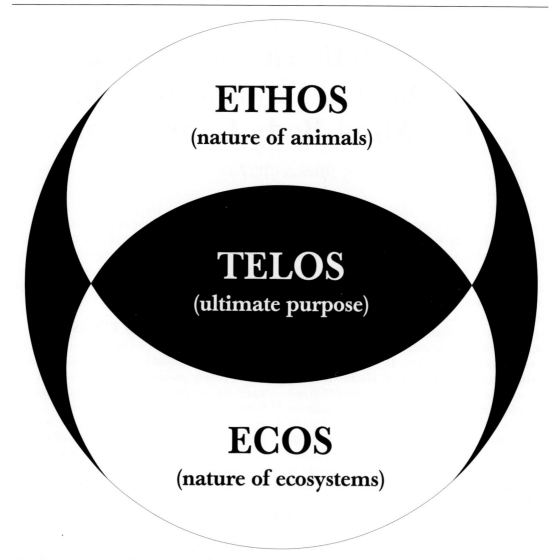

Figure 8.1. Interrelationships between the nature and natural purpose of animals and the ecosystem with which they have co-evolved. Domestication and other human influences have affected *ethos*, *telos*, and *ecos*, often with harmful consequences to both animals and ecosystems (from Fox 1999).

dominion surely need not have to be victims of such mind-body-environment dislocations that result in suffering and distress.

Only in the past 50 years have scientists, bioethicists, and veterinarians begun to consider the stress, distress, and suffering of animals under conditions of extreme and chronic confinement and environmental deprivation, often coupled with inconceivably high stocking densities (as with the intensive production of farmed animals). Such mistreatment creates pathogenic conditions, especially as a result

of stress and immunosuppression, for the proliferation of infectious and contagious "domestogenic" and production-related diseases (Fox 1984, 1986). These animal health and welfare problems are significant economic and public health concerns that will not be rectified by new vaccines, stronger antibiotics, and other drugs that are not all environmentally friendly and consumer-safe. Neither can the answer lie in selectively breeding and genetically engineering animals for food, fiber, and biomedical purposes. Nor is it to be found in the pet industries designed to enhance the animals' utility, productivity, and adaptability. This is because there are biological limitations that should translate into ethical limitations in how we should alter the *ethos* and *ecos* of animals for our own pecuniary and other, purely human, ends (Fox 1992, 1999).

Before reviewing some landmark studies, old and new, of the mind-body connection and the influence of emotional and cognitive states and environment on animals' health and well-being, I wish to summarize the above overview of principles of optimal animal care. The following five bioethical principles combine to make a simple formula to help ensure animals' health and well-being: *Right Environment + Right Genetics and Breeding + Right Understanding + Right Relationship + Right Nutrition = Animal Health and Well-being.*

Applying these principles within the holistic paradigm that addresses the animals' *ethos*, *ecos*, and *telos* facilitates the objective determination of animal health (which is not simply the absence of disease); the assessment of stress and distress using established physiological, neurochemical, and behavioral indices; and the identification of welfare parameters and basic standards of animal husbandry that meet animals' physical, as well as psychological and behavioral, needs.

STEPS TOWARD UNDERSTANDING

Significant advances have been made in the science of applied animal ethology and welfare assessment and improvement since the first English language book—*Abnormal Behavior in Animals* (Fox 1968)— on this interdisciplinary subject was published. This book included essays by veterinarians, ethologists, neuropsychologists, clinical and experimental psychologists, and Pavlovian physiologists. One chapter by L. Chertok, "Animal Hypnosis" (an intriguing mind-body phenomenon in vertebrate and invertebrate animals), was reprinted from a 1964 book—the first book ever published, to my knowledge, addressing animals' emotional states and behavioral (psychogenic) and psychosomatic diseases associated with stress and distress from a primarily veterinary perspective. This book, edited by two French veterinarians, was called *Psychiatrie Animale* (Brion & Ey 1964).

Between the 1960s and 1980s, interest grew in comparative psychiatry, from Harlow's maternally-deprived caged macaques to other experimental psychologists' often-gruesome studies of learned helplessness in rats repeatedly half-drowned. Other work included numerous studies of restrained dogs being given inescapable shock (Overmeier 1981), the end product being a proposed model of human coping in the presence of hopelessness and depression. It was believed that such research might be of value in testing the new anti-depressant psychotropic drugs that were being developed around that time (see also Seligman 1975).

Disturbing, but not devoid of some value in awakening our understanding of the similarities in how humans and laboratory animals manifest distress and psychological suffering, these experiments should never be, nor need ever be, repeated. Nor should those of Pavlovian—classical conditioning—that resulted in much animal suffering, especially of dogs; yet like the Nazi medical experiments on concentration-camp prisoners, these experiments provided empirical evidence affirming the mind-body connections of stress and distress, as well as various psychogenic, psychosomatic, traumatic, and infectious disease processes (Pavlov 1928, Gantt 1944, Lidell 1956).

Using Pavlovian conditioning, researchers were able to identify and characterize different animal (dog) temperaments and went on to demonstrate how these various psychomorphs responded to pain, conditioned fear (anxiety, terror), infections, trauma (such as having a leg broken), and total body radiation (Figure 8.2), the details of which were provided by Prof. I.T. Kurtsin and published (along with a review of Harlow's infant monkey maternal deprivation research by Gene Sackett) in *Abnormal Behavior in Animals.*

DOMESTICATION EFFECTS

The seminal and less invasive research findings of another Soviet scientist, Prof. D.K. Belyaev, were first published in the West in another book that I edited—*The Wild Canids: Their Systematic Behavioral Ecology and Evolution* (1975). Belyaev and Trut (1975) reported changes in reproductive activity that they regarded as a "destabilization" process in captive silver foxes after several generations of selectively breeding the most tractable and docile. Thereafter, generations of foxes developed floppy ears and piebald coats, and females became bi-estrus rather than having one heat per year. Belyaev and Trut showed how the domestication process (of selectively breeding the most docile animals) affected the animals' morphology and physiology, notably their reactivity to ACTH injections and psychological stress. American researcher Curt Richter had come to similar conclusions in his earlier

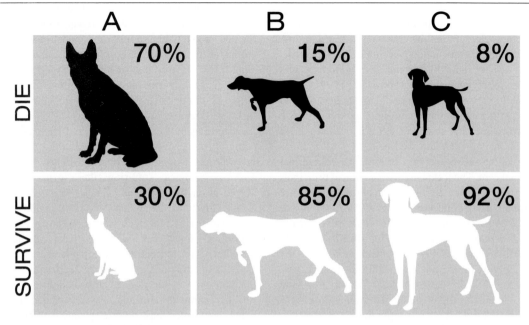

Figure 8.2. Drawings showing the influence of the type of nervous system on the percentage of dogs that die as a result of radiation sickness. **(A)** in a dog with a weak nervous system; **(B)** in a dog with a strong, unbalanced nervous system; **(C)** in a dog with a strong, balanced nervous system. The percentage of dogs making up each group is shown in the upper right of each box (from Kurtsin 1968).

(1954) research on the effects of domestication on the Norway rat, concluding that the laboratory rats were relatively hypergonadal and hypoadrenal compared to their wild counterparts, such endocrine changes being attributed to artificial selection for high fertility and docility. Domestication, according to Belyaev and Trut, influences the hypothalamo-pituitary-adrenal-gonadal systems; the selection from docile, tractable behavior leads to the dramatic emergence of new forms (phenotypes) and the destabilization of ontogenesis manifested by the breakdown of correlated systems (adrenal-pituitary, gonadal-pituitary) created originally under stabilizing (i.e., natural) selection. (For some of the earliest original thinking and research in this area, see Stockard 1941).

Experimental psychologist E. Gellhorn (1968) (who made cats more docile by eliminating their senses of smell, sight, and hearing to make them more trophotropic- or parasympathetic-system-dominant—they slept more) was coming to conclusions similar to those of Belyaev and Trut (although by a less ethical and humane path), which he felt had implications for neuropsychiatry. The tuning of the parasympathetic and adrenergic systems, the latter being linked with the neurohy-

pophysis-pituitary-gonadal and other neuroendocrine and immune-system modulating mind-body connections, became the focus of converging and diverging animal studies during this time that helped further our understanding of the mind-body and environment connections, as well as the effects of domestication.

Robert Ader, in 1981, put several authors together in a book that supported his thesis that mental states (emotions), distress, and stress affect the body, especially the immune system. It was appropriately titled *Psychoneuroimmunology* (Ader 1981).

This was a major turning point in demonstrating how social, emotional, and environmental stimuli, events, and experiences can influence the animal's neuroendocrine system, stress tolerance, and disease susceptibility. This new understanding demanded a more holistic approach in veterinary practice to the diagnosis, treatment, and prevention of domestogenic diseases and syndromes in farmed, laboratory, zoo, and companion animals. A holistic approach to animal health and welfare in the biomedical and intensive factory farm environments was particularly important for scientific and financial reasons, as well as on moral grounds (Fox 1984,

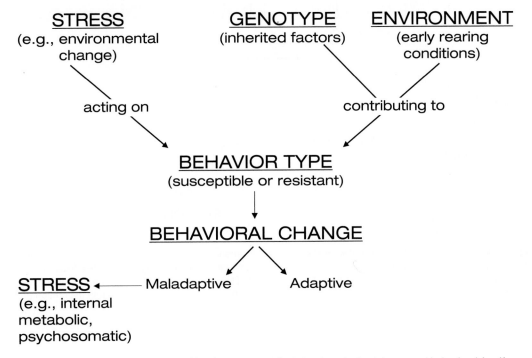

Figure 8.3. Schema of interrelated variables that may contribute to phenotypic variance and behavioral (and/or physiological) changes (from Fox 1986).

1986). The holistic, interdisciplinary approach to addressing mind-body-environment dislocations (Figure 8.3) that may cause animals to suffer and become diseased called for applying ethology, the study of animal behavior, to the science and art of veterinary medicine and comparative medicine, which I stressed in the Wesley W. Spink Lectures on Comparative Medicine at the University of Minnesota (Fox 1974).

The British Veterinary Ethology Society was established around this time and, after only a few years, became the International Society of Applied Ethology, encouraging veterinary colleges and animal science departments to offer courses and conduct research on this subject. Since these encouraging beginnings, several benchmark studies, symposia, and texts have been published, (Katcher & Beck 1983, Davis & Balfour 1992, Lawrence & Rushen 1993, Dodman & Shuster 1998, Panksepp 1998, Moberg & Mench 2000).

A more holistic understanding of animals' *ethos* and welfare requirements has also come from research in *cognitive ethology*, the field of study that investigates animal consciousness; mental states; and the *umvelt*, or animals' perceptual world (Griffin 1977, Bekoff 2002).

The British Brambell (1965) report on farm animal welfare included the following statement by the eminent neurologist Lord Brain:

> I personally can see no reason for conceding mind to my fellow men and denying it to animals. Mental functions, rightly viewed, are but servants of the impulses and emotions by which we live, and these, the springs of Life, are surely diencephalic in their neurological location. Since the diencephalon is well developed in animals and birds, I at least cannot doubt that the interests and activities of animals are correlated with awareness and feelings in the same way as my own, and which may be, for ought I know, just as vivid.

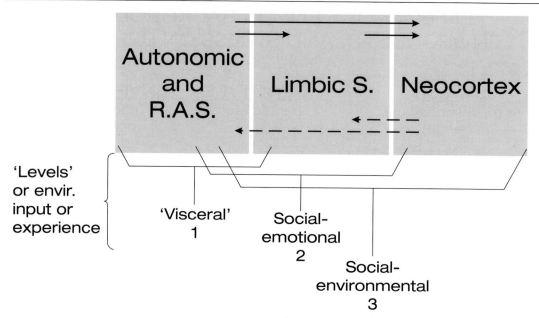

Figure 8.4. Schema of relationships between stages of development of the central nervous system and the times when various types of environmental influence have their greatest effects. **1.** Handling early in life affects the adrenal-pituitary, autonomic, and reticular activating systems. **2.** Development of social attachments correlates with the development of limbic (emotional) centers. **3.** Social and environmental influences affect brain maturation (from Fox 1986).

McMillan (2003) has stressed the clinical and animal welfare importance of considering more than physical pain and relief of same, because "emotional pain" (as fear, panic, anxiety, helplessness, and depression) is a welfare-related concern in addition to physical pain per se.

DEVELOPMENTAL EFFECTS

Further understanding of developmental processes that influence the behavioral phenotype come from studies of early experiences, both pre- and postnatally (Figure 8.4), that entailed various handling procedures of pregnant animals—mainly mice—and of the offspring soon after birth. Gentle handling on a regular basis was found to affect emotional reactivity, learning ability, stress resistance, and disease susceptibility, which had profound implications in animal husbandry and pointed to an epigenetic, neo-Lamarkian phenomenon of inherited, intergenerational environmental influences on animals' physiology and behavior (Levine & Mullins 1966, Denenberg 1967). As a consultant in Biosensor Research for the Walter Reed Army Medical Center in the early 1970s, I applied some of

these findings in developing a socialization and rearing program that provided selected beneficial experiences to puppies during their formative weeks. This Superdog project, which I made available to puppy owners and breeders in my 1972 book *Understanding Your Dog*, was aimed at enhancing in-field performance, stress-tolerance, and disease resistance in adult German Shepherd dogs under combat conditions in Vietnam.

This field of developmental psychobiology showed that heredity and pre- and early postnatal experiences influenced animals' physiology, behavior, temperament, learning ability, and stress and disease resistance when early handling, socialization, and environmental enrichment were provided during critical or sensitive periods of development (Scott & Fuller 1965; Fox 1971; McMillan 1999c, 2002). Such profound consequences of external stimulation and experiences on the mind-body connection are now more widely recognized, providing a scientific basis for the value of tender loving care (TLC). Spitz (1949) first pointed out how the lack of TLC can cause marasmus, growth retardation, and increased morbidity and mortality in orphaned,

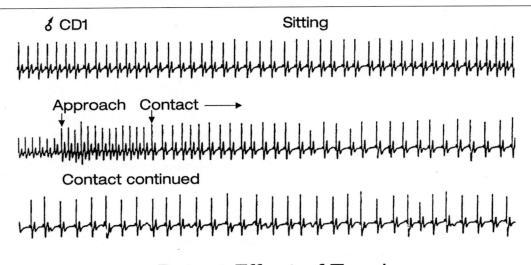

Potent Effect of Touch

Figure 8.5. Heartbeats in a dog (recorded with a biotelemeter) showing how petting, stroking, grooming, etc. slows the heart rate to a rate lower than when sitting and during contact (from Fox 1986).

institutionalized human infants. The relevance of these findings to improving the husbandry, health, and productivity of farmed animals was realized in particular by Hemsworth and Coleman (1998), who went on to demonstrate that sows that had been gently handled and socialized early in life had more offspring than sows not given such early experience.

The attitudes of animal caretakers toward the animals under their care are significantly influenced by the conditions under which they work and the conditions under which the animals are kept (Seabrook 1984), which underscores yet another variable in assessing animals' welfare and in setting optimal husbandry standards for various animal species. An animal caretaker's gentle handling can affect heart rate and other physiological indices (Figure 8.5). The petting of rabbits can significantly mitigate the harmful effects of a high fat and cholesterol diet, reducing the incidence of artherosclerosis by some 60 percent compared to non-handled rabbits fed the same diet (Nerem et al. 1980). This research further underscores the importance of recognizing the interactive nature of animals' social environment, emotional state, nutrition, and health.

The research of veterinarian W.B. Gross, now Professor Emeritus, Virginia and Maryland College of Veterinary Medicine, has shown the complexities of genotype-environment interactions—the mind-body connection—on the development, behavior, stress resistance, and disease susceptibility in poultry (Gross & Siegel 1981,1983; Gross 1982; Gross et al. 2002), the clinical and husbandry implications of which are indeed profound. He has also shown the benefits of vitamin C in blocking the adrenal stress response in the clinical setting of dogs presented with various forms of cancer, with promising results (Gross et al. 2001). These findings indirectly support the claimed clinical benefits of corticosteroid replacement therapy for a variety of chronic degenerative diseases in companion animals documented in practice by Plechner and Zucker (2003). As with Gross' lines of poultry, different breeds of dogs, cats, pigs, cattle, and other domesticated animals and hybrids with different temperaments and emotional reactivity respond differently to stress and other social and environmental stimuli. This can result in different disease profiles in animals raised under similar conditions. Adaptation and "fitness" under natural conditions call for a set of organismic responses that evolve over millennia. Animals under unnatural conditions of captivity and domesticity, to which they are not adapted, often show maladaptive responses. Further, being unable to adapt, they may suffer physically and psychologically.

PSYCHOPHARMACOLOGY

With the discovery of cholinergic, serotonergic, dopaminergic, and other neurochemical pathways and opioid, benzodiazepine, and other neural receptor sites that mediate and modulate various subjective, cognitive, and affective states, the field of behavioral psychopharmacology has opened a new door into the mind-body connections of human and nonhuman animals.

The mind-body connections of neuropeptides (e.g., the opiates) centered in the limbic system (the "seat" of the emotions) form a regulatory matrix of emotional, behavioral, and physiological processes that help promote animals' survival and well-being. Neuropeptide receptors have also been found in lymphocytes and spleen monocytes (which secrete ACTH and endorphin), creating a linkage with the immune system and central nervous system (CNS). Receptors for immunopeptides such as lymphokines, cytokines, and interleukins have been found in the CNS, and opiate and other receptors in the gastrointestinal tract and throughout most body organs and tissues. This means that bidirectional communication exists among mind and body, brain, and immune system such that mood and other mental states are linked with cellular defense and repair mechanisms (for a review, see McMillan 1999a).

The health benefits of companion animals to their human guardians, and vice versa, are associated at this molecular level with beneficial changes in levels of neurochemicals such as endorphin, prolactin, oxytocin, dopamine, and phenylethylamine in both humans and dogs during friendly contact (Odendaal & Meintjes 2003). This mind-body linking of neuropeptides and other chemical receptor systems makes it possible to lower an animal's blood pressure and enhance its immune response through classical and operant conditioning, biofeedback, and regular gentle petting. As Seligman (1975) has shown, control and predictability are important elements of coping for human and nonhuman animals in environments where having little or no control or predictability can lead to helplessness, depression, and immune-system impairment.

The thyroid gland can also be involved in stress and distress reactions; captive wild rabbits exposed to dogs, for example, may die from acute thyrotoxicosis (Kracht 1954). Loneliness and separation anxiety may be manifested as colitis-like diarrhea and bloody stools in dogs precisely because of these environment-mind-body connections, a greater understanding of which calls for the practice of holistic medicine. Stress-free understimulation (i.e., social isolation) leading to boredom vices (Wemelsfelder 1990) and higher mortalities can be as detrimental as overstimulation (as through overstocking). This means that an optimal level of stimulation and stress—called eustress—exists for individuals, breeds, and species, which helps maintain psychophysical homeostasis. Distress (caused by too little or too much stimulation) leads to *dystasis* (i.e., behavioral, metabolic, and cellular disruption of homeostatic systems).

The increasing spectrum of psychotropic drugs, analgesics, tranquilizers, anxiolytics, dissociatives, and skeletal muscle relaxants is of considerable value in veterinary practice (see Marder & Posage, this volume). They are especially valuable in reducing stress and fear in wild animals needing veterinary attention and in dealing with the obsessive-compulsive and separation-anxiety afflicted companion animals, but they should never become a matter of routine prescription for animals suffering from emotional, behavioral, or cognitive disorders to the exclusion of providing the right understanding, relationship, and environment, which are the best preventives of many behavioral anomalies, psychogenic disorders (such as self-mutilation in bored and anxious captive parrots), and psychosomatic diseases (such as ulcerative colitis in high-strung, i.e., highly empathic or extremely fearful, German Shepherd dogs).

The cage stereotypies of animals in barren environments may be associated with developmental abnormalities in the brain and impaired basal ganglia activity (Garner & Mason 2002). As these authors conclude from their evidence for a neural substrate for cage stereotypy, animals with stereotypies may experience novel forms of psychological distress, and the observed stereotypy might well represent a confound in many behavioral experiments. The effects of the impoverished laboratory cage environment and of environmental enrichment on brain development, neurochemistry, and behavior have been long recognized (Rosenzweig et al. 1962, Diamond et al. 1967). These effects can compromise both animals' welfare and their utility for research (introducing uncontrolled experimental variables), as emphasized by Fox (1986) and more recently by Wurbel (2001) and Markowitz and Timmel (this volume).

A new perspective on stereotypic behavior in horses has been given by Marsden (2002), who looks at various treatments from an ethological and

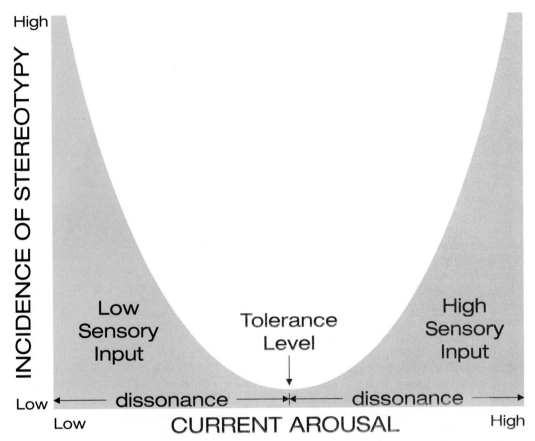

Figure 8.6. Relationships between arousal level and degree of stereotypy illustrate the homeostatic function (or ethostasis) of stereotyped behavior patterns. With low arousal (e.g., in isolation) or intense arousal, the frequency of stereotyped actions increases (from Fox 1986).

animal welfare perspective, identifying those treatments that can be detrimental when the underlying motivation and/or frustration is not addressed. Stereotypic behavior can be interpreted as a maladaptive response to hypostimulation or hyperstimulation (Fox 1986), the environmental dissonance between stimulus-input and the animal's arousal level being homeostatically regulated by increased or decreased activity (Figure 8.6). A bored, understimulated animal may groom excessively, sometimes to the point of self-mutilation, and behave similarly when stressed by fear or anxiety and frustration when confined in a strange place, or in the presence of strangers. Such self-comforting behav-

ior associated with hypostimulation and hyperstimulation can be correctly interpreted as obsessive-compulsive behavior, but should be distinguished from schizoaffective disorder that can manifest similar clinical signs but have a different etiology and motivation. One example is the dog who self-mutilates after displaying agonistic behavior, the self-mutilation being a consequence of self-directed aggression, sometimes accompanied by psychogenic hallucinations, such as fly-snapping and staring at one spot.

The effects of living alone in a cage, pen, or room on millions of dogs, cats, birds, and other pets for long periods of time, devoid of social contact with humans and, all too often, other animals, is a veterinary medical and ethical problem. Reliance on psychotropic drugs to alleviate these adverse effects is neither an appropriate medical nor ethical solution.

Another group of chemicals influencing mind-body reactions that are generally much safer, if not cheaper, than psychotropic drugs are the pheromones, or animal essences, and the plant essences, or essential oils derived from various herbs, flowers, trees, and other vegetative life forms. These phytochemical substances of plants have co-evolved neurochemical affinities with the mammalian brain and other systems of the body. One example of this is the endogenous opioid beta-endorphin pain-alleviating receptor system that is present even in earthworms. Some of these essential oils may affect serotonergic, gamma-aminobutyric acid, and dopaminergic neurotransmission, or have anticholinergic, antispasmodic, and other mind-body effects that may prove beneficial to animals suffering from a variety of behavioral problems. Horses and other animals that develop stress- and boredom-related stereotypies and other obsessive-compulsive disorders develop elevated dopamine and opioid levels that may be inhibited by dopaminergic and opioid agonists. More research in the veterinary and animal husbandry applications of plant essences, popularly known as aromatherapy, is needed in this clinically promising but scientifically little-understood area of alternative-complementary medicine (Bell 2002).

It might be rewarding to evaluate the euphoric, mood-elevating properties of essential oils such as Bergamot and Clary Sage. After all, many cats enjoy mood-altering catnip. Clinical studies of a synthetic pheromone that is chemically similar to that emitted from the sebaceous glands on the mammary region of nursing dogs have shown that the odor has a calming effect on many dogs suffering from separation-anxiety and fear of fireworks (Sheppard & Mills 2003).

SOCIAL INFLUENCES

Animal well-being includes happiness and playfulness, which will, however, require more direct human involvement than magical oils and the offerings of behavioral pharmacology. I know farmers who play with their chickens, pigs, steers, cows, and ewes, like the Indian villagers who play and sleep with young goats and calves. These animals are healthier and more productive. Similarly, in families where there is no intra- or inter-species play pro-

vided for live-alone dogs, cats, parrots, and other pets, there are more health and behavioral problems than in families where the animals are happy because they can play (see Horwitz et al. 2002). Inter-species play, as between a billy goat and a young bull, a calf and two young dogs, a lamb and ten dogs, a monkey with a pack of more than thirty dogs, and a herd of twenty cattle and a band of more than ninety donkeys, that I have witnessed at the India Project for Animals and Nature's (IPAN) Hill View Farm Animal Refuge, is a sight to behold. It is the essence of the joy of life that heals, makes whole, and inspires and affirms the will to be. Play is the best of all natural therapies, and it is a cardinal animal welfare science indicator of animal welfare and well-being.

The use of massage therapy and the healing touch (Fox 1990) can also be valuable in reducing animals' tension, fear, and distrust and can help speed recovery from various conditions.

Pavlov's demonstration that dogs can be conditioned to respond to injections of normal saline as though they had been injected with morphine raises the question of conditioned and associative learning as well as anticipation and expectation in relation to positive and negative placebo-like effects in animal patients. As McMillan (1999b) proposes, the goal of clinical application of placebo effects should not be the substitution of placebo treatments for standard treatments, but rather the use of placebo effects to accentuate the efficacy of such treatments.

Animals engage in mutual greeting displays and self-care and mutual-care behaviors, including grooming, making contentment sounds, and various intention-movements or displays (like lip-smacking in macaques) of epimeletic (caregiving) and et-epimeletic (care-seeking) motivational and behavioral systems. Mimicking such species-specific caregiving behavior is a prerequisite for veterinarians and animal handlers who need to enter an animal's personal space and make physical contact. Giving a treat as a caregiving gesture is often the first step.

Some animals are highly motivated caregivers; as Chief Consultant and Veterinarian with IPAN, I have witnessed at our refuge how the recovery of many frightened, sick, or injured animals is enhanced by the reassuring presence and attentions of our caregiving resident dogs, ponies, and cows. Being isolated from conspecifics, especially for sheep and most young animals, can be extremely stressful. The staff are trained to feed animals treats and to groom or stroke the animals during various treatments such as changing a dressing on a lacerated limb, be the animal a horse, half-wild bullock, or captive elephant. Epimeletic behavior and empathy make for good animal handlers. The handlers also sleep with dogs, calves, baby elephants, and other animals, monitoring their conditions, checking IV drips, etc., when emergency cases requiring intensive care come in for treatment. Most importantly, the handlers are instructed to encourage the animals in recovery to play, engage with healthy resident animals, and engage in natural behaviors in a free but safe environment rather than remain confined all the time in a small cage or pen.

CONCLUSIONS

I am glad of the opportunity to contribute to this important book that I see as a high watermark for the veterinary profession in helping accomplish what I have advocated my entire professional life: healing and enhancing the human-nonhuman animal bond through sound science, understanding, empathy, and respect. Through this, compassionate action will enhance the establishment of a mutually beneficial human-animal bond. My friend and mentor Thomas Berry (1999) put it this way: The universe is not a collection of objects, it is a community of subjects. Compassion will be absolute, or it is not at all.

The communion of subjects that I examine in my book *The Boundless Circle* (1996) creates what I call the empathosphere, a realm of empathic feeling that Sheldrake (2000), in his studies of dogs and cats who somehow seem to know when their human companions are coming home, calls the morphic field. It is a realm of in-feeling that, without further scientific study, will regrettably continue to be regarded as psychic or illusory to the rationally minded. Fortunately, some controlled experiments have demonstrated the beneficial effects of healing-directed prayer as well as distant or remote mental intentionality on such nonhuman subjects as bacteria, plants, chicks, gerbils, cats, and dogs (Grad 1965, Dossey 2001). These findings undermine scientism's belief in consciousness as an epiphenomenon of brain neurochemistry and support a holistic paradigm of consciousness as a fundamental principle that is irreducible to anything more basic, and which is both co-inherent and omnipresent, particular and universal.

Be this as it may, I urge all veterinary students, as well as children and adults who have animals in their lives, to take time out, suspend all judgment, and simply *be* with animals, ideally in situations where they have behavioral freedom and can be with their own kind. Observe them, feel with them and for them, and become them. Perhaps the animals may then welcome you to the empathosphere like many before you who became shamans, healers, good husbanders, and stewards of the land.

REFERENCES

Ader R (ed). 1981. *Psychoneuroimmunology*. New York: Academic Press.

Bekoff M (ed). 2002. *The cognitive animal*. Boston: MIT Press.

Bell KE. 2002. *Holistic aromatherapy for animals*. Forres, Scotland: Findhorn Press.

Belyaev DK, Trut LN. 1975. Some genetic and endocrine effects of selection for domestication in silver foxes. In: Fox MW (ed), *The wild canids: Their systematics, behavioral ecology and evolution*. New York, Van Nostrand Reinhold:416–426.

Berry T. 1999. The great work: Our way into the future. New York: Bell Tower.

Brambell RWR. 1965. Report of the technical committee to enquire into the welfare of animals kept under intensive livestock husbandry systems, (Cmnd. 2836). London: HM Stationery Office.

Brion B, Ey H. 1964. Psychiatrie Animale. Paris: Brouwer.

Darwin C. 1920. The expression of emotions in man and animals. New York: Appleton.

Davis H, Balfour D (eds). 1992. The inevitable bond: Examining the scientist-animal interactions. Cambridge, UK: Cambridge University Press.

Denenberg VH. 1967. Stimulation in infancy emotional reactivity and exploratory behavior. In: Glass DC (ed), *Neurophysiology and emotion*. New York, The Rockefeller University Press:161–190.

Descartes R. 1970. *Philosophical letters*. Oxford, UK: Oxford University Press.

Diamond MC, Linder B, Raymond A.1967. Extensive cortical depth measurements in neuron size increases in the cortex of environmentally enriched rats. *J Comp Neurol* 131:357–364.

Dodman NH, Shuster L (eds). 1998. *Psychopharmacology of animal behavior disorders*. Malden, MA: Blackwell Science.

Dossey L. 2001. *Healing beyond the body: Medicine and the infinite reach of the mind*. Boston, MA: Shambala Press.

Fox MW. 1962. Observations on paw raising and sympathy lameness in the dog. *Vet Rec* 74:895–896.

Fox MW (ed). 1968. *Abnormal behavior in animals.* Philadelphia, PA: W.B. Saunders.

Fox MW. 1971. *Integrative development of brain and behavior in the dog.* Chicago, IL: University of Chicago Press.

Fox MW. 1972. *Understanding your dog.* New York: St. Martin's Press.

Fox MW. 1974. *Concepts in ethology: Animal and human behavior, Vol. 2, The Wesley W. Spink lectures in comparative medicine.* Minneapolis: University of Minnesota Press.

Fox MW. 1984. *Farm animals: Husbandry, behavior and veterinary practice.* Baltimore, MD: University Park Press.

Fox MW. 1986. *Laboratory animal husbandry: Ethology, welfare and experimental variables.* Albany: SUNY Press.

Fox MW. 1990. *The healing touch.* New York: New Market Press.

Fox MW. 1992. *Superpigs and wondercorn: The brave new world of biotechnology and where it all may lead.* New York: Lyons and Burford.

Fox MW. 1996. *The boundless circle: Caring for creatures and creation.* Wheaton, IL: Quest Books.

Fox MW. 1997. Veterinary bioethics. In: Schoen AM, Wynn SG (eds), *Complementary and alternative veterinary medicine.* St. Louis, MO, Mosby:673–678.

Fox MW. 1999. *Beyond evolution: The genetically altered future of plants, animals, the earth and humans.* New York: Lyon's Press.

Fox MW. 2001. *Bringing life to ethics: Global bioethics for a humane society.* Albany: SUNY Press.

Gantt WH. 1944. Experimental basis for neurotic behavior. *Psychosomatic medicine monographs*, Vol. 3. New York: Woeber.

Garner JP, Mason GJ. 2002. Evidence for a relationship between cage stereotypies and behavioral disinhibition in laboratory rodents. *Behav Brain Res* 136:83–92.

Gellhorn E. 1968. Central nervous system tuning and its implications for neuropsychiatry. *J Nerv Ment Dis* 147:148–162.

Grad BR. 1965. Some biological effects of laying-on-of-hands: A review of experiments with animals and plants. *J Am Soc Psychical R* 59:95–127.

Griffin D. 1977. *The question of animal awareness.* New York: Rockefeller Press.

Gross WB, Siegel PB. 1982. Socialization as a factor in resistance to infection, feed efficiency and response to antigens in chickens. *Am J Vet Res* 43:2010–2012.

Gross WB, Roberts KC, Gogal R. 2001. Ascorbic acid as a possible treatment for canine tumors. *J Am Holistic Vet Med Assoc* 20:35–40.

Gross WB, Siegel PB. 1981. Long term exposure of chickens to three levels of social stress. *Avian Dis* 25:312–325.

Gross WB, Siegel PB. 1983. Evaluation of the heterophil/lymphocyte ratio as a measure of stress in chickens. *Avian Dis* 27:972–979.

Gross WB, Siegel PB, Pierson FW. 2002. Effects of genetic selection for high or low antibody response on resistance to a variety of disease challenges and the relationship to resource allocation. *Avian Dis* 46:1007–1010.

Hemsworth PH, Coleman GJ. 1998. *Human livestock interactions: The stockperson, productivity and welfare of intensively farmed animals.* New York: CAB International.

Horwitz D, Mills D, Heath S. 2002. *BSAVA Manual of canine and feline behavioral medicine.* Quedgeley, UK: British Small Animal Veterinary Association.

Katcher AH, Beck AM. 1983. *New perspectives on our lives with companion animals.* Philadelphia: University of Pennsylvania Press.

Kracht J. 1954. Fright-thyrotoxicosis in the wild rabbit, a model of thyrotropic alarm-reaction. *Acta Endocrinol* 15:355–367.

Kurtsin IT. 1968. Physiological mechanisms of behavioral disturbances and corticovisceral interrelations in animals. In: Fox MW (ed), *Abnormal behavior in animals.* Philadelphia PA., W.B. Saunders:107–116.

Lawrence BB, Rushen J (eds). 1993. *Stereotypic animal behavior: Fundamentals and applications to welfare.* Tucson, AZ: CAB International.

Levine S, Mullins RF. 1966. Hormone influences on brain organization in infant rats. *Science* 152:1585–1592.

Lidell HS. 1956. *Emotional hazards in animals and man.* Springfield, IL: Charles C. Thomas.

Marsden D. 2002. A new perspective on stereotypic behavior problems in horses. *Vet Rec, In Practice* Nov/Dec:558–569.

McMillan FD. 1999a. Influence of mental states on somatic health in animals. *J Am Vet Med Assoc* 214:1221–1225.

McMillan FD. 1999b. The placebo effect in animals. *J Am Vet Med Assoc* 215:992–999.

McMillan FD. 1999c. Effect of human contact on animal well-being. *J Am Vet Med Assoc* 215:1592–1598.

McMillan FD. 2002. Development of a mental wellness program for animals. *J Am Vet Med Assoc* 220:965–972.

McMillan FD. 2003. A world of hurts—is pain special? *J Am Vet Med Assoc* 223:183–186.

Moberg GP, Mench JA (eds). 2000. *The biology of animal stress: Basic principles and implications for animal welfare*. New York: CAB International.

Nerem RM, Levesque MJ, Cornhill JF. 1980. Social environment as a factor in diet induced atherosclerosis. *Science* 208:1475–1476.

Odendaal JSJ, Meintjes RA. 2003. Neurophysiological correlates of affiliative behavior between humans and dogs. *Vet J* 165:296–301.

Overmeier JB. 1981. Interference with coping: An animal model. *Acad Psychol B* 3:105–118.

Panskepp J. 1998. *Affective neuroscience: The foundations of human and animal emotions*. New York: Oxford University Press.

Pavlov JP. 1928. *Lectures on conditioned reflexes* (WH Gantt, Trans). New York: International Publishers.

Plechner AJ, Zucker M. 2003. *Pets at risk: From allergies to cancer, remedies for an unexpected epidemic*. Troutdale, OR: New Sage Press.

Richter C. 1954. The effects of domestication and selection on the behavior of the Norway rat. *J Natl Cancer I* 5:727–738.

Rosenzweig MR, Krech D, Bennett EL, et al. 1962. Effects of environmental complexity and training on brain chemistry and anatomy: A replication and extension. *J Comp Physiol Psych* 55:429–437.

Scott JP, Fuller JL. 1965. *Genetics and social behavior of the dog*. Chicago: University of Chicago Press.

Seabrook MF. 1984. The psychological interaction between the stockman and his animals and its influence on performance of pigs. *Vet Rec* 115:84–89.

Seligman ME. 1975. *Helplessness: On depression, development and death*. San Francisco: W. H. Freeman.

Sheldrake R. 2000. *Dogs that know when their owners are coming home—and other unexplained powers of animals*. New York: Crown Publishing Group.

Sheppard G, Mills DS. 2003. Evaluation of dog-appeasing pheromone as a potential treatment for dogs fearful of fireworks. *Vet Rec* 152:432–436.

Spitz R. 1949. The role of ecological factors in emotional development. *Child Dev* 20:145–155.

Stockard CR. 1941. *The genetic and endocrine basis for differences in form and behavior*. Philadelphia: Wistar Institute Press.

Wemelsfelder F. 1990. Boredom and laboratory animal welfare, In: Rollin BE, Kesel ML (eds), *The experimental animal in biomedical research*. Boca Raton, FL, CRC Press:243–372.

Wurbel H. 2001. Ideal homes? Housing effects on rodent brain and behavior. *Trends Neurosci* 24:207–211.

9

Mental Illness in Animals—The Need for Precision in Terminology and Diagnostic Criteria

Karen L. Overall

INTRODUCTION

In the 1980s, orthopedic surgeons at the University of Pennsylvania School of Veterinary Medicine were teaching that "pain is a great immobilizer." Two decades later we are appalled by this notion, yet our change in attitude has been accompanied by painstakingly obtained, yet only moderate, progress in understanding and definitively assessing pain (Lees et al. 2003, Pascoe 2003, Short 2003, Taylor 2003, Webb 2003). Human physicians also struggle with assessment of pain, but they often rely on patient self-reports while acknowledging the gaps between perception, complaint, and the underlying biological processes (Scholz & Woolf 2002). Although we cannot directly measure or accurately characterize pain, we no longer deny its existence or that of the nociceptive processes associated with it. The same cannot be said for another class of problems where measurement and terminology are also issues: behavioral concerns.

While the field of physical pain assessment and management is ascending, the field of veterinary behavioral medicine, which deals with equally invisible and equally real pain, is still struggling for acceptance. The vast majority of veterinary schools in North America, where a specialty college in the discipline exists, still offer no full-time, integrated, clinical, and didactic training by full-time, faculty-level specialists. Rather than asking if we can understand behavioral problems as a form of behavioral pain and suffering, or "mental illness," the vast majority of clients and veterinarians, wittingly or not, engage in a terminology and thought process rooted in an adversarial relationship with the animals who share their lives. Physical pain is deemed as "real," afflicting innocent patients; behavioral pain is often thought to be someone's fault or the result of a deeply flawed character. Fortunately,

when done correctly, science provides us with paradigms by which we can learn whether something is true. Behavioral problems are still the most common reasons pets are relinquished or euthanized in the typical veterinary practice in the United States, Australia, and Canada, countries for which adequate data exist (Houpt et al. 1996; Salman et al. 1998, 2000; New et al. 1999; Scarlett et al. 1999, 2002). Accordingly, it is incumbent on us to impose science on a field that has long resisted its advance and to begin to understand the mental pathology of behavioral problems in domestic animals.

APPROACHING COMPLEX SITUATIONS

Diagnoses are not diseases; correlation is not causality. The logic for using very specific phenomenological diagnoses is to (a) identify the particular behavioral manifestation that needs to be altered or assessed and (b) identify areas where specific behavioral intervention can be useful (Table 9.1) (Overall 1997a, 1997b).

Behavioral diagnoses are made largely on the basis of constellations of nonspecific signs. Signs or descriptors are often erroneously or carelessly used as a diagnosis. By viewing a diagnosis mechanistically as a hypothesis to be tested it is possible to begin to define and understand abnormal behaviors at a variety of levels that include, but are not restricted to, the phenotypic, functional, and phenomenological diagnoses that are most commonly employed (Table 9.2; Figures 9.1 and 9.2).

The first step in this process is to define the *necessary* and *sufficient* criteria for making the diagnosis. Once this is done, separate clusters of phenotypes may exist that are characterized by shared nonspecific signs. In human psychiatry, these are often called "endophenotypes" (Gottesman &

Table 9.1. Understanding patterns of behavior within levels of a mechanistic approach.

Note that none of these levels are independent, the first 4 are very dynamic, an action can originate at any level that then affects the other levels, and the extent to which they interact is a function of the genetic response surface and learning. All levels other than phenotypic interact to produce mechanistic grouping of phenomenological diagnoses.

  A. Phenomenological, phenotypic, functional diagnoses: must meet necessary and sufficient terminological criteria
    B. Neuroanatomical diagnoses
      C. Neurochemical/Neurophysiological diagnoses
        D. Molecular diagnose
          E. Genetic diagnoses

Table 9.2. Example for Consideration of Interaction of Phenotypic Level of Mechanism with Others

Table 9.2a

Phenotype	A Abnormal Variant A	B Abnormal Variant B	C Abnormal Variant C	D Normal
Neuroanatomical variant	I	I	I	I
Neurochemistry	a	b	a	b
Molecular products	I'	II'	II'	II'
Genotype	a'	b'	b'	b'

In this example the variants in the condition are due to some difference in environmental response. This could be a purely phenotypic effect (Abnormal variant B). Alternatively, the effect could be due to learning and long-term potentiation (in which case the molecular level is affected - Abnormal variant A); this molecular effect also affects neurochemistry. The effect could also be one of neurochemistry, without affecting the molecular level (Abnormal variant C).

Table 9.2b

Phenotype	A Abnormal Variant A	B Abnormal Variant B	C Normal
Neuroanatomical variant	I	I	I
Neurochemistry	a	b	b
Molecular products	I'	II'	II'
Genotype	a'	b'	b'

In this example the variants in the condition are due to some difference in environmental response. This could be a purely phenotypic effect, as presented. Alternatively, the effect could be due to learning and long-term potentiation (in which case the molecular level is affected) or the effect could be one of neurochemistry. The two latter choices are reflected as (**).

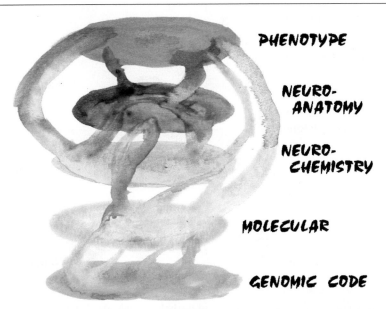

PHENOTYPE

NEURO-
ANATOMY

NEURO-
CHEMISTRY

MOLECULAR

GENOMIC CODE

Figure 9.1 This graphic illustrates the relative 'response surfaces' that exist for each of the mechanistic diagnostic levels discussed in the text. Note that phenotype can be affected directly or indirectly. The extent to which the different levels interact directly or indirectly could be a function of intensity, duration, or type of stimulus. There is no way to know these effects in the absence of specific data collection. Here, the genomic code provides that set of choices that could, but may not necessarily, affect the molecular and neurochemical expression of behavioral phenotypes. In essence, the genomic response surface acts to define boundary conditions.

Shields 1972). For example, once the definitional criteria are met, condition A could sort into 2 phenotypic groups based on treatment response. In the simplest scenario, group 1 responds only to drug 1 and group 2 responds only to drug 2, although behaviorally, the groups are indistinguishable. A pattern like this would hint that two underlying mechanisms are functioning (Figure 9.2). In another variant of this example, the definitional criteria are met, but group 1 most commonly displays signs 1–3 and group 2 displays signs 3–5. The question now becomes whether shared or separate mechanisms contribute to these clusters (Figure 9.2). If these clusters are truly wholly separate at all levels of mechanism, one could rationally argue that these are two truly phenotypically separate diagnostic conditions and that sign 3 is a truly nonspecific, non-informative sign for this level of inquiry.

The implementation of "necessary and sufficient" criteria, using the terms as they are used in logical and mathematical applications, is a refinement over descriptive definitions of terms. The imposition of necessary and sufficient diagnostic criteria acts as qualitative, and potentially quantitative, exclusion criteria. They allow for uniform and unambiguous

assessment of aberrant, abnormal, and undesirable behaviors. A *necessary* criterion or condition is one that must be present for the listed diagnosis to be made. A *sufficient* criterion or condition is one that will stand alone to singularly identify the condition. Sufficiency is an outcome of knowledge; the more we learn about the genetics, molecular response, neurochemistry, and neuroanatomy of any condition and its behavioral correlates, the more succinctly and accurately we will be able to define a sufficient condition.

Definition of necessary and sufficient conditions is *not* synonymous with a compendium of signs associated with the condition. The number of signs present and the intensity of those signs may be a gauge for the severity of the condition or may act as a flag when there can be variable, non-overlapping presentations of the same condition. The pattern by which the signs cluster will help in defining heterogeneity of the underlying afflicted population, will identify potentially important endophenotypes, and will permit epidemiological studies to be executed and tests of multiple causality of underlying mechanisms to be conducted.

Implicit in this approach is that no known underlying physical or physiological reason exists for the

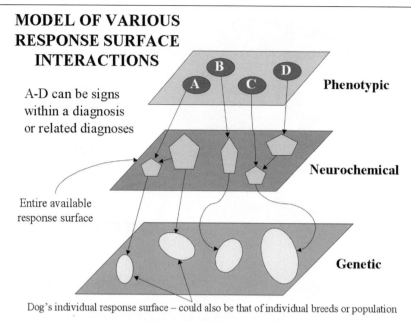

MODEL OF VARIOUS RESPONSE SURFACE INTERACTIONS

A-D can be signs within a diagnosis or related diagnoses

Phenotypic

Neurochemical

Entire available response surface

Genetic

Dog's individual response surface – could also be that of individual breeds or population

Figure 9.2 In this schematic only 3 of 5 discussed mechanistic levels are represented as 3 different response surfaces. Situation B is the one everyone hopes to find: here 1 gene is responsible for 1 neurochemical change and that change maps uniquely onto the problem behavior. The real world is a bit more complex that this. In example D, one set of genes gives rise to one set of neurochemical responses that then changes into another neurochemical response set. Each set of neurochemical responses gives rise to 2 separate phenotypes (C & D). Therefore, in this case, the same genetic background can produce 2 diagnostic groups acting through 2 neurochemical mechanisms. For phenotype A 2 neurochemical mechanisms are also involved, but they are each the result of 2 separate genes that then produce 2 neurochemical responses that interact.

behavioral problem *and* that physical and physiological "causes" have been ruled out. In other words, the way we recognize illness in animals often involves a change in behavior; the cat either vomits or she doesn't. However, behaviors that have proximal physical "causes" (e.g., the cat was poisoned) may act as nonspecific signs (e.g., vomiting) and should be recognized as such rather than being forced into an interpretation that requires a nonproximal "cause" (e.g., feline bulimia) when this is not the most parsimonious explanation. It is also important to remember that classifications as discussed in this chapter represent diagnoses of problem behaviors, not just descriptions of a behavioral event (i.e., impulse control aggression can be *only* a diagnosis for an abnormal behavior, but interdog aggression can be both a diagnosis and a description). The proposed terminology represents an attempt to create a terminology that is internally consistent, easily used because of its descriptive utility, and informative because of the manner in which it allows data (e.g., demography, associated nonspecific signs, etc.) to be collected and used to test ideas about various levels of mechanism, while

concurrently avoiding psychological jargon. This is harder than it sounds.

This approach is similar to that taken by the American Psychiatric Association for the Diagnostic and Statistical Manual (most recent edition, DSM-IV), the World Health Organization diagnostic guidelines, and other sources, but is not based on them. If one reads descriptions of human psychiatric diagnoses, one will see that the required criteria—the necessary and sufficient equivalents—are actually imbedded within. Because numbers of patients examined are huge in human psychiatry, however, subgroups of patients can be characterized by nonspecific signs, demography, treatment responses, etc. Instead of these patterns being used to learn about variability in underlying mechanisms, these groupings have become the basis for diagnosis. In other words, many diagnoses in human psychiatry are now based on nonspecific signs and then attached a label that may not reflect the biological reality. This failure is due, at least in part in the USA, to the need to have a diagnostic code to receive payment, and it is one reason that genome scans utilizing diagnostic codes have produced so little useful information. We need to realize that behavioral medicine is one area where veterinary medicine could take a leading role. The field is so new that diagnostic biases are not deeply entrenched, yet the field is developing at a time when neurobehavioral, molecular, and genetic tools have never been more accessible. The conditions that are of interest in veterinary behavioral medicine do not have to be exact analogues of human conditions for this type of attempt at classification to be meritorious. The approach provides for a mechanism to collect behavioral data from a variety of populations across time and compare the data.

The set of necessary and sufficient conditions for behavioral diagnoses are detailed elsewhere (see Appendix F in Overall 1997a; Overall 2004a). These descriptions provide veterinarians with the information with which they can gain some first-hand experience with the complexity of thought involved in behavior. The first publication of these criteria in the American Veterinary Society of Animal Behavior (AVSAB) Newsletter in 1994 (Overall 1994) was intended to provoke a discussion, not to set a standard. The silence was deafening. Subsequent compilations (Overall 1997a, 1997b, 1997c; Overall et al. 2001; Overall & Dunham 2002; Overall 2004a) have produced some

discussion, but the focus of that discussion has unfortunately been on largely irrelevant topics such as philosophical schools of thought (Mills 2003) rather than on biology. This approach has been taken in more-profitable directions in human psychiatry in response to frustration about "treatment failures" in complex conditions (Castellanos & Tannock 2002). That said, comparisons of data predicated on the classification below should engender revisions and refinements of the classification. The classification itself is not important; the extent to which it provides a structured, logical, heuristic tool for the development of thought in the field *is* important.

PITFALLS ABOUT LABELS

If what we call something affects the way we think about it, then what we call it is essential; yet we in behavior have been incredibly careless and in so being, have done harm. Behavioral medicine can only advance when the descriptors we use have clear and agreed-on definitions, when those definitions are amended by developing data, and when none of the terms are culturally or sociologically loaded (Table 9.3). We can no longer leave unaddressed the dangers of employing a terminology

Table 9.3 General definitions (from Overall 1997c, used with permission from the North American Veterinary Conference)

Abnormal behavior – Activities which show dysfunction in action and behavior.

Anxiety – The apprehensive anticipation of future danger or misfortune accompanied by a feeling of dysphoria (in humans) and, or somatic symptoms of tension (vigilance and scanning, autonomic hyperactivity, increased motor activity and tension). The focus of the anxiety can be internal or external.

Fear – A feeling of apprehension associated with the presence or proximity of an object, individual, social situation, or class of the above. Fear is part of normal behavior and can be an adaptive response. The determination of whether the fear or fearful response is abnormal or inappropriate must be determined by context. For example, fire is a useful tool, but fear of being consumed by it, if the house is one fire, is an adaptive response. If the house is not on fire, such fear would be irrational, and, if it was constant or recurrent, probably maladaptive. Normal and abnormal fears are usually manifest as graded responses, with the intensity of the response proportional to the proximity (or the perception of the proximity) of the stimulus. A sudden, all-or-nothing, profound, abnormal response that results in extremely fearful behaviors (catatonia, panic) is usually called a phobia.

Phobia – A sudden, all-or-nothing, profound, abnormal response that results in extremely fearful behaviors (catatonia, panic) is usually called a phobia. An immediate, excessive anxiety response is characteristic of phobias. Phobias usually appear to develop quickly, with little change in their presentation between bouts; fears may develop more gradually, and within a bout of fearful behavior, there may be more variation in response than would be seen in a phobic event. It has been postulated that once a phobic event has been experienced, any event associated with it or the memory of it is sufficient to generate the response. Phobic situations are either avoided at all costs, or if unavoidable, are endured with intense anxiety or distress.

that may be unfounded. We must also consider that behavior is a dynamic process, yet the roles of time, repeated exposure, and learning are all but ignored. By the time most true behavioral problems are recognized by the clients, the behaviors and social relationships between the participants have changed. We can further change these relationships—and in the wrong direction—if we continue to operate within the flawed context that results from adherence to inapplicable and wrong terminologies.

Consider, for example, the issue of "dominance" in dogs. Two broad contexts exist in which the term "dominance" is used with respect to dogs: when describing interactions between dogs and when describing the role the client is recommended to take in interactions with the dog. Neither of these approaches are valid.

The modern and evolving understanding of complex social behaviors is going to require that we relinquish simplistic and damaging labels; the concept of a "dominant" dog is not useful in these situations, and asking clients and practitioners to identify and then exhibit behaviors that encourage or discourage the "dominant" dog can cause morbidity and mortality for dogs and humans. For example, in a review of dozens of cases involving interdog aggression between household dogs, we (Overall & Dunham 2004) found that most clients had been advised to support or reinforce the "dominant" dog, and that when they did so, the aggression worsened. One could accordingly argue that the clients are not correctly identifying the "dominant" dog, but if a label is causing such difficulties, the time may have come to just let the label go. The issues of "dominance" and social rank on group interactions compose one of the oldest, most confusing, and most hotly debated areas in behavioral literature. It is important that we understand why this concept has caused problems in the practice of veterinary behavioral medicine.

The existence of a hierarchy has been postulated to be a stress-reducing device (Collias 1953); however, situations in which hierarchies are most rigidly maintained are also ones in which measures of stress are high (Rowell 1966). In the traditional scheme, the dog who "submits" (generally undefined) or gives way to another as a result of prior interactions is considered the "subordinate" while the individual inducing such behavior is usually considered the "dominant" animal in the pairing. "Dominance" has been traditionally defined as an individual's ability, generally under controlled situations, to maintain or regulate access to some

resource (Landau 1951; Hinde 1967, 1970; Rowell 1974). Given that the definition of "dominance" can be further refined as a description of winning or losing staged contests over resources (Archer 1988, Horwitz et al. 2002) and that a winning outcome needn't confer priority of access to those resources (Archer 1988), we must accept that variable distributions of resources (e.g., access to attention, beds, resting sites, toys, food dishes, etc.) will lead to variable hierarchal classifications.

My concerns about such terminology primarily focus on two related issues: (1) the extent to which the labeling of an event, interaction, or pattern of interactions may interfere with our ability to truly understand behaviors and signals in the relevant context and (2) the extent to which, if we subscribe to a hierarchical system, we are then tempted or constrained to force all interpretations of behaviors into that system. Such practices have encouraged humans to treat dogs inhumanely under the guise of being "dominant" to them, which has likely resulted in the injury or death of many dogs. In the case of interdog aggression, such logic leads to "reinforcing" a truly pathological animal as "dominant." These concerns are not new; the potential to mislead was Rowell's primary concern when she published her groundbreaking study on the intricacies of baboon social interactions (Rowell 1967). In fact, when free-ranging baboon interactions were classified by behavioral types (e.g., friendly, approach-retreat) and then analyzed according to specific behaviors of the participants, no "dominance" system was noted. In fact, a much more complex, elegant system of interactions that reflected relatedness, age, sex, social history, and other factors became apparent.

Most social behaviors, when fully examined, are not characterized by agonistic encounters but by fluid, context-specific, deferential behaviors (Overall 1997a, 2004b). Deference is not analogous to submission or subordination; deference is about relative status that is freely given, not imposed, and it may vary with context. The animal to which most others defer is the animal that behaves most appropriately given the context, not the animal that must always be at the door first or must eat first. In fact, a need to control regardless of context can be neither adaptive nor normal. The central and organizing role for deferential behaviors is supported by authors who have looked extensively at social interactions (e.g., Crowell-Davis et al. 2004) when they discuss the variability in the behavior of high-ranking animals. These findings are supported by others who emphasize the importance of understanding when the behaviors are about normal, of learning about relative and fluid roles in changing social environments, and of understanding when the behaviors are pathological. Because learning works by altering neurochemistry (see Overall 2001), we need to understand that both early intervention designed to avert anxiety associated with underlying aggression and pharmacological intervention can help, but neither approach will be used appropriately until the clients can understand the signaling and interactions from the dogs' viewpoints (Rooney et al. 2001).

In this worldview, diagnosis and treatment is about both understanding the neurochemical changes that occur with learning and repeated exposure and about becoming humane. To do this we must begin to see the world from our patient's point of view, which requires that we understand normal ethology and behavioral ontogeny of that species. Heuristically, this approach minimally requires that we let go of labels that may say more about us and our needs than about the behavior. As the field of veterinary behavioral medicine advances, we should become more mindful of terminology, issues, and approaches that can inadvertently do more harm than good.

One key factor that we often neglect is the role of ontogeny and learning in any behavioral problem. The blurring of the lines between normal (the aggressor is truly at risk, and aggressive behavior is adaptive) and abnormal aggression (there is no risk to the aggressor) are real; they are a function of our lack of knowledge about how behavioral conditions develop. In fact, the extent to which an animal deviates from "normal" in aggression or any other suite of behaviors may depend on ontogeny, multiple gene effects, and pleiotropic environmental effects (Nijhout 2003) (Figures 9.3, 9.4, 9.5). If anxiety-based aggression has a causal pattern similar to other anxiety-based conditions such as obsessive-compulsive disorder (OCD), both a familial or genetic "predisposition" and a social stressor play roles in the development of the aggression (Overall & Dunham 2002).

UNDERSTANDING DIFFERENT LEVELS OF MECHANISTIC INTERACTION

Identification of a diagnosis using definitional criteria represents an algorithmic approach that clusters behaviors of patients that are more similar to each

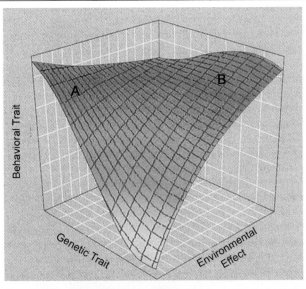

Figure 9.3 A model, complex, non-linear response surface that predicts what a trait or phenotype will look like given the effect of a certain gene and the effect of a certain environment. Note that at some points on this response surface the phenotype would be indistinguishable, even given wildly different environment and gene effect, whereas in other regions of the response surface a small environmental or genetic change can, by itself, have a huge effect. This is the question we are always asking when we seek to understand temperament in dogs; for example: to what extent does the environment in which the dog lives display any genetic liability for any behavior? Simple but specific examples for the outcome of this question are shown in Figures 9.4 and 9.5 (modified from Nijhout 2003, used with permission).

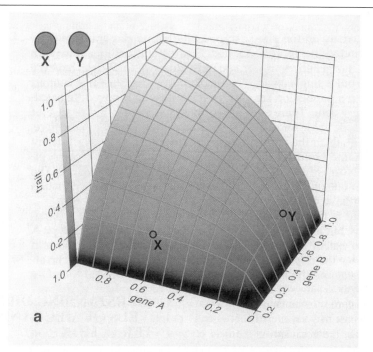

Figure 9.4 This figure illustrates the specific circumstance where 2 factors can be very different (in fact, here the effects of each gene are the opposite of the other), but still have an equal and indistinguishable phenotypic effect, given the shape of the response surface. Here the phenotypes / diagnoses / behaviors are represented by X and Y (from Nijhout 2003, used with permission).

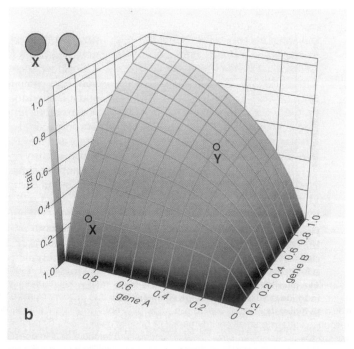

Figure 9.5 The specific circumstance where one factor changes, but the other remains constant. Here only the effects of gene A are changed. A change in 3 units for gene A does not change phenotype X from Figure 9.4, above, but the effect of a 3 unit change on phenotype Y is profound. This is the effect of the complex genetic interactions that define the non-linear response surface (from Nijhout 2003, used with permission).

other and separates them from those less similar. This clustering, or labeling as a diagnosis, does not mean that patients will be equally afflicted or that they are all exhibiting the same underlying pathology even if their behavior is the same (Table 9.2; Figure 9.3). The beauty of this logic-based approach is that it acknowledges variability in cause, variability in presentation, and the fact that they may not represent a unitary mapping. This algorithmic approach also allows us to understand variants of normal behaviors. We seldom discuss a definition of normal, but it may be best characterized as the ability to recover and respond normally after a provocative stimulus. If we define "normal behavior" as the ability to be fluid in response, given the context, and to recover when provoked, we are able to qualitatively and quantitatively compare behaviors exhibited by both normal and abnormal animals. This is the only way we are going to be able to link behavioral response surfaces to genetic ones.

The value of a phenotypic diagnosis should be to help both the clinician and client understand the provocative circumstances that can induce a worsening or improvement in the behavior and the distress that goes with it. That said, how important are diagnostic subsections and associations between nonspecific signs? Examples from three sets of conditions in which adequate clinical data exist to answer this question can help: canine impulse control aggression, canine separation anxiety and associated noise/thunderstorm phobia, and canine and feline OCD (see Table 9.4).

THE EVOLVING STORY OF IMPULSE CONTROL AGGRESSION

Aggression is best defined as an appropriate or inappropriate inter- or intra-specific challenge, threat, or contest resulting in deference or combat and resolution (Archer 1988, Overall 1997a). The importance of context cannot be overemphasized in any evaluation of aggression. Most abnormal aggressions are the result of underlying anxiety (Overall 1997a, 2000; King et al. 2000). Canine and feline anxieties, particularly those involving more-extreme responses, appear to have a genetic component. Because of the use of breeds of dogs for certain types of work, more is known about both canine aggression and the putative genetic mechanisms that underlie it than about feline aggression. The probability that any dog will be afflicted with a profoundly anxious or panicky response is associated, in part, with breed. In the large but overwhelmingly non-experimental literature on working dogs, the single best predictor

of failure in any working dog is fear, and the factor that prohibits most dogs from completing training programs is their aggressive/fearful/anxious/uncertain response to novel or complex environments (Weiss & Greenberg 1997, Slabbert & Odendaal 1999, Koda 2001, King et al. 2003). Any tests that can help identify early aspects of fear and anxiety and their effects on aggression will lead to future research on intervention for, and effects of intervention on, learning.

Some of our knowledge of canine aggression, in particular, will come from similar studies in humans. Dogs share both foraging mode and a virtually identical social system with humans (Overall 1997a) and have co-evolved for cooperative work with humans for approximately 135,000 years with intense selection for specific suites of behavioral traits (e.g., the development of breeds) occurring in the last 12,000–15,000 years (Geffen et al. 1996; Vilà et al. 1997, 1999; Wayne & Vilà 2001; Leonard et al. 2002). Dogs mirror humans in hallmarks of social development (Overall 1997a). Also, like humans, dogs suffer from what we recognize as maladaptive anxiety—that which interferes with normal functioning—which was selected against during the co-evolution of dogs and humans.

Paradoxically, some of the best data for aberrant or abnormal aggression involves one of the most controversial canine behavioral diagnoses: impulse control aggression (formerly called "dominance aggression"). This aggression is about control or access to control in direct social situations involving humans. This is a discrete definition of impulse control aggression and has the advantage of not coupling the challenge to food (food-related aggression), toys (possessive aggression), or space (territorial aggression). These aggressions can all be correlates of impulse control aggression and when associated with it, may be indicative of a more severe situation. This diagnosis cannot be made on the basis of a one-time event. This definition is radically different from the common descriptions of this aggression that specify that the dog will often react to being pushed on, to being corrected with a leash, or to being pushed from a sofa or a person. The number of situations in which the dog reacts inappropriately or the intensity with which he or she reacts does not affect the necessary and sufficient conditions, although these factors may affect ability to treat the condition, the prognosis, and the risk to people.

The range of behaviors manifest in this condition includes postural threats and stares to sudden stiff-

Table 9.4. Necessary and sufficient conditions for selected behavioral diagnoses discussed in the text (adapted from Overall 1997b, 2004a).

Behavioral Diagnosis	Necessary Condition	Sufficient Condition
Impulse control aggression	Abnormal, inappropriate, out-of-context aggression (threat, challenge, or attack) consistently exhibited by dogs towards people under any circumstance involving passive or active control of the dog's behavior or the dog's access to the behavior	Intensification of any offensive - aggressive response from the dog upon any passive or active correction or interruption or control of the dog's behavior or the dog's access to the behavior
Noise phobia	Sudden and profound, non-graded, extreme response to noise, manifest as intense, active avoidance, escape, or anxiety behaviors associated with the activities of the sympathetic branch of the autonomic nervous system; behaviors can include catatonia or mania concomitant with decreased sensitivity to pain or social stimuli; repeated exposure results in an invariant pattern of response	
Obsessive-compulsive disorder	Repetitive, stereotypic motor, locomotory, grooming, ingestive, or hallucinogenic behaviors that occur out-of-context to their "normal" occurrence, or in a frequency or duration that is in excess of that required to accomplish the ostensible goal	As for Necessary Condition, in a manner that interferes with the animal's ability to otherwise function in his or her social environment
Separation anxiety	Physical or behavioral signs of distress exhibited by the animal *only* in the absence of, or lack of access to, the bonded human companion	Consistent, intensive destruction, elimination, vocalization, or salivation exhibited *only* in the virtual or actual absence of the bonded human companion; behaviors are most severe close to the separation, and many anxiety-related behaviors (autonomic hyperactivity, increased motor activity, and increased vigilance and scanning) may become apparent as the client exhibits behaviors associated with leaving

ening and bites (Podberscek & Serpell 1996, 1997; Overall 1997a). This is the primary category of canine aggression in which no warning is given (Borchelt 1983). The classically afflicted dog growls, lunges, snaps, or bites if it is stared at, physically manipulated—often when a human reaches over the animal's head to put on a leash, physically disrupted, or moved from a resting site—no matter how gently this is done, or physically or verbally

"corrected." Otherwise, clients report that these are perfectly wonderful and charming dogs for well over 95% of the time. Clients are further puzzled by the observation that the dog often seeks them out for attention and then bites them when they give it. As for most other behavioral conditions, this aggression commonly develops during social maturity, when neurochemistry undergoes changes that will result in the individual's adult neurochemical profile. However, dogs exhibiting this behavioral abnormality at social maturity tend to be male, whereas when females are affected, they exhibit the behavioral pathology in puppyhood, suggesting that this is a multi-factorial disorder with different underlying mechanisms leading to similar pheno-types (Overall 1995, Overall & Beebe 1997). The average age of onset is approximately 12 months for affected males and 8 months for affected females, a statistically significant difference.

THE SEPARATION ANXIETY/NOISE AND THUNDERSTORM PHOBIA LINK

Anxiety disorders are among the most common health concerns in human medicine (Narrow et al. 2002), as they are for pet dogs. Like humans, dogs with one anxiety-related diagnosis frequently have other anxiety-related diagnoses (Overall et al. 2001, Overall & Dunham 2002), suggesting the existence of some putative genetic or neurochemical liability (Smoller & Tsuang 1998, Scherrer et al. 2000). Neuroanatomical studies of panic disorder are closely linked to those pertaining to fear and to peripheral responses. The extent to which learning and memory play roles in fear, anxiety, phobias, and OCD has been poorly studied because it is difficult to study, given the complexity of the neurochemical systems involved. What is known is that (1) a func-tioning amygdala is required to learn fear, (2) a functioning forebrain is required to unlearn fear (i.e., to effect habituation), and (3) many human abnormalities involving fear appear to be the result of the inability to inhibit a fear response. Accordingly, it has been hypothesized that fear is, in part, due to chronic amygdala overreaction, failure of the amygdala to turn off after the threat has passed, or both. The specific neuroanatomy of a fear response involves the locus ceruleus (LC), the prin-cipal norepinephrinergic (noradrenergic) nucleus in the brain. Dysregulation of the LC appears to lead to panic and phobias in humans (Charney & Heninger 1984). The LC directly supplies the limbic systems and may be responsible for many correlated "lim-bic" signs. Patients with true panic and phobic responses are more sensitive to pharmacologic stim-ulation and suppression of the LC than are controls (Ko et al. 1983, Charney & Heninger 1984, Pyke & Greenberg 1986).

Although few quantitative clinical studies on anx-ious dogs exist, those focusing on separation anxi-ety (Overall et al. 2001) and OCD (Overall & Dunham 2002) have shown that a high percentage of affected patients experience other, co-morbid

anxiety disorders (~90% and 75%, respectively). In the case of separation anxiety, the co-morbid diag-nosis is usually noise or thunderstorm phobia. Although the data are few, owing to the nature of retrospective studies, we know that heightened noise reactivity or fear as a young dog may predis-pose the individual to the later development of sep-aration anxiety (Overall et al. 2001). If so, this strongly suggests that associations between various anxiety and "mood" conditions (e.g., depression and anxiety, panic and social phobias, etc.) may be the result of an increased risk that is either the direct result of a shared underlying cause of the initial dis-order or the indirect result of neurochemical changes, molecular changes, or both that occur because of the initial disorder.

Separation anxiety occurs significantly more often as a solitary diagnosis than would be expect-ed under random conditions, and noise phobias occur significantly less often as a solitary diagno-sis under the same conditions. These findings sup-port the concept that although they share nonspe-cific signs, the diagnoses are separate entities. Furthermore, the finding that the observed fre-quency of a diagnosis of separation anxiety + thun-derstorm phobia and of separation anxiety + noise phobia was significantly lower than expected were they independent, but that the observed frequency of a diagnosis of thunderstorm phobia + noise phobia and of separation anxiety + noise phobia + thunderstorm phobia is significantly higher than expected were the diagnoses independent, supports two important conclusions (Overall et al. 2001). First, noise and thunderstorm phobia are different from each other and affect the frequency and inten-sity of related behaviors in co-morbid diagnoses differently. Second, the interaction of multiple pathological responses to noise likely either reflects an altered, dysfunctional, underlying neu-rochemical substrate or is the result of one.

OCD IN DOGS AND CATS—A CASE STUDY IN VARIATION

Although the underlying etiology of OCD is unclear for both dogs and humans, the symptomology and pathophysiology are striking. OCD is characterized by repetitive, ritualistic behaviors in excess of that required for normal function, the execution of which interferes with normal daily activities and functioning. Inherent in this description is a behav-ior that is exaggerated in form as well as duration. The behavior can be perceived by the human patient as abnormal and may be controlled to the extent that the behavior is performed only minimally or not at all in the presence of others. This is probably also true for domestic animals. Dogs who flank suck or tail chase may, after frequent reprimands and corrections, remove themselves from view and then commit the behavior elsewhere. When a person approaches the behavior ceases, to be begun again when no one is watching or when the animal removes himself from view. The existence of this evasive behavior pattern is supported for dogs and cats (Overall & Dunham 2002). The presence of this cognitive component suggests that the problem is rooted at a higher level than the behavior alone may indicate (i.e., the dog is flank-sucking, but not because anything is "wrong" with his flank). Such examples support that obsessions are a valid component of OCD. We evaluate obsessions in humans by asking the individuals about ruminant, invasive thoughts.

Not all dogs and cats fit a volitional pattern in which they can at least temporarily stop their compulsive behaviors. Some animal patients exhibit continuous stereotypic and ritualistic behavior regardless of training; distraction; or canine, feline, or human companionship. This is an important point because clients and veterinarians may attribute the nonspecific signs associated with OCD to boredom. Boredom is an often-invoked and seldom-proven "cause" of OCD. In situations involving minimal stimulation and exercise, such as some laboratory and other confinement conditions, animals may spin or chase their tails because they are "bored" or under-stimulated. In such cases, increased stimulation through exposure to human or canine companions, toys, music, exercise, or rooms with views of activity should diminish or stop this behavior.

It is not necessary that the behavior be continuously witnessed for the animal to have OCD, but it is requisite that the offending behavior substantially interfere with normal functioning in the absence of physical restraint. If the desire to exhibit the behavior is present despite restraint because of punishment, training, or physical incarceration, the condition is present. The key is that if such control is removed and the animal could commit the behavior, he would commit the behavior. Ignoring this crucial point will result in under-diagnosis of OCD and underestimation of its frequency in canine and feline populations.

Obsessive-compulsive disorder in humans frequently appears in adolescence at the onset of social maturity and continues through midlife. Human patients are generally clustered into four major groups: washers, checkers, ruminators, and an indistinct group of primary obsessive slowness. In dogs and cats, OCD also appears during this indistinct period of social maturity (Range for dogs: 12–36 months, average ~18–24 months; Range for cats: 24–48 months, average ~30–36 months); left untreated, whether by behavioral or pharmacologic intervention, it worsens (Overall & Dunham 2002). Given the relatively early age at which this condition develops and the probability of profound deterioration when left untreated, young animals should be routinely screened for OCD and treated appropriately early. Dogs and cats from families having a history of OCD should be carefully watched for its appearance, albeit possibly a different form than that exhibited by their relatives.

Of 23 cats studied, 10 manifested their particular form of OCD after some physical trauma or social upheaval, and the OCD in these cases may have occurred with intercat aggression or elimination complaints (Overall & Dunham 2002). Siamese were ranked as the second most-common breed in this study. Although this does not differ substantially from their rank in the overall VHUP population (3rd), it is dramatically different from the breed rank in the VHUP Behavior Clinic population (22nd), suggesting that when a Siamese cat is seen in the Behavior Clinic, it is likely to be because of behaviors associated with OCD. Siamese cats were most often involved in ingestion of fabric, supporting other findings regarding increased prevalence of OCD in Oriental-breed cats (Seksel & Lindeman 1998), but there were too few members of each breed on which to base broad, feline breed-related conclusions. It is interesting that the one Bengal cat in this study showed self-mutilation and urine marking; these are both anxiety-related conditions and may have some association with the relatively recent domestication history of this breed. Most cats affected with OCD exhibit self-mutilation or excessive grooming. No cats were reported to hallucinate; however, "hallucinations" may have been associated with tail chasing. Most clients with these cats reported that the cats acted as if something were on or near the cat's tail and that the cat was either trying to chase this entity or escape it. Accordingly, feline hallucinations may not have been adequately identified in this study.

Unlike cats, few dogs in the study exhibited OCD following trauma or social/situational distress or upheaval. The two cases of trauma involved abusive training: hanging by a choke chain collar. That 2% of this self-selected population of patients for whom clients were seeking treatment for OCD was subject to such abuse should give us all pause.

One pet store dog exhibited profound coprophagia, eating his own feces while also seeking out and eating the feces of others, suggesting that at some point, coprophagia represented a nutritional strategy. Of the 103 dogs in the study, few (~10%) had a putative neurological disorder, physical condition, or potentially painful disorder associated with their OCD, which could either be primary or secondary to the OCD. One dog had a diagnosis of "irritable bowel syndrome," a diagnosis that may be simply a nonspecific sign of an anxiety-related condition. This finding supports the hypothesis that OCD in dogs is based in some primary neurochemical/neurogenetic dysfunction and that mechanisms driving OCD may differ between dogs and cats.

Obsessive-compulsive disorder affects at least 2% of the human population, and this is believed to be an underestimate (Robins et al. 1984, Flamment et al. 1988, Karno et al. 1988). Some forms of OCD have a familial genetic component (Pauls et al. 1995, Nestadt et al. 2000b, Grados et al. 2001); however, most instances of human OCDs appear to be sporadic. It is important to recognize that the development of specific breeds and the practice of inbreeding within those breeds suggests that the incidence of OCDs in dogs could be higher than that reported for humans.

Based on client interviews and complaints, the breeds of dogs in which OCD appears to run in family lines may include at least Great Danes, German short-haired pointers, German Shepherds, bull terriers (Moon-Fanelli & Dodman 1998), Jack Russell terriers, Dalmatians, Bouvier de Flanders, salukis, Cairn terriers, basset hounds, and soft-coated Wheaton terriers. The tight correlations between canine breeds and form of OCD (German shepherds: tail chasing; Rottweilers, Dalmations, Bulldogs: hallucinations) strongly supports a genetic basis for OCD, albeit, in part, as the result of genetic canalization associated with breed.

As is true for humans, first-degree relatives usually have a different manifestation of OCD than does the proband. These features support the above hypotheses of a neurochemical basis for OCD. That 50% of the dogs in this study for whom familial data were known had a relative affected with some form of OCD strongly suggests two important points: (1) purebred dogs appear to have a high incidence of OCD, perhaps higher than that in the human population and (2) a larger percentage of canine family members are affected than appears true for humans.

This frequency of familial occurrence strongly suggests a genetic component of OCD that should be further investigated.

Recent research strongly suggests that OCD in humans is the result of genetically controlled dysfunction of genes involving regulatory systems (Nestadt et al. 2000a, Greer & Capecchi 2002). Such complex regulatory functions that have a genetic, heritable basis have also been reported for dogs (Mignot 2001) and warrant further investigation in dogs and cats affected with OCD.

ROLES FOR AROUSAL AND REACTIVITY

The roles played by arousal and reactivity cannot be ignored if we are to understand dogs with anxiety-related conditions such as separation anxiety, noise phobia, and thunderstorm phobia. Some dogs respond either more quickly or more intensely to a given stimulus than other dogs. At some level, this "hyper-reactivity" is probably truly pathological and represents yet another phenotypical manifestation of some neurochemical variation associated with anxiety. If so, the more frequently the dog reacts to the anxiety-provoking stimulus, the worse and more rapid the response. At some point, any exposure can result in a full-blown, non-graduated anxious reaction in which true panic may be involved. Accordingly, anticipation and early treatment are critical for these individuals, again supporting the concept that behavioral phenotype and underlying neurochemical response are linked dynamically. Early intervention can only be accomplished by understanding the spectrum of signs exhibited in related conditions.

ROLES FOR DOING HARM— STANDARD VETERINARY CARE AND ANTICIPATORY GUIDANCE

It should be clear from the above discussion that problematic behaviors can develop because of a genetic, molecular, or neurochemical liability or an environmental liability. The answer to the classic nature-or-nurture question is "Yes." All response surfaces of all factors interact (Figures 9.1–9.5). Because this is true, veterinarians may wish to consider whether they change the way they practice veterinary medicine. This change would be driven by a belief in the mental health benefits of meeting the patients' needs and in understanding our complicit—albeit unintentional—role in creating anxiety and distress in our patients.

If veterinarians wish to pursue this approach, they will have to address every aspect of what they do from the size and design of their waiting rooms to accommodate individual response and approach distances to the order and style in which they conduct examinations. The average animal approach distance before one enters the space in which the dog or cat may feel uncertain and uncomfortable is 1–1.5 body lengths. If the animal is already distressed or experiences fear or anxiety when approached by or unable to escape from another animal or a human, it will exhibit physiological, neurochemical, and behavioral signs of anxiety, distress, or both. Addressing this concern can be accomplished by providing larger waiting rooms with more-flexible furniture arrangements, enlarging exam rooms and always having one available for anxious pets, conducting some examinations outside in more-relaxed environments where some animals may be more comfortable, and scheduling patients so the animals do not have to wait for appointments. House-calls can provide a greater level of comfort for many pets, but this is not always so. Furthermore, house-calls are often used by clients to avoid addressing the behavioral problems that their pet is exhibiting—not because the clients are lazy or negligent, but because they have no recourse to the information and treatment that could improve the quality of everyone's life. In the late 1980s, I conducted an informal study at a veterinary teaching hospital and private practices and asked clients to whom they would go if they had behavioral questions. No one chose veterinarians first or second. In fact, veterinarians were the last choice or not listed. Clients provided reasons for their selections and felt that veterinarians were not interested in and did not know anything about behavior. There is a lesson here that we should heed and for which we, as alumni of veterinary schools, should campaign using our alumni donations.

Physical and philosophical changes in how we practice medicine will also decrease anxiety and distress in clients. Given that interactions between people and their dogs appear to be mutualistic in terms of neurochemical and physiological changes (Odendaal & Meintjes 2003), it's not sufficient just to address sources of distress and anxiety for one member of the pair, but this is what's usually done: redress usually focuses on the partner who pays the bill.

That said, most recommendations are ones that manage the distress and anxiety after it is apparent.

If we wish to promote good behavioral health, we need to alter a lot more than the behaviors we encourage in our waiting rooms. We need to change how we do things.

Puppies and kittens represent an opportunity for veterinarians to learn to do it differently, and if they are lucky, to finally get it right. Puppies and kittens should be vaccinated at the end, not at the beginning, of the visit, and pediatric appointments should be among the longest, not the shortest. This is the chance to teach the young animal that veterinary practices are fun places to come and that the staff doesn't hurt them. Plunking an unfamiliar infant animal on a cold metal table and jabbing it after sticking a rod up its rectum is unlikely to produce this desired response.

Puppies and kittens also represent an opportunity for the clinicians, nurses, and support staff to have fun. If they have fun, the pets have fun and learn—at the most profound molecular level—that the vet's office and staff are not threats. These visits should start out with play, which provides a golden opportunity to discuss normal signaling, normal play, and appropriate ways to play with dogs and cats, and to react when the pet exhibits a potentially problematic, worrisome behavior (e.g., biting). If the staff plays long enough with the pet, the pet—being a baby—will make a mistake. There is no better way to convince clients that they don't have to hit, kick, squeeze, thump, flick, or shriek at their canine and feline companions than by demonstrating an alternate technique. For example, if the kitten nips, all play stops; no interaction with humans occurs until the cat looks at someone for information, and then play with a toy designed to redirect the behavior is resumed. This is repeated as necessary. If we want clients to have humane skills, we must have them ourselves and we must teach them.

Those who wish more information about twenty-first-century suggestions for greater involvement of other professional staff in behavioral issues should contact the Society of Veterinary Behavior Technicians (SVBT: www.svbt.org) and the Association of Pet Dog Trainers (APDT: www.apdt. org).

SUMMARY

In this chapter I have discussed how to think about behavioral conditions and diagnostic criteria for these conditions. Additionally, I have provided examples of three broad sets of conditions that emphasize how important discrete diagnoses are, how reliance on nonspecific signs can be treacherous, and how interactions of conditions can both go unnoticed unless we are rigorous *and* suggest more appropriate treatments. I have discussed how this mechanistic approach to thinking about the cause of behavioral concerns can be applied to a radically new, preventative, "holistic," humane approach for veterinary care. Finally, I have discussed the definitions for behavioral diagnoses (see Appendix F, Overall 1997a, 2004a) to (a) demonstrate to veterinarians how clear thinking can tell us what we don't know and (b) help veterinarians better diagnose and understand the behavioral concerns of their patients. In doing so, I have tried to provide a window into what I think is the future and the cutting edge of both human and veterinary medicine: neurobehavioral genetics.

Because what we call something affects how we think about it, we can do considerable harm. The association between labels and thought processes is considerably less damaging for traditional somatic conditions in which we can all recognize a hole in the heart, an intestinal worm, a broken bone. When what is broken is intangible, dynamic, and affects all other organ system responses, our terminology can blind us to what we need to know and stop us from acknowledging what we don't know. Paradigms that appear to work for purely "organic" conditions don't work for behavioral ones, in part because of changes in neuronal function that are induced by the behavior itself. As we learn more, we will see that these diagnostic and treatment paradigms really work only for the most obvious of medical conditions. By exploring the complex response surface interactions that define neurobehavioral genetics, we may also be able to introduce an understanding of complexity and mechanism into all areas of medicine and shed archaic paradigms. In veterinary behavioral medicine, in particular, this paradigm shift may also represent our last best chance to become more humane.

REFERENCES

Archer J. 1988. *The behavioural biology of aggression*. Cambridge, UK: Cambridge University Press.

Borchelt PL. 1983. Aggressive behavior in dogs kept as companion animals: Classification and influence by sex, reproductive status, and breed. *Appl Anim Behav Sci* 10:54–61.

Castellanos FX, Tannock R. 2002. Neuroscience of attention-deficit/hyperactivity disorder: The search for endophenotypes. *Nat Neurosci* 3:617–628.

Charney DS, Heninger GR. 1984. Abnormal regulation of noradrenergic function in panic disorders. *Arch Gen Psychiat* 43:1042–1058.

Collias NE. 1953. Social behaviour in animals. *Ecology* 34:810–811.

Crowell-Davis SL, Curtis TM, Knowles RJ. 2004. Social organization in the cat: A modern understanding. *J Feline Med Surg*: in press.

Flamment M, Whittaker A, Rapoport J, et al. 1988. Obsessive compulsive disorder in adolescence: An epidemiological study. *J Am Acad Child Adolesc Psychiatry* 27:764–771.

Geffen E, Gompper ME, Gittleman JL, et al. 1996. Size, life-history traits, and social organization in the canidae: A reevaluation. *Am Nat* 147:140–160.

Gottesman II, Shields J. 1972. *Schizophrenia and genetics: A twin study vantage point*. New York: Academic Press.

Grados MA, Riddle MA, Samuels JF, et al. 2001. The familial phenotype of obsessive-compulsive disorder in relation to tick disorders: The Hopkins OCD family study. *Biol Psychiat* 50:559–565.

Greer JM, Capecchi MR. 2002. Hoxb8 is required for normal grooming behavior in mice. *Neuron* 33:23–34.

Hinde RA. 1967. The nature of aggression. *New Society* 9:302–304.

Hinde RA. 1970. *Animal behaviour*, 2nd ed. New York: McGraw-Hill.

Horwitz D, Mills D, Heath S. 2002. *BSAVA manual of canine and feline behavioural medicine*. Gloucestershire: BSAVA.

Houpt KA, Honig SU, Reisner IL. 1996. Breaking the human-companion bond. *J Am Vet Med Assoc* 208:1653–1659.

Karno M, Golding I, Sorenson S, et al. 1988. The epidemiology of obsessive compulsive disorder in five U.S. communities. *Arch Gen Psychiat* 45:1094–1099.

King J, Simpson B, Overall KL, et al. 2000. Treatment of separation anxiety in dogs with clomipramine. Results from a prospective, randomized, double-blinded, placebo-controlled clinical trial. *J Appl Anim Behav Sci* 67:255–275.

King T, Hemsworth PH, Coleman T. 2003. Fear of novel and startling stimuli in dogs. *Appl Anim Behav Sci* 82:45–64.

Ko GN, Elsworth JD, Roth RH, et al. 1983. Panic-induced elevation of plasma MHPG levels in phobic anxious patients. *Arch Gen Psychiat* 40:425–430.

Koda N. 2001. Inappropriate behavior of potential guide dogs for the blind and coping with the behavior of human raisers. *Appl Anim Behav Sci* 72:79–87.

Landau HG. 1951. On dominance relations and the structure of animal societies. I. Effects of inherent characteristics. *B Math Biophys* 13:1–19.

Lees P, Taylor PM, Landoni FM, et al. 2003. Ketoprofen in the cat: Pharmacodynamics and chiral pharmacokinetics. *Vet J* 165:21–35.

Leonard JA, Wayne RK, Wheeler J, et al. 2002. Ancient DNA evidence for old world origin of new world dogs. *Science* 298:1613–1616.

Mignot E. 2001. A commentary on the neurobiology of the hypocretin/orexin systems. *Neuropsychopharmacol* 25:S5–S15.

Mills DS. 2003. Medical paradigms for the study of problem behaviour: A critical review. *Appl Anim Behav Sci* 81:265–277.

Moon-Fanelli AA, Dodman NH. 1998. Description and development of compulsive tail chasing in terriers and response to clomipramine treatment. *J Am Vet Med Assoc* 212:1252–1257.

Narrow WE, Rae DS, Robins LN, et al. 2002. Revised prevalence estimates of mental disorders in the United States: Using a clinical significance criterion to reconcile 2 surveys' estimates. *Arch Gen Psychiat* 59:115–123.

Nestadt G, Lan T, Samuels JF, et al. 2000a. Complex segregation analysis provides compelling evidence for a major gene underlying obsessive-compulsive disorder (OCD) and heterogeneity by gender. *Am J Hum Genet* 67:1611–1616.

Nestadt G, Samuels JF, Riddle M, et al. 2000b. A family study of obsessive-compulsive disorder. *Arch Gen Psychiat* 57:358–363.

New JG Jr, Salman MD, Scarlett JM, et al. 1999. Moving: Characteristics of dogs and cats and those relinquishing them to 12 U.S. animal shelters. *J Appl Anim Welf Sci* 2:83–96.

Nijhout F. 2003. The importance of context in genetics. *Am Sci* 91:416–423.

Odendaal JS, Meintjes RA. 2003. Neurophysiological correlates of affiliative behaviour between humans and dogs. *Vet J* 165:296–301.

Overall KL. 1994. Proposal for diagnostic criteria. *AVSAB Newsletter* 16:3.

Overall KL. 1995. Sex and aggression. *Canine Pract* 20:16–18.

Overall KL. 1997a. *Clinical behavioral medicine for small animals*. St. Louis: Mosby.

Overall KL. 1997b. Terminology in behavioral medicine: Diagnosis, necessary and sufficient conditions, and mechanism. Proceedings of the First International Conference on Veterinary Behavioural Medicine: European Society of Veterinary Clinical Ethology. Birmingham, UK:14–19.

Overall KL. 1997c. Neurobiology and neurochemistry of fear and aggression. NAVC Proceedings 11:33–39.

Overall KL. 2000. Natural animal models of human psychiatric conditions: Assessment of mechanism and validity. *Prog Neuro-psychoph* 24:727–776.

Overall KL. 2001. Pharmacological treatment in behavioral medicine: The importance of neurochemistry, molecular biology, and mechanistic hypotheses. *Vet J* 62:9–23.

Overall KL. 2004a. *Manual of small animal clinical behavioral medicine*. St. Louis, Elsevier: in press.

Overall KL. 2004b. Commentary for special issue on feline behavior. *J Fel Med Surg*: in press.

Overall KL, Beebe AD. 1997. Dominance aggression in young female dogs: What does this suggest about the heterogeneity of the disorder? Proceedings of the First International Conference on Veterinary Behavioural Medicine: European Society of Veterinary Clinical Ethology. Birmingham, UK:58–63.

Overall KL, Dunham AE. 2002. Clinical features and outcome in dogs and cats with obsessive-compulsive disorder: 126 cases (1989–2000). *J Am Vet Med Assoc* 221:1445–1452.

Overall KL, Dunham AE. 2004. Unpublished data.

Overall KL, Dunham AE, Frank D. 2001. Frequency of nonspecific clinical signs in dogs with separation anxiety, thunderstorm phobia, and noise phobia, alone or in combination. *J Am Vet Med Assoc* 219:467–473.

Pasco PJ. 2003. Better therapies for everyday pain: Exciting advances in pain management. *Vet J* 166:215–217.

Pauls DL, Alsobrook JP, Goodman W, et al. 1995. A family study of obsessive-compulsive disorder. *Am J Psychiat* 152:76–84.

Podberscek AL, Serpell JA. 1996. The English cocker spaniel: Preliminary findings on aggressive behavior. *Appl Anim Behav Sci* 47:75–89.

Podberscek AL, Serpell JA. 1997. Aggressive behaviour in English cocker spaniels and the personality of their owners. *Vet Rec* 141:73–76.

Pyke T, Greenberg H. 1986. Norepinephrine challenge in panic patients. *J Clin Psychol* 6:279–285.

Robins LN, Helzer JE, Weisman MM. 1984. Lifetime prevalence of specific psychiatric disorders in three sites. *Arch Gen Psychiat* 41:949–958.

Rooney NJ, Bradshaw JWS, Robinson IH. 2001. Do dogs respond to play signals given by humans? *Anim Behav* 61:715–722.

Rowell TE. 1966. Hierarchy in the organization of a captive baboon group. *Anim Behav* 14:430–443.

Rowell TE. 1967. A quantitative comparison of the behaviour of a wild and a caged baboon group. *Anim Behav* 15:499–509.

Rowell TE. 1974. The concept of social dominance. *Behav Biol* 11:131–154.

Salman MD, Hutchison J, Ruch-Gallie R, et al. 2000. Behavioral reasons for relinquishment of dogs and cats to 12 shelters. *J Appl Anim Welf Sci* 3:93–106.

Salman MD, New JG Jr, Scarlett JM, et al. 1998. Human and animal factors related to the relinquishment of dogs and cats in selected animal shelters in the United States. *J Appl Anim Welf Sci* 1:207–226.

Scarlett JM, Salman MD, New JG Jr, et al. 1999. Reasons for relinquishment of companion animals in U.S. animal shelters: Selected health and personal issues. *J Appl Anim Welf Sci* 2:41–57.

Scarlett JM, Salman MD, New JG, et al. 2002. The role of veterinary practitioners in reducing dog and cat relinquishments and euthanasias. *J Am Vet Med Assoc* 220:306–311.

Scherrer JF, True WR, Xian H, et al. 2000. Evidence for genetic influences common and specific to symptoms of generalized anxiety and panic. *J Affect Disorders* 57:25–35.

Scholz J, Woolf CJ. 2002. Can we conquer pain? *Nat Neurosci* Suppl 5:1062–1067.

Seksel K, Lindeman MJ. 1998. Use of clomipramine in the treatment of anxiety-related and obsessive-compulsive disorders in cats. *Aust Vet J* 76:317–321.

Short CE. 2003. The management of animal pain—where have we been, where are we now, and where are we going? *Vet J* 165:101–103.

Slabbert JM, Odendaal JSJ. 1999. Early prediction of adult police dog efficiency—a longitudinal study. *Appl Anim Behav Sci* 64:269–288.

Smoller JW, Tsuang MT. 1998. Panic and phobic anxiety: Defining phenotypes for genetic studies. *Am J Psychiat* 155:1152–1162.

Taylor P. 2003. Pain management in dogs and cats—more causes and locations to contemplate. *Vet J* 165:186–187.

Vilà C, Maldonàdo JE, Wayne RK. 1999. Phylogenetic relationships, evolution, and genetic diversity of the domestic dogs. *J Hered* 90:71–77.

Vilà C, Savolainen P, Lamdonado JE, et al. 1997. Multiple and ancient origins of the domestic dog. *Science* 276:1687–1689.

Wayne RK, Vilà C. 2001. Phylogeny and origin of the domestic. In: Ruvinsky A, Sampson J (eds), *The genetics of the dog*. New York, CABI International:1–14.

Webb AA. 2003. Potential sources of neck and back pain in clinical conditions in dogs and cats: A review. *Vet J* 165:193–213.

Weiss E, Greenberg G. 1997. Service dog selection tests: Effectiveness for dogs from animal shelters. *Appl Anim Behav Sci* 53:297–308.

10

Treatment of Emotional Distress and Disorders—Non-Pharmacologic Methods

John C. Wright, Pamela J. Reid, Zack Rozier

DOMESTICATION AND COMPANION ANIMAL BEHAVIOR

Domestication in animals can be viewed as a form of evolutionary process that proceeds over generations within the context of associations with humans. The complex interplay among genotype, experience, and environment (e.g., captivity) results in changes in gene allele frequencies, which in turn lead to developmental changes in morphology, physiology, and behavior. Physiological changes include increases or decreases in hormonal and neurotransmitter activity that contribute to the expression of aggressiveness, earlier maturation of sensory systems, and later onset of fear responses to novelty (Morey 1994, Price 1998). Distinctive behavioral changes (e.g., for *Canis familiaris*) include whining, barking, submissiveness, and friendliness toward people (Morey 1994).

Not only is the genotypic milieu different for domestic species relative to their wild counterparts, but so are the environmental stressors (Price 1984). Less important and even risky for domesticated species' survival are "wild-counterpart" bio-behavioral mechanisms that increased fitness in the wild but that no longer support anthropocentric living. Adaptations to environmental stressors that were once important to canids but are less important for domesticated companion animals include those related to foraging (predator-prey relationships), intra-specific fighting (for access to food and a mate), emotional reactivity (for avoidance of predators), and problem-solving in a natural environment (Bradshaw & Nott 1995, Coppinger & Coppinger 1998).

Human-centered factors constitute the most salient environmental stressors that co-act with genes to shape domesticated dogs' biology and behavior. Companion animals' well-being is dependent on their ability to remain in proximity to man because most domesticated dogs must rely on humans to satisfy their biological, social, and behavioral needs. Thus, dogs' survival depends on their symbiotic relationship with people, and among the most important outcomes of the differential selection process inherent in domestication are biobehavioral adaptations that support human-centered care-seeking and caregiving.

Whether dogs' genetic and behavioral divergence is a result of purposive selection (e.g., Clutton-Brock 1995) or a result of differential mortality of wild ancestors that reproduced and thrived in the presence of people (e.g., Coppinger & Coppinger 1998), it is clear that domesticated dogs are no longer wolves. Developmental changes and changes in the timing of ontogenetic events have been suggested to account for important behavioral differences between dogs and their ancestors (see Morey 1994), as have changes in response thresholds above or below normal levels of stimulation (see Price 1998).

Regardless of the specific mechanisms of change, domestication has resulted in increased tameness, ease of handling, and reduced responsiveness to environmental change (Price 1998). Thus, domesticated dogs do better than wolves at following human signals such as pointing regardless of their rearing experience with people (Hare & Tomasello 1999, Call et al. 2003), but they do worse at solving problems independently (they tend to give up more quickly and await human help [Frank & Frank 1985]), and almost fail to thrive when left alone in the absence of human care (Hubrecht 1995).

It is not surprising, then, that many serious behavioral problems referred to veterinary and applied animal behaviorists have as their primary focus an association with people, in the acquisition of a distressed behavior, its maintenance, or resolution. Just as evolved human behaviors and propensities can lead to serious psychological and physical maladies in the modern environment (Buss 2000), so too can emotional behaviors exhibited by dogs become manifest in undesirable ways. Extreme cases such as serious and fatal bites toward people or conspecifics can result in pet euthanasia and severe legal consequences for dog owners (Blackshaw 1991). When dogs display motivated behaviors to "fight" or "flee" from a perceived threat to their survival (whether in the evolutionary sense or as a learned association), negative feelings of distress are first elicited, followed by recruitment of behavioral mechanisms that restore predictability and control. Prime examples of these emotional/behavioral systems include conditioned fear, separation anxiety, and aggression, all of which are associated with emotions experienced as negative and distressful. This behavioral trio and its emotional components alone account for a large proportion of the problem behaviors reported by dog owners (Wright 1991, Overall 1997).

It is probably not a coincidence that domesticated animals exhibit emotional behavior in contexts that have something to do with their relationships with people. Domestication has increased the likelihood that companion animals will react negatively, both emotionally and behaviorally, when their psychosocial needs are not met. Animals also run into trouble when their attempts to control a situation to their benefit involves resorting to ancestrally prepared emotional behaviors that include biting other animals or people. Fortunately, veterinary and applied animal behaviorists have treatment programs that include non-pharmacological intervention to reduce emotion-laden behavior problems in pets. We identify the properties of stressors that commonly elicit unacceptable emotional behavior in companion animals followed by the tools—the treatment procedures—that are used to bring about significant change.

STRESSORS AND DISTRESS

A definitive definition of the term stress is difficult to arrive at because of its surplus meaning in the scientific and lay literatures. Stress has been defined at different times as a stimulus, a response to a stimulus, and as a consequence. Thus, for the purposes of this chapter, we will avoid any attempt to sort out the definitional problems with the term, but instead provide a working definition of the term *stressor*, the component of stress most relevant to the experience of distress, and proceed to a discussion of procedures for the reduction of distress. Stressors, or stressful experiences, consist of situations that threaten the attainment or maintenance of a goal and include threats to one's physical or psychological well-being (Lazarus & Folkman 1984). Characteristics of different kinds of stressful experiences for companion animals include threats to basic needs and resources of a biological, psychological, and social nature. Distress, then, is a negative psychological response to a stressful experience that may be physically or psychologically threatening and that leads to a variety of cognitive-emotional states such as fear, anxiety, anger, or helplessness (Maier & Watkins 1998).

Part and parcel to a discussion of treatment procedures that lead to a reduction in companion animal distress is an identification of the properties of stressors that contribute to distress. Properties of circumstances (stressors) that can lead to distress include those that are novel, ambiguous, unpredictable, and uncontrollable (Averill 1973, McGrath 1977, Weinberger & Levine 1980, Thompson 1981, Mineka & Hendersen 1985). Distress may be associated with any one of these properties, although exposure to all four kinds of stressors increases the likelihood that conditions are right for the experience of distress. Because distress is a property of the animal and not of the circumstance, objectively similar activities or events may contribute to negative emotional experiences (distress) in one dog and positive emotional responses in another. For example, an adult dog may be inoculated to the *novelty* of moving to a new home if she had successfully moved with her human to new homes several times in the past. Although the new home may certainly be novel, the outcome of moving to a new home is predictable. Further, the dog may experience little distress associated with the move if other significant life events remain unchanged or seem familiar, including her daily routine, social relationships (with other dogs and family members), furniture and bedding, brand of food, and even the sound of her caretaker's car's engine indicating that exercise and other psycho-social perks are close at hand. However, if it were the dogs' first move, other things being equal, the experience of distress might be more likely.

Circumstances that increase the likelihood of distress include changes in daily routine, lifestyle, and social relationships. Animals organize their behavior around significant bio-psycho-social events. A dog reared alone in a quiet home for six years by a soft-spoken person would be at risk for distress if placed in an overcrowded, noisy shelter. Potential problems for the dog include the *novelty* of a new location and unfamiliar people (experienced as a cacophony of sensory inputs, each potentially novel); the disruption of her existing daily routine and social relationship and the *unpredictability* of knowing how or when her needs will be met; the *ambiguity* of her role or job in the shelter (is the shelter's ten-year-old volunteer someone to protect or to be protected from?); and the inability to *control* or know how to bring about change in any of the above circumstances (due to an insufficient behavioral repertoire, inadequate socio-behavioral skills, or circumstances beyond her control). Increasing the duration of exposure to these properties may increase the severity of the psychological response (McEwen 1998).

Distress Is Subjective

Distress results when the demands in a specific circumstance are perceived to outweigh the resources (Thoits 1983, Blascovich & Tomaka 1996). The extent to which distress is experienced is a perceptual phenomenon based on whether one has the responses available to affect the properties of threat (i.e., to oneself, one's resources) or the outcome of the properties. Appraisals of threat are subjective, and perceptual filtering of stressors may result in large differences in the amount of distress experienced across animals; thus, the same threatening situation may elicit quantitatively—or in some cases, qualitatively—different emotional experiences for an animal that has developed a number of effective coping strategies than for an unprepared animal. Both animals may be distressed by the situation, but one animal may experience mild anxiety, and the other, dread.

It may be that the primary task of an applied animal behaviorist in changing behavior associated with negative emotion is to determine ways to change distressful circumstances into those leading to emotionally positive life experiences. Put another way, we should be about creating ways to elicit positive psychosocial responses to stressors that previously resulted in negative appraisal and the experience of distress.

EMOTIONS AND BEHAVIOR

Dogs' reactions to stressful situations range from ones of withdrawal and depression (one extreme), to aggressive and highly aroused or agitated (another extreme). Dogs that freeze and crouch low to the floor in reaction to an intense, unpredictable stimulus (e.g., a loud noise) may be showing behaviors indicative of acute stress (Beerda et al. 1997). A careful description of the emotional behavior and an identification of the contexts and stimuli that elicit the emotional behavior are necessary steps in any behavior modification program.

Separating emotional behavior into its affective and behavioral components is helpful in conceptualizing how to assess and treat a behavioral problem. The behavioral component can be described by its predominant form, either defensive or offensive. The defensive component consists of those behaviors that disengage, including escape, freezing, (defensive) threat, avoidance, or other behaviors designed to decrease proximity to a stimulus or circumstance. The offensive component consists of behaviors that engage or that are designed to increase proximity to a stimulus or circumstance. Offensive behavior may range from active greeting and play to aggressive bite, hold, and shake.

The affective component of emotional behavior can be described by the quality of cognitive-emotional experience, either negative or positive (inferred from the dog's communicative signals and postures and the stimulus circumstance). Negative affect includes arousal labeled as fear, anger (for lack for a better descriptor), and anxiety, and positive affect may be described as happiness, euphoria, or joy. (To what extent dogs' experience of these emotional states is similar to ours is not the focus of this chapter.)

Each form of behavior and emotion can be further characterized by its arousal. By quantifying the "amount" of each component that contributes to emotionally disordered behavior on a scale from 1 (not at all) to 7 (extremely) one can determine initial baselines and, in many cases, the severity of emotional behavior. Weekly changes in emotional state (e.g., from negative to positive) and behavior (e.g., from defensive to submissive approach) can be used as an assessment tool for the amount of change realized in the treatment program. Graphically plotting the weekly changes can give an indication of the slope of change.

Parceling out emotional state from emotional behavior can be most helpful in assessing serious behavior problems such as aggression. For example, dogs that are more likely to bite seem to be those who inhibit neither their emotionality nor their behavior in the presence of mild threat. Further, they do not quickly decrease their negative arousal once the "stimulus" has been removed (they stay overly aroused [Wright & Lockwood 1987]). Thus, for many dogs, bite likelihood increases with the size of the emotional component accompanying the behavior and with the inability to restrain the aggressive behavior in the presence of stimulation.

COMPONENTS OF TREATMENT

Non-pharmacological procedures designed to reduce emotional distress and disorders in companion animals consist of two components: management and treatment. The purpose of management is to decrease the opportunities for the expression of negative, emotion-laden behaviors. The objectives of management are to (1) reduce the likelihood that the animal will continue to experience distress and/or damage to itself; (2) reduce the strengthening of any associations and patterns of responding that may result from the animal's repeated exposure to negative circumstances; (3) reduce the likelihood that the animal's display of emotional behavior will result in damage to people, other animals, or property; and (4) empower family members with one strategy they can use to reduce the risks associated with their companion animal's negative behaviors. Clients may be more willing to embark on a treatment program if they can be provided with at least some degree of respite from the distress of experiencing their pet's unpredictable and often dangerous behavior.

The purpose of the treatment component is to reduce negative emotional behaviors and in many cases overall arousal and replace them with positive emotional behaviors. An effective treatment procedure can be conceptualized as affecting both negative and positive responding, whereby negative streams of responding are reduced while incompatible, positive patterns of emotional behaviors are elicited and strengthened. Weekly assessments of each pattern of responding can be used to help determine the relative success of the treatment procedure in bringing change. Daily fluctuations of change relative to baseline are less important than weekly, directional slopes of change (e.g., negative slopes for emotional distress, positive slopes for positive emotional behaviors, from week to week). Successful treatment should result in stable responding that appears to be a pattern of positive emotional behavior exhibited in the presence of a stressful situation that once elicited distress. Time frames for the assessment of treatment effectiveness vary, although six-month follow-ups are not uncom-

mon. Initial patterns of negative reactivity may resurface in time because they are not "unlearned" and are subject to recovery. Conditions that may facilitate the recovery of initial negative responding and ways to reduce the likelihood of their occurrence are addressed below.

TREATMENT OPTIONS FOR DISTRESSFUL DISORDERS

Although behaviorists use a variety of modification techniques to alter the behavior of companion animals, the one most commonly applied to the treatment of distress disorders is desensitization and counterconditioning (DSCC) (Voith 1979, Hetts 1999, Landsberg et al. 1997). According to Wolpe and Lazarus (1966), DSCC involves the "breaking down of neurotic anxiety-response habits, employing a physiological state incompatible with anxiety to inhibit the anxiety response to a stimulus that evokes it weakly, repeating the exposure until the stimulus loses completely its anxiety-provoking ability." That statement packs a wallop! First of all, DSCC works to change an animal's response to a stimulus by repeatedly presenting the stimulus at such a low level that the animal's arousal is kept to a minimum, thereby setting the animal up to habituate (or "desensitize") to the stimulus. At the same time, however, the stimulus is paired with the presentation of a second stimulus that elicits responses motivationally and/or physically incompatible with the distress responses. The distress responses originally exhibited by the animal to the stimulus are "countered" by this new and very different association.

In practical applications, the components of desensitization and counterconditioning can be utilized together or separately. Analyses of counterconditioning applications reveal that there are two similar, but theoretically and procedurally distinct, methods in use. We describe how desensitization and counterconditioning procedures work and outline their benefits and limitations below.

DESENSITIZATION AND COUNTERCONDITIONING

The first report of the clinical use of DSCC, also known as graduated exposure therapy (Antony & Barlow 1997), described eliminating fear in children (Jones 1924). Children temporarily housed in an institution were assessed for their reactions to a variety of stimuli, including a snake, a rat, a rabbit, a frog, loud noises, and scary faces. Jones (1924) subjected children, who responded with extreme distress to one or more of the stimuli, to procedures designed to eradicate their fear. The most successful intervention consisted of the therapist bringing the child to the cafeteria, placing the feared stimulus sufficiently far away that it did not interfere with the child's desire to eat, and feeding the child a favorite food, like ice cream. While the child ate, the stimulus was slowly brought nearer the table, then placed on the table, and, finally, brought close enough for the child to touch. In one instance, the child ate ice cream while a rabbit, which initially had terrified the child, sat in the child's lap. Increasing the child's hunger enhanced the effectiveness of the method.

Wolpe (1958) reported on the eradication of conditioned fear in cats using DSCC. He established "experimental neurosis" in hungry cats by associating the act of feeding with the delivery of electric shock. After the initial conditioning, the cats refused to eat in the experimental room, despite one to two days of food deprivation. This inhibition of feeding generalized to rooms that were similar to the experimental room. Wolpe identified a room that was sufficiently unlike the experimental room to enable the cats to eat. The cats were still visibly anxious, but they ate. Successive feedings in the new room eliminated all signs of distress. The cats were then moved to a room slightly closer in appearance to the experimental room and offered food. The same routine was repeated in a series of rooms of increasing similarity to the experimental room, remaining in each room until distress was no longer visible. In some cases, Wolpe paired an auditory stimulus with the delivery of shock, and the same procedure was successful for eliminating fear of the sound. The cat was moved away from the source of the sound until it was able to feed. Much the same as in Jones's study with the children, the cat was gradually moved closer to the sound until it no longer elicited fear and inhibited feeding.

A classic application of DSCC in clinical animal behavior can be provided through the example of a dog that fears the sound of thunder. First, there has to be a way of presenting the noise at a volume so low that it fails to evoke a distress response in the dog. For instance, the dog could be exposed to a very quiet recording of thunder. While the dog hears the recording, it is fed especially tasty food so the dog learns the new association of thunder and food. Anticipation of the food elicits responses that are motivationally incompatible with fear, and these responses eventually come to replace distress responses. In other words, the dog comes to expect food when it hears thunder at low volume.

Gradually, the intensity of the stimulus is increased while the animal's arousal is maintained at a low level. Distress responses continue to decline while appetitive behaviors predominate. Eventually, the dog can tolerate the sound of thunder at realistic volumes without becoming afraid. Theoretically, the dog would be expected to salivate upon hearing thunder.

Pets that become distressed when in the presence of strangers can be treated in much the same way as Jones treated her children. For example, imagine a dog that tucks its tail and trembles at the sight of an unknown person. If the person ventures too close, the dog will retreat or, if escape is not possible, bark and lunge. To employ DSCC, the dog is positioned, on leash or otherwise contained, at one end of a room or hallway while a stranger stands far enough away that the dog is willing to eat. Variations that might be required include having the person lower his or her head, sit, or stand facing away from the dog to further lower the dog's arousal. In some cases, the person may need to stand behind a blind or be covered with a sheet during the initial sessions. The dog is fed especially tasty food continually while the person is present. When the person leaves, the food is removed. The session can consist of one period of exposure, as Jones did, or of a series of discrete exposures (trials), in which the person appears in view for a short time while the dog is fed, then the person disappears for a time during which the dog is not fed. As with any type of conditioning, the time between stimulus presentations (the inter-trial interval) should be lengthy (Mackintosh 1974).

DESENSITIZATION ALONE

The use of desensitization (DS) alone relies on the processes of habituation to the feared stimulus and/or extinction of an association between two stimuli that historically were linked. In a typical study of habituation, a stimulus is repeatedly presented alone. Over presentations, there is a relatively permanent decline in responding to the stimulus, presumably reflecting a general reduction in the animal's attention to the stimulus. In a typical study of extinction, the animal first undergoes a series of conditioning trials to establish an association between a stimulus and an outcome, and then that link is subsequently abolished. For instance, Wolpe's cats first learned an association between food and shock, and later, food was repeatedly presented alone without shock until the animals ceased showing distress when exposed to food.

In a clinical application of desensitization alone, the animal experiences repeated presentations of the feared stimulus, but at such a low intensity that it does not elicit distress responses. No attempt is made to countercondition by pairing the stimulus with an unconditioned stimulus (UCS) such as food. For instance, the dog that fears the sound of thunder could be constantly bombarded with a recording of thunder played at a very low volume. The dog would likely initially alert to the sounds but eventually learn to ignore it. Gradually, probably over the course of several days, the volume is increased. The dog is observed to cease alerting to the sound or showing any signs of distress before each increase.

Aside from the fact that it is logistically simpler to implement, the authors see no reason to use desensitization alone to treat distress disorders. The addition of counterconditioning invariably makes behavior change more probable.

COUNTERCONDITIONING

Counterconditioning involves an explicit attempt to counter the animal's distress by associating the feared stimulus with a second stimulus that elicits an incompatible motivational state and/or physical response. When counterconditioning is used alone, the feared stimulus is presented at full intensity. Sometimes desensitization is simply not possible, as there is no way to lower the intensity of the stressor (e.g., fear of flying in an airplane).

For an example of counterconditioning alone, consider a dog that has learned to fear children because of a history of punishment whenever children were present. Whenever a child is nearby, the dog attempts to hide. The dog could be counterconditioned by associating the presence of a child with a game of fetching a ball. The motivational state elicited by ball playing is incompatible with the distress elicited by the child. *If the desire to play ball is stronger than the motivation to hide*, anticipation of play will come to replace the original anticipation of punishment. If it is not, the fear association will remain intact. In classic opponent-process style, the desire to play and the motivation to hide are assumed to exert antagonistic influences on each other until arousal in one system inhibits arousal in the opposing system and interferes with its motivating, reinforcing, and response-producing capabilities (Lovibond & Dickinson 1982).

The importance of identifying powerful reinforcement cannot be underestimated when it comes to treating distress disorders. Laboratory examples of counterconditioning invariably involve food as the appetitive stimulus, but Premack (1965) clarified that any pleasurable activity can function as reinforcement in the right circumstances. Therapists use a variety of activities, such as martial arts, relaxation, book reading, and inducing laughter, to successfully treat anxiety, fear, and anger in human patients (Spiegler & Guevremont 1993). Tortora (1998) argues that play should be preferred over food when treating distress in animals because he believes play is more emotionally incompatible with fear than feeding. Indeed, the author's (PR) dog exhibited extreme distress in the car when going through an automated car wash. Several repetitions of car wash and the dog's favorite treats had no discernible impact on the dog's fear. The dog ate the food but still shivered in terror. A switch to play had an immediate and dramatic effect. The use of certain phrases that had already been conditioned to predict games like tug and fetch completely changed the dog's affect and behavior so that within one session, the dog was barking with glee and chasing the water spraying on the windows. Furthermore, the change was permanent. Years later, the dog still wags his tail at the sight of a car wash. Clients can often identify a hierarchy of phrases (i.e., "walkies!", "wanna go for a car ride?", etc.) that reliably produce changes in their pets' affects to be used as reinforcement in a counterconditioning application.

Classical Counterconditioning

The literature on counterconditioning can be confusing because the term is used to describe two theoretically and procedurally distinct approaches. In the examples presented thus far, the feared stimulus (the conditioned stimulus [CS]) is linked with a pleasant UCS (such as food) in an attempt to replace distress responses with appetitive conditioned responses. This is more accurately called *classical counterconditioning* because the two stimuli are presented contiguously, with no explicit conditioning of behavior. In other words, presentation of the UCS (food) is presented in conjunction with the CS (the feared stimulus), regardless of the animal's behavior. Presentation of the stimuli is not contingent on behavior. The objective is to change behavior, of course, but this is expected to occur through a change in the animal's emotional or motivational state. For instance, in the example presented in the previous section, the dog is exposed to a child, and shortly thereafter, the dog is engaged in play. The play is offered regardless of the dog's behavior toward the child; the dog might initially be trembling, panting, pacing, growling, barking, or any number of behaviors designed to increase distance between the dog and the child. With sufficient repetitions, the dog will ideally come to associate play, rather than fear, with the presence of children, and so the responses elicited by the stimulus of a child will come to reflect this new association—responses that are elements of the play behavior system. In a nutshell, classical counterconditioning focuses on altering the affect or emotive state of the animal with the assumption that the form of behaviors elicited by the emotions will also change.

Classical counterconditioning is an extremely powerful agent for behavior change. Laboratory studies of classical counterconditioning are often referred to as cross-motivational transfer experiments. In most demonstrations, an initially neutral stimulus is first paired with one UCS such as shock, and then, at a later time, the stimulus is paired with a motivationally disparate UCS such as food. In other demonstrations, though, two biologically relevant but incompatible UCSs are paired together. For instance, Erofeeva (1921) used a strong electric shock to signal the delivery of food to hungry dogs. Erofeeva reported that the dogs initially responded with defensive behaviors such as struggling and yelping. Yet, as conditioning progressed, the dogs began to show typical appetitive responses in response to the shock, including lip licking and salivation. Even more surprising, Dearing and Dickinson (1979) found that after counterconditioning an aversive stimulus to signal an appetitive one, the aversive stimulus was incapable of functioning as a punishing stimulus in an instrumental paradigm. This supports the interpretation that classical counterconditioning actually produces a change in the motivational and reinforcing properties of a UCS.

Operant Counterconditioning

An alternative approach is to explicitly condition a volitional behavior that is physically incompatible with the undesirable distress behavior. Tarpy and Bourne (1982) define counterconditioning as a form of training in which "a new behavior, counter to the original response, is reinforced, while at the same time the original response is not rewarded." Defined as such, this counterconditioning is the result of instrumental contingencies and should correctly be referred to as operant counterconditioning. The focus is on replacing behaviors rather than emotions. Operant counterconditioning, although identi-

fied simply as counterconditioning, is the method often described in the applied animal behavior literature. For instance, Overall (1997) writes that "in counterconditioning . . . the dog is taught to engage in a behavior that competitively inhibits the performance of the undesirable behavior." Overall provides an example of operant counterconditioning in the treatment for submissive urination: "as soon as the dog's rump touches the ground without any leakage, the treat is released. Clearly, if the dog rolls, grovels, or leaks, it does not get the food." In this example, delivery of the UCS (food) *is contingent on* the dog displaying or inhibiting a specific response. Contrast that with a classical counterconditioning approach to submissive urination. Suppose the CS (the stressor) is identified as direct eye contact from a person. The dog experiences direct eye contact from a person, followed immediately by the delivery of a treat regardless of whether the dog urinates. With sufficient pairings, the dog will come to associate eye contact with treats and, if the dog finds the treats pleasurable, then urinating should be replaced with solicitous behaviors such as approaching, lip licking, and tail wagging.

Differentiating Operant and Classical Counterconditioning

Why is this distinction between classical and operant counterconditioning important? To start, a significant difference exists in how these procedures play out in an applied setting. Take, for instance, the example of a dog that experiences fear at the sound of the vacuum cleaner. This negative emotion prompts the dog to flee under the bed, where it pants and trembles. Is it more effective to expose the dog to the stimulus (the vacuum) and simply present an appetitive reinforcer (treats) or to require that the dog perform a behavior incompatible with avoidance (such as sit-stay) to earn the appetitive reinforcer? In the first instance, classical counterconditioning, the behaviorist's task is to identify a UCS, such as food or play, that is affectively incompatible with the original emotion, fear, and pair the sound of the vacuum with the new UCS. This pairing can be accomplished every time: present the vacuum, present the food. If the food is sufficiently appealing, the expectation of food will come to replace the fear associated with the sound of the vacuum, and as a result, approach behavior will take the place of avoidance behavior.

In contrast, the second instance uses an operant counterconditioning procedure in which the dog is required to sit-stay before receiving the UCS. The dog hears the vacuum and is then cued to sit-stay. If it does, it gets a treat. If it does not, it does not get a treat (no UCS). With classical counterconditioning, a correlation of 1.0 exists between CS presentation (vacuum) and UCS presentation (food). With operant counterconditioning, the correlation between CS and UCS may be < 1.0, because it is up to the animal whether to perform the requisite behavior. If the animal does not perform the behavior, the UCS is not presented in conjunction with the feared stimulus. Conditioning is always stronger with a greater contingency between CS and UCS (Mackintosh 1974).

The second reason why it is necessary to differentiate between classical and operant counterconditioning is critical. Because emotion "drives" most serious behavior problems such as aggression and separation anxiety, conditioning procedures that elicit changes in a dog's emotional state should be more effective in reducing negative emotional behaviors than are procedures that attempt to treat the behavior directly. Thus, classical counterconditioning should be most effective in reducing these behavior problems by changing the quality and intensity of the emotion that surrounds the behavior. Instrumental contingencies may produce a change in the animal's behavior but are less likely to result in a shift in affective state. In other words, while the animal's behavior may be altered, the underlying motivational state remains unchanged, and the original problematic behavior is likely to reappear. Barlia (1988) provides an illustration of this limitation in his report of a dog that behaved aggressively toward unfamiliar people. The client trained the dog to adopt specific postures (sit, down) with such high reliability that the dog would remain in position even when approached directly by a stranger. Barlia noted that the dog remained stiff and tense during interactions, however, despite the extensive training and exposure to people. Although the dog's responses toward the feared stimulus had been transformed through operant counterconditioning, the underlying affective state remained intact. Likewise, it is not uncommon for human subjects to report that although they are able to function more effectively in the presence of a feared stimulus, such as sitting through an airplane flight, they still experience extreme anxiety and fear (Hersen 1973).

Voluntary and Involuntary Behavior

Not only is classical counterconditioning better at getting to the core source of problematic behavior, involuntary emotionally linked behaviors such as escape and aggression are easily classically conditioned but far less sensitive to instrumental contingencies (Skinner 1957, Thompson 1958). Specific behaviors can be thought of as ranging on a continuum of voluntary–involuntary. Certain behaviors, such as sit and down, are under good volitional control, while behaviors such as trembling or freezing are closely linked to underlying emotional states and are much more difficult, if not impossible, for an animal to control. Other behaviors are more likely to fall somewhere in the middle. For instance, a dog's bark can be highly emotive, yet still, the dog may exercise some control over whether to bark. Although it is recognized that emotionally charged behaviors are sometimes placed under operant control (Salzinger 1962), the typography of the behavior is altered and the response becomes emancipated from the emotion. A prime example of this is the dog that has been taught to bark on cue. The sound of the bark is noticeably different from the bark produced by the dog in response to an intruder. Likewise, a dog taught to growl for the reward of a tidbit can do so, but the growl sounds quite different from a growl the same dog produces when it is experiencing the associated affect.

The fact that behaviors are differentially sensitive to classical and operant contingencies goes unrecognized by some behaviorists and trainers, forming the basis for a basic misconception about treating distress disorders in animals. Widespread reluctance to use classical counterconditioning exists because of the belief that the undesired behavior will be inadvertently reinforced, that "coddling" the dog will reward timid or fearful behavior (see, for example, Aloff 2001, Miller 2001, Price 2001). It is exceedingly difficult to instrumentally condition anxiety-related behaviors, and even if a client were particularly adept at teaching his or her dog to react as though afraid of a stimulus, the resulting behaviors would be unfettered by the underlying emotion of fear.

Perhaps the best way to conceptualize the infeasibility of reinforcing distress behaviors is to examine classical counterconditioning in the laboratory. The procedure typically consists of two phases. In Phase 1, a neutral stimulus, such as a tone, is paired with an aversive UCS, usually shock. Conditioning continues until the animal reacts fearfully in response to the tone by itself. Animals typically freeze because the shock is unavoidable. In Phase 2, the animal learns that the exact same tone now reliably precedes the delivery of food. At first, the animal reacts by freezing when it hears the tone, despite the fact that food is delivered. From an instrumental conditioning perspective, the animal receives reinforcement for the behavior of freezing; however, the behavior of freezing *does not* increase in frequency, as would be expected if the behavior were susceptible to the instrumental contingency. Instead, freezing at the sound of the tone *decreases* in intensity while orienting to the feeder and salivating become predominant. Thus, the new association between the tone and the food is more powerful than the adventitious reinforcement of the animal's fearful behavior. This is true even when the conditioned responses are not mutually exclusive—for instance, if the animal can freeze and eat in the same location (Scavio 1974).

WHICH PROCEDURE IS BEST?

The concurrent use of DSCC is considered to more effectively facilitate behavior change than either desensitization or counterconditioning by itself. Poppen (1970) contrasted four procedures for eliminating rats' fearful responses to a tone that had previously been paired with shock. In the *extinction* condition, rats were exposed to repeated presentations of the full-volume tone in the absence of shock (also called flooding or implosion therapy). In the *desensitization* condition, rats were presented with graded presentations of the tone in the absence of shock; the volume of the tone was increased only when the rats no longer showed a fearful reaction at the current volume. In the *counterconditioning* condition, rats were exposed to the tone at full volume, followed by the delivery of food. In the *DSCC* condition, the rats experienced graded tones paired with the delivery of food, with an increase in the volume of the tone only when the rats no longer showed a fearful reaction at the current volume. The DSCC condition was superior to the other conditions, although all four conditions were effective to varying degrees in eliminating the rats' fear of the tone.

Although classical counterconditioning is clearly superior to instrumental counterconditioning for altering emotionally-linked behavior, is it possible that also conditioning a behavior that is physically incompatible with the distress response might facilitate treatment? Gambrill (1967) explored this question by first teaching rats to run on a wheel to avoid shock. Once wheel running was well established, shocks were no longer delivered. One group of rats was then permitted to run on the wheel until the behavior extinguished. The other group had similar access to the wheel, but they were also taught to press a bar to obtain food. Did this group, with the

opportunity to engage in a physically incompatible response, learn more quickly not to bother running on the wheel? Both groups extinguished the wheel running response at roughly the same rate. Providing an incompatible response did not facilitate elimination of the avoidance behavior.

For most types of distress disorders, we recommend the use of desensitization wherever possible, combined with classical counterconditioning, during initial treatment. For instance, consider a dog that becomes disturbed when approached by other dogs during leashed walks. Desensitization is achieved by maintaining sufficient distance from passing dogs. As soon as the dog detects the oncoming stimulus (the other dog), the client delivers a constant stream of tasty food until the stimulus disappears from view. The food is delivered regardless of the dog's behavior. If the procedure proves successful, the first observable change in behavior is likely to be that the dog orients toward the client when in the presence of another dog. This is a new conditioned response, generating from the expectation of food. At this point we generally recommend switching to operant counterconditioning, thereby requiring that the dog perform the orienting response to earn the treats. This further strengthens the conditioned response, which continues to supersede the original fearful reactions even as proximity to the passing dog increases.

PROCEDURAL CONSIDERATIONS

Classical counterconditioning is certainly easier for most clients to implement than is operant counterconditioning because no response-dependent contingencies exist. It is helpful to identify for clients in advance the types of conditioned responses likely to appear. As we mentioned previously, behavior change is more likely to occur when desensitization (graded exposure) is used with either classical or operant counterconditioning. Desensitization is not only more effective but also more humane. Human patients report more comfort with graded exposure than with exposure to stimuli at full intensity (Antony & Barlow 1997). Both DSCC and counterconditioning alone are more likely to be successful if sessions are long (prolonged exposure is better) and if treatment sessions are scheduled frequently (Antony & Barlow 1997). Pearce and Dickinson (1975) showed that the effectiveness of counterconditioning is a function of the level of activation of the defensive system. Counterconditioning was less successful if the neutral stimulus was initially paired with a high intensity shock than when paired with a low intensity shock; thus, animals showing extreme distress behavior are more resistant to counterconditioning than those showing mild distress. Dickinson and Pearce (1977) provide evidence to support that when food is used as the UCS, greater food deprivation leads to more effective counterconditioning. The hungrier the animal, the more likely the appetitive association replacing the aversive association.

The most serious limitation of counterconditioning is that the resulting behavior change is highly susceptible to relapse. After a great deal of effort to countercondition a switch from a fearful association to an appetitive one, the undesired fearful responses can easily be re-acquired. Bouton and Peck (1992) demonstrated spontaneous recovery of the original association simply by allowing time to pass after counterconditioning. A client might spend weeks successfully counterconditioning a cat to tolerate stroking, but the cat's fearful response to being touched could reappear if, for example, the client left the cat alone for a few days. Renewal of the original association is an even more daunting problem (Peck & Bouton 1990). If counterconditioning always takes place in one context—for instance, the cat learns to tolerate stroking in the bedroom—renewal is likely to occur if the client attempts to stroke the cat in the kitchen. Finally, Brooks et al. (1995) demonstrated reinstatement of the original association after counterconditioning. If something occurs to frighten the cat—for instance, the cat sniffs the client and receives a static shock—the cat may regress and react fearfully when being stroked.

OTHER TECHNIQUES FOR TREATING DISTRESS DISORDERS

A number of other procedures that are quite similar to operant counterconditioning exist.

1. *Countercommanding* is a technique that serves as a precursor to operant counterconditioning. The animal is presented with the feared stimulus and then explicitly cued to perform an incompatible behavior. For instance, the client cues the dog to back away from a stranger rather than lunge forward. This is often the way operant counterconditioning begins; however, the eventual outcome is for the stranger to function as the discriminative stimulus, cueing the new behavior without the aid of the client. Countercommanding never progresses to this level of conditioning (Borchelt 1987). *Competing response training* presents the animal with the feared stimulus, so as to elicit a full-blown distress response, and then focuses on teaching the animal to perform a specific behavior. Much the same as operant counterconditioning, this technique trains the animal to respond with a new behavior when fearful responses are elicited. The main difference is that users of competing response training emphasize generalization of the new behaviors to a realistic range of stimuli (Schwartz & Robbins 1995). *Differential reinforcement of incompatible behavior* (DRI) is a procedure that consists of identifying a specific incompatible response and reinforcing it when it occurs while ignoring unwanted behavior. No effort is made to elicit the incompatible response, so it must be a behavior that has some probability of occurring on its own. For instance, suppose the dog typically vacillates between hiding under the bed and peering around the doorway when a guest is in the home. If the client were to implement a DRI schedule, the dog would be reinforced each time it pokes its head around the doorway, and if the schedule is effective, the frequency of peering out will increase while the frequency of hiding will decrease. Any of these related procedures could be as efficacious as operant counterconditioning in the right circumstances.

2. The *Summation* procedure involves presenting an appetitive stimulus and an aversive stimulus in combination. A classic example of the summation procedure is conditioned suppression. An animal is conditioned to expect a shock when it hears a tone. Following successful conditioning, the tone is sounded while the animal is responding for food. Typically, the animal ceases responding for a period of time after hearing the tone. The influence of the tone, an aversive CS, on responding reveals the relative activation levels of the aversive and appetitive systems. More relevant to clinical applications, presenting an appetitive conditioned stimulus (such as a tone that signals food), overlaid during avoidance responding (pacing while strangers are in the home), usually inhibits responding (Grossen et al. 1969). Barlia (1988) described how he used summation to inhibit fear-motivated aggressive behavior in a dog. The dog was conditioned to view a leather glove as an appetitive stimulus by pairing the glove with a variety of pleasing experiences (e.g., tactile contact, play, feeding). After the dog had established a strong conditioned response to the glove, the glove was worn by approaching strangers (an aversive stimulus). Barlia reported a desirable affective change in the dog, as judged by a reduction in muscular tension and a willingness to interact in a friendly manner with gloved strangers.

3. *Backward chaining* can be used to establish new sequences of behavior in a distressing situation (Martin & Pear 1996). This technique is most useful for teaching animals to move through frightening environments, such as conditioning an agoraphobic dog to go for walks. Backward chaining starts with the final link of the behavioral chain so that the animal is always moving toward a familiar, safe place. In the case of a dog that is frightened to go for walks, the final link is returning to the home. The owner begins by carrying or driving the dog a very short distance from home and walking back. The dog is motivated to walk because it is moving toward the safety of home. Each day, the dog is taken a bit farther from home and required to walk back. Each step along the way is reinforced because the dog is moving closer to safety, along an increasingly familiar route, as the context comes to take on appetitive properties. Eventually, the dog can be taken out the front door and walked along the prescribed route. From the dog's perspective, it is always walking home, even though it is now starting from home. Clients need to be made aware that they must stick to the same route in order for the dog to remain comfortable. Backward chaining is also useful for treating animals that are afraid to traverse stairways or are reluctant to walk on certain substrates, such as tiled floors.

4. *Clicker training* is a technique that can facilitate the replacement of distress behaviors with desirable ones. Technically, clicker training means operant conditioning, using the clicker as an auditory conditioned reinforcer. Through classical conditioning, the animal is taught to associate the sound of the clicker (the CS) with food (the UCS) until the clicker comes to take on secondary reinforcing properties. The clicker is then inserted into the training sequence to mark the desired behavior and bridge the time between the behavior and the delivery of the food reinforcement. Use of a conditioned reinforcer has been shown to enhance learning when compared to the same training without a conditioned reinforcer (Williams & Dunn 1991); however, clicker training is often a euphemism for a hands-off form of operant conditioning that involves shaping new behavior topographies by differentially reinforcing successive approximations (SBSA) to the desired behavior. SBSA is extremely helpful when working with animals suffering from distress disorders because of the hands-off nature of the technique, as handling can sometimes interfere with a fearful animal's ability to learn. For example, a dog that displays hand shyness can be shaped, with the use of a clicker, to approach, and even touch, an outstretched hand without the person making any movement toward the dog. SBSA is also helpful for teaching an animal to perform certain behaviors such as entering a crate or wearing a muzzle. Many animals show reluctance or even fear during crating or muzzling. Because the use of SBSA never involves forcing or even tempting the animal with treats to enter the crate or accept the muzzle, fear is not elicited, and training therefore proceeds at a level that is comfortable for the animal.

CONCLUSION

The non-pharmacologic treatment of emotional distress and disorders in physically healthy companion animals involves a careful assessment of the problem behaviors, the eliciting stimuli, and contexts within which the behavioral event is exhibited. Treatment programs leading to a reduction of emotional behaviors consist of both behavior management and exposures to triggering stimuli, which reduce negative emotional states and negative behaviors and replace them with positive emotions and behaviors. Classical conditioning procedures, such as systematic desensitization and classical counterconditioning, should be most effective in changing emotional distress. Once changed, behaviors can be maintained and strengthened with the use of operant strategies.

REFERENCES

Aloff B. 2001. *Positive reinforcement: Training dogs in the real world*. Neptune City, NJ: T. F. H. Publications.

Antony MM, Barlow DH. 1997. Social and specific phobias. In: Tasman A, Lieberman JA (eds), *Psychiatry*. Philadelphia, PA, WB Saunders:1037–1059.

Averill JR. 1973. Personal control over aversive stimuli and its relationship to stress. *Psychol Bull* 80:286–303.

Barlia E. 1988. A case study on aggression in dogs. In: Wright JC, Borchelt PL (eds), P. L. Animal Behavior Consultant Newsletter, Vol. 5, #4, p. 2.

Beerda B, Schilder BH, van Hoof JA, et al. 1997. Manifestations of chronic and acute stress in dogs. *Appl Anim Behav Sci* 52:307–319.

Blackshaw J. 1991. An overview of types of aggressive behavior in dogs and methods of treatment. *Appl Anim Behav Sci* 30:351–361.

Blascovich J, Tomaka J. 1996. The biopsychosocial model of arousal regulation. *Adv Exp Soc Psychol* 28:1–51.

Borchelt PL. 1987. Counterconditioning and counter-commanding. *Animal Behavior Consultant's Newsletter* 4:3.

Bouton ME, Peck CA. 1992. Spontaneous recovery in cross-motivational transfer counterconditioning. *Anim Learn Behav* 20:313–321.

Bradshaw JWS, Nott HMR. 1995. Social and communication behaviour of companion dogs. In: Serpell J (ed), *The domestic dog: Its evolution, behaviour, and interactions with people*. Cambridge, UK, Cambridge University Press:115–130.

Brooks DC, Hale B, Nelson JB, et al. 1995. Reinstatement after counterconditioning. *Anim Learn Behav* 23:383–390.

Buss DM. 2000. The evolution of happiness. *Am Psychol* 55:15–23.

Call J, Brauer J, Kaminski J, et al. 2003. Domestic dogs are sensitive to the attentional states of humans. *J Comp Psychol* 117:257–263.

Coppinger R, Coppinger L. 1998. Differences in the behavior of dog breeds. In: Grandin T (ed), *Genetics and the behavior of domestic animals*. New York, Academic Press:167–202.

Clutton-Brock J. 1995. Origins of the dog: Domestication and early history. In: Serpell J (ed), *The domestic dog: Its evolution, behaviour, and interactions with people*. Cambridge, UK, Cambridge University Press:7–20.

Dearing MF, Dickinson A. 1979. Counterconditioning of shock by a water reinforcer in rabbits. *Anim Learn Behav* 7:360–366.

Dickinson A, Pearce JM. 1977. Inhibitory interactions between appetitive and aversive stimuli. *Psychol Bull* 84:690–711.

Erofeeva MN. 1921. Additional data on nocuous conditioned reflexes. *Investiga Petrogradskogo Nauchnago Instituta im. P. F. Lesgafta.* 3:69–73.

Frank H, Frank MG. 1985. Comparative manipulation-test performance in ten-week-old wolves (*Canis lupus*) and Alaskan malamutes (*Canis familiaris*): A Piagetian interpretation. *J Comp Psychol* 99:266–274.

Gambrill E. 1967. Effectiveness of the counterconditioning procedure in eliminating avoidance behavior. *Behav Res Ther* 5:263–274.

Grossen NE, Kostansek DJ, Bolles RC. 1969. Effects of appetitive discriminative stimuli on avoidance behavior. *J Exp Psychol* 81:340–343.

Hare B, Tomasello M. 1999. Domestic dogs (*Canis familiaris*) use human and conspecific social cues to locate hidden food. *J Comp Psychol* 113:173–177.

Hersen M. 1973. Self-assessment of fear. *Behav Ther* 4:241–257.

Hetts S. 1999. Pet behavior protocols: What to say, what to do, when to refer. Lakewood, CO: American Animal Hospital Association Press.

Hubrecht R. 1995. The welfare of dogs in human care. In: Serpell J (ed), *The domestic dog: Its evolution, behaviour, and interactions with people*. Cambridge, UK, Cambridge University Press:179–198.

Jones MC. 1924. The elimination of children's fears. *J Exp Psychol* 7:382–390.

Landsberg GM, Hunthausen W, Ackerman L. 1997. *Handbook of behavioural problems of the dog and cat*. Oxford, UK: Butterworth-Heinemann.

Lazarus RS, Folkman S. 1984. *Stress, appraisal and coping*. New York: Springer.

Lovibond PF, Dickinson A. 1982. Counterconditioning of appetitive and defensive CRs in rabbits. *Q J Exp Psychol* 34:115–126.

Mackintosh NJ. 1974. *The psychology of animal learning*. London, UK: Academic Press.

Maier SF, Watkins LR. 1998. Cytokines for psychologists: Implications of bidirectional immune-to-brain communication for understanding behavior, mood, and cognition. *Psychol Rev* 105:83–107.

Martin G, Pear J. 1996. *Behavior modification: What it is and how to do it*, 5th ed. Upper Saddle River, NJ: Prentice Hall.

McEwen BS. 1998. Protective and damaging effects of stress mediators. *New Engl J Med* 338:171–179.

McGrath JE. 1977. Settings, measures and themes: An integrative review of some research on social-psychological factors in stress. In: Monat A, Lazarus RS (eds), *Stress and coping: An anthology*. New York, Columbia University Press:67–76.

Miller P. 2001. *The power of positive dog training*. New York: Hungry Minds.

Mineka S, Hendersen RW. 1985. Controllability and predictability in acquired motivation. *Ann Rev Psychol* 36:495–529.

Morey DF. 1994. The early evolution of the domestic dog. *Am Sci* 82:336–347.

Overall KL. 1997. *Clinical behavioral medicine for small animals*. St. Louis, MO: Mosby.

Pearce JM, Dickinson A. 1975. Pavlovian counterconditioning: Changing the suppressive properties of shock by association with food. *J Exp Psychol Anim B* 1:170–177.

Peck CA, Bouton ME. 1990. Context and performance in aversive-to-appetitive and appetitive-to-aversive transfer. *Learn Motiv* 21:1–31.

Poppen R. 1970. Counterconditioning of conditioned suppression in rats. *Psychol Rep* 27:659.

Premack D. 1965. Reinforcement theory. In: Levine D (ed), *Nebraska symposium on motivation*. Lincoln: University of Nebraska Press:123-180.

Price C. 2001. *Understanding the rescue dog.* Bristol, UK: Broadcast Books.

Price EO. 1984. Behavioral aspects of animal domestication. *Q Rev Biol* 59:1–32.

Price EO. 1998. Behavioral genetics and the process of animal domestication. In: Grandin T (ed), *Genetics and the behavior of domestic animals.* New York, Academic Press:31–66.

Salzinger K. 1962. The operant control of vocalization in the dog. *J Exp Anal Behav* 5:383–389.

Scavio MJ Jr. 1974. Classical-classical transfer: Effects of prior aversive conditioning upon appetitive conditioning in rabbits (*Oryctolagus cuniculus*). *J Comp Physiol Psych* 86:107–115.

Schwartz B, Robbins SJ. 1995. *Psychology of learning and behavior,* 4th ed. New York: W. W. Norton.

Skinner BF. 1957. *Verbal behavior.* New York: Appleton-Century Crofts.

Spiegler MD, Guevremont DC. 1993. *Contemporary behavior therapy,* 2nd ed. Pacific Grove, CA: Brooks/Cole.

Tarpy RM, Bourne LE Jr. 1982. *Principles of animal learning and motivation.* Glenview, IL: Scott, Foresman.

Thoits PA. 1983. Dimensions of life events that influence distress: An evaluation and synthesis of the literature. In: Kaplan HB (ed), *Psychosocial stress: Trends in theory and research.* New York, Academic Press:33–103.

Thompson SC. 1981. Will it hurt less if I can control it? A complex answer to a simple question. *Psychol Bull* 90:89–101.

Thompson WR. 1958. Social behavior. In: Roe A, Simpson G (eds), *Behavior and evolution.* New Haven, CT: Yale University Press:291-310.

Tortora DF. 1998. Personal communication. New Jersey City University.

Voith VL. 1979. Treatment of phobias. *Mod Vet Pract* 60:721–722.

Weinberger J, Levine S. 1980. Psychobiology of coping in animals: The effects of predictability. In: Levine S, Ursin H (eds), *Coping and health.* New York, Plenum Press:39–59.

Williams BA, Dunn R. 1991. Substitutability between conditioned and primary reinforcers in discrimination acquisition. *J Exp Anal Behav* 55:21–35.

Wolpe J. 1958. *Psychotherapy by reciprocal inhibition.* Stanford, CA: Stanford University Press.

Wolpe J, Lazarus AA. 1966. *Behavior therapy technique.* New York: Pergamon Press.

Wright JC. 1991. Canine aggression toward people: Bite scenarios and prevention. *Vet Clin N Am-Small* 21:299–314.

Wright JC, Lockwood R. 1987. Behavioral testing of dogs implicated in a fatal attack on a young child. Animal Behavior Society Meeting, Williamstown, MA, June.

11

Treatment of Emotional Distress and Disorders—Pharmacologic Methods

Amy R. Marder and J. Michelle Posage

People who live with animals consider their animals' behavior to be a problem when the behavior interferes with their lifestyle and as a result, the human household members suffer emotional distress. At the same time, the animal may suffer emotional distress not only from the behavior "problem" but also from their caretaker's response to the problem. For example, a cat who is eliminating outside of the litter box may be anxious because of conflict caused by a dirty litter box and the "normal" search for an alternative elimination area. This anxiety may be compounded by a caretaker's punishment of the cat for eliminating in inappropriate areas. Because of this combination, most behavior problems result in anxiety and emotional distress for the animal.

When people see animals in emotional distress, they often assume that the animals are feeling the same as they do when they are distressed. Unfortunately, this may not be true. It is possible that animals experience emotions differently than human beings. Because animals most likely live in the present, without worrying about the future or reliving the past, their emotional feelings may be less complicated than ours. Furthermore, an animal's response to a stressor may be very effective in reducing the animal's anxiety but very disturbing to a human caretaker. For example, a dog that jumps into the bathtub during a thunderstorm may be feeling much less anxious while in the bathtub. The human, however, becomes distressed at the sight and demands therapy.

A treatment program for a specific behavior problem and the concomitant emotional distress must address both the animal's behavior and the human caretaker's behavior toward the animal. The program may consist of a combination of avoidance, environmental manipulation, behavior modification, and drug therapy. Due to recent developments over the past decade, behavioral pharmacotherapy is now commonly prescribed as part of veterinary behavioral therapy programs. Effective drug therapy may not only ease the implementation of a behavior modification but may also help to alleviate the emotional distress that an animal is experiencing.

IMPORTANT CONSIDERATIONS REGARDING THE USE OF PHARMACOTHERAPY IN TREATING EMOTIONAL DISTRESS

1. As with any disease, in order to choose the most effective treatment protocol, it is essential that a veterinarian make a diagnosis. A diagnosis of an emotional disorder requires a very thorough behavioral history concentrating on behavioral signs. The existence of behavioral signs of distress is currently the most feasible means to evaluate emotions in animals.

2. In easing emotional distress, drug therapy is most effective when used as *part* of a behavioral therapy program (see Wright et al., this volume). Just as in people, although drug therapy alone can greatly alleviate the suffering of unpleasant emotions such as that associated with separation anxiety, maximal relief is achieved when drug therapy and behavior modification are combined. A danger exists that drug therapy may depress behavioral signs while not truly reducing emotional distress. The use of combination programs may treat the individual cause of a problem and not simply reduce behavioral signs.

3. All drugs have potential side effects. Clinicians should be thoroughly familiar with indications, mechanisms of action, dosages, contraindications,

and side effects before prescribing drug therapy. We want to make every effort to prevent the production of new forms of discomfort in striving to alleviate unpleasant emotional feelings. Daily health and behavioral monitoring is required to prevent and respond to serious medical, behavioral, and emotional side effects.

4. Although some studies have been made of the use of drug therapy to treat behavioral problems (e.g., barking, destruction, elimination caused by separation anxiety), virtually none have carefully followed the signs of emotional distress (e.g., panting, pacing, trembling). Because animals cannot tell us how they are feeling, careful monitoring of behavioral signs is essential to determining the effectiveness of drug therapy on emotional well-being.

5. Many drugs require one month or more of treatment to reach stable therapeutic blood levels. This is an important concept for owners to understand, as people usually want the distress their animals are experiencing to be alleviated as soon as possible. They must understand that the relief provided by pharmacotherapy may not be instantaneous.

6. Psychotropic drugs are expensive. Even those that are available in generic forms can still cost one to two dollars per dose, depending on the size of the animal.

7. Most psychotropic drugs are not approved for use in dogs and cats. To enhance the safe use of these drugs, a baseline CBC and blood chemistry profile is recommended. This is an additional expense.

WHEN DRUG THERAPY SHOULD BE CONSIDERED

Most animals that are exhibiting behavior problems experience emotional distress to some degree. The distress may be obvious, as in a dog with separation anxiety or loud noise phobia, or subtle, as in a cat with an elimination problem. Even dogs who are aggressive to humans or other dogs often display dilated pupils and stiff bodies during aggressive events, both which may be interpreted as unpleasant emotional feelings. Every behavior problem should not be treated with medication just because an emotional component is involved. Although an animal may be experiencing some emotional discomfort, other less-invasive procedures (e.g., avoidance, behavior modification) may effectively improve the animal's emotional well-being(see Wright et al., this volume). Some cases exist when an animal's

emotional state interferes with the implementation of behavior modification, however; in these cases, drug therapy is indicated. For example, a dog with separation anxiety who becomes uncontrollably anxious at the first hint that the owner is leaving, thus impeding the initiation of behavior modification, should be treated with an anti-anxiety drug. For a cat who has developed an intense fear of the litter box or another animal, drug therapy may help to "jump-start" a behavior modification program.

Human studies have revealed that psychotherapy used with or without drug therapy is more effective than drug therapy alone for the treatment of some conditions. When used alone, problems recur after the drug is discontinued. Relapse rates are much lower when psychotherapy is a part of treatment. The same may be true for animals.

Several outcome studies and reports on the effectiveness of drug therapy to treat behavior problems in animals are available. Although some address the behavioral signs of emotional discomfort, few, if any, directly address emotional well-being. Because of our lack of knowledge in the treatment of emotional disorders in animals, it is safest for us to consider drug therapy only when outcome data is available. A thorough review of the literature should be pursued before "experimenting" with pharmacotherapy. Table 11.1 describes the indications, side effects, and references for pharmacologic agents commonly used in animals with emotional distress and/or behavior problems.

PHEROMONE THERAPY

Recently, the use of synthetic pheromone preparations has been promoted for the treatment of some behavior problems. Feline spraying and transport anxiety, canine separation anxiety, noise phobia, and anxiety during veterinary exams have been successfully treated with pheromone therapy. Investigators believe that pheromones' effects on individual behaviors can be explained by stress reduction. If this is true, they are promising safe alternatives for the treatment of emotional disorders (Paget & Gaultier 2003).

Unlike drug therapy, synthetic pheromones have no toxicity or side effects. Administration is external, through either an environmental spray or diffuser, making dispensing simple. Feliway® (Veterinary Products Laboratories) is a mixture of synthetic feline facial pheromones. Dog Appeasing Pheromone® (Veterinary Products Laboratories) is a synthetic analogue of a calming pheromone secreted by nursing bitches.

Table 11.1. Pharmacologic agents commonly used in animals with emotional distress and/or behavior problems.

Drug Name	Canine Dose	Feline Dose	Uses	Relative Cost	Side Effects
Acepromazine	0.55–2.2 mg/kg (Fort Dodge 2001)	1.1–2.2 mg/kg (FortDodge 2001)	Chemical restraint	$	Hypotension, CNS stimulation, contradictory responses. Use with caution in boxers and greyhounds
Alprazolam	0.02–0.1 mg/kg q 8–12h (Landsberg et al. 1997)	0.125–0.25 mg/cat q 12h (Marder 1991)	Anxiety, noise phobias, canine submissive urination, feline urine marking	$	Sedation, ataxia, increased appetite, paradoxical excitation
Amitriptyline HCl	2.2–4.4 mg/kg q 12–24h (Juarbe-Diaz 1997a, 1997b)	5–10 mg/cat q 24h (Marder 1991, Papich 2002) 2.5–5.0 mg/cat q 12–24h (Sawyer et al. 1999)	Anxiety, canine and feline fear aggression, feline urine marking, feline displacement grooming, canine stereotypy	$	Sedation, gastrointestinal effects, dry mouth, increased thirst, urinary retention
Buspirone HCl	2.5–10 mg/dog q 12–24h or 1.0–2.0 mg/kg q 12h (Papich 2002) 1.0 mg/kg q 8–12h (Crowell-Davis et al. 2001)	2.5–7.5 mg/cat q 12h (Crowell-Davis et al. 2001) 2.5–5.0 mg/cat q 8–12h (Marder 1991)	Phobia, anxiety, feline urine marking	$$$$	Uncommon, not sedating
Chlorpheniramine Maleate	0.22 mg/kg q 8h (Overall 2000)	1–4 mg/cat q 12–24h (Overall 2000)	Sedation	$	Sedation, anticholinergic effects, GI effects

(continues)

Table 11.1. Continued

Drug Name	Canine Dose	Feline Dose	Uses	Relative Cost	Side Effects
Clomipramine HCl	2–4 mg/kg q 24h or divided q 12h (Novartis 2000)	0.5–1 mg/kg q 24h (Reisner & Houpt 2000)	Canine separation anxiety, feline urine marking, compulsive disorder, feline hyperesthesia syndrome, feline psychogenic alopecia, canine acral lick dermatitis, phobia	$$	Sedation, GI effects, anticholinergic effects, cardiac effects
Clorazepate Dipotassium	2 mg/kg q 12h (Papich 2002) 0.55–2.2 mg/kg q 4h (Overall 1997)	0.5–1.0 mg/kg q 12–24h (Overall 1997)	Anxiety, noise phobias, canine submissive urination, feline urine marking	$$	Sedation, ataxia
Cyproheptadine HCl	No published dose	2 mg/cat q 12h (Schwartz 1999)	Feline urine marking	$	Anticholinergic effects, sedation
Diazepam	0.55–2.2 mg/kg prn (Crowell-Davis et al. 2001)	1–4 mg/cat q 12–24h (Papich 2002) 0.2–0.4 mg/kg q 12–24h (Cooper & Hart 1992)	Canine and feline phobia, feline urine marking	$	Rare cases of acute liver failure in cats, sedation, paradoxical excitation, muscle relaxation, increased appetite

Drug Name	Canine Dose	Feline Dose	Uses	Relative Cost	Side Effects
Doxepin HCl	3–5 mg/kg q 12h (max dose 150 mg/ dog q 12h) (Crowell-Davis 1999)	0.5–1.0 mg/kg q 12–24h (Crowell-Davis et al. 2001)	Compulsive disorders resulting in self-mutilation, feline psychogenic alopecia	$$	Hyperexcitability, GI effects, lethargy
Fluoxetine HCl	1.0–1.5 mg/kg q 24h (Crowell-Davis 1999)	0.5–1.0 mg/kg q 24h (Crowell-Davis 1999, Crowell-Davis et al. 2001)	Aggression, canine separation anxiety, compulsive disorders, feline urine marking	$$$	Lethargy, inappetence, anorexia, GI effects
Hydrocodone Bitartrate	0.25–1.0 mg/kg q 8–12h (Marder & Bergman 1999)	1.25–5.0 mg/cat q 12–24h (Marder & Bergman 1999)	Compulsive disorders resulting in self-mutilation	$	Sedation, constipation, GI effects
Imipramine HCl	2–4 mg/kg q 12–24h (Papich 2002)	0.5–1.0 mg/kg q 12–24h (Crowell-Davis et al. 2001)	Canine submissive urination	$	Sedation, anticholinergic effects
Medroxyprogesterone Acetate	5–10 mg/kg SQ, IM; do not exceed 3 treatments per year (Voith & Marder 1998)	10–20 mg/kg SQ (Voith & Marder 1998)	Treatment of last resort for aggression and feline urine marking	$	Polyphagia, polydipsia, sedation, diabetes mellitus, pyometra, mammary hyperplasia, endometrial hyperplasia, carcinoma
Megestrol Acetate	1.1–2.2 mg/kg q 24 for 2 wks, then 0.5–1.1 mg/kg q 24 for 2 wks (Voith & Marder 1998)	5 mg/cat q 24h x for 2 months (Hart & Eckstein 1998)	Treatment of last resort for aggression and urine marking	$	Same as medroxyprogesterone acetate

(continues)

Table 11.1. Continued

Drug Name	Canine Dose	Feline Dose	Uses	Relative Cost	Side Effects
Melatonin	0.1 mg/kg q 8–12h (with amitriptyline) (Aronson 1999)	No published dose	Canine fear, phobia	$	Side effects appear to be minimal, but not well studied
Methylphenidate HCl	5 mg (small dog) – 20 mg (large dog) q 8–12h; do not give near bedtime (Crowell-Davis et al. 2001) 2–4 mg/kg q 12–24h (Marder & Bergman 1999)	No published dose	Canine hyperkinesis	$$$$	CNS arousal, GI effects, inappetence, cardiac effects, hypertension, stranguria
Naltrexone HCl	2.2 mg/kg q 12h (Papich 2002)	25–50 mg/cat q 24h (Crowell-Davis et al. 2001)	Canine acral lick dermatitis, canine stereotypic behavior, compulsive disorders	$$$$	GI effects, insomnia, nervousness
Paroxetine HCl	0.5–1.0 mg/kg q 24h (Papich 2002)	0.5–1.0 mg/kg q 24h (Crowell-Davis et al. 2001) 1.25–2.5 mg/cat q 24h (Mills & Simpson 2002)	Aggression, canine separation anxiety, compulsive disorders, feline urine marking	$$$	Lethargy, GI effects, inappetence, constipation

Drug Name	Canine Dose	Feline Dose	Uses	Relative Cost	Side Effects
Phenobarbital	2–8 mg/kg q 12h (Papich 2002) 1.5–2.0 mg/kg q 12h (Dodman et al. 1992)	2–3 mg/kg prn (Overall 2000)	Canine and feline compulsive tail chasing, unprovoked canine rage aggression	$	Lethargy, ataxia, polyuria, polydipsia, polyphagia
Phenylpropanolamine HCl	1.1 mg/kg q 8h (Plumb 1988)	No published dose	Canine submissive/ excitement urination	$	Restlessness, hypertension, anorexia
Propranolol HCl	5–40 mg/dog q 8h (Crowell-Davis 1999)	0.25 mg/kg prn (Crowell-Davis 1999)	Canine fear aggression, noise phobia	$	Bradycardia, lethargy, hypotension, syncope
Selegiline HCl	0.5–1.0 mg/kg q 24h in AM (Pfizer 2000)	No published dose	Canine cognitive dysfunction syndrome	$$$$	GI effects, restlessness or lethargy, anorexia
Sertraline	0.5–4.0 mg/kg q 24h (Crowell-Davis et al. 2001)	0.5–1.0 mg/kg q 24h (Crowell-Davis et al. 2001)	Anxiety, fear, aggression	$$$	Sedation, GI effects

All doses are per os unless otherwise indicated.

Abbreviations: prn, as needed; h, hours.

Relative cost: $ inexpensive, $$ moderate cost, $$$ relatively costly, $$$$ most expensive.

REFERENCES

Aronson L. 1999. Animal behavior case of the month: Extreme fear in a dog. *J Am Vet Med Assoc* 215:22–24.

Cooper L, Hart BL. 1992. Comparison of diazepam with progestin for effectiveness in suppression of urine spraying behavior in cats. *J Am Vet Med Assoc* 200:797–801.

Crowell-Davis S. 1999. *Behavior psychopharmacology*. Kansas City: Central Veterinary Conference.

Crowell-Davis SL, Curtis T, Murray T, et al. 2001. Pharmacology for veterinarians: Knowing which drug to use and when to use it. Lecture Notes, College of Veterinary Medicine, University of Georgia.

Dodman NH, Miczed KA, Knowles K, et al. 1992. Phenobarbital-responsive compulsive tail chasing in a dog. *J Am Vet Med Assoc* 201:1580–1583.

Fort Dodge. 2001. Prom Ace®, Package Insert. Madison, NJ: Wyeth.

Hart BL, Eckstein RA. 1998. Progestins: Indications for male-typical behavior problems. In: Dodman NH, Shuster L (eds), *Psychopharmacology of animal behavior disorders*. Malden, MA, Blackwell Science:255–263.

Juarbe-Diaz SV. 1997a. Social dynamics and behavior problems in multiple dog households. *Vet Clin N Am-Small* 27:497–514.

Juarbe-Diaz SV. 1997b. Assessment and treatment of excessive barking in the domestic dog. *Vet Clin N Am-Small* 27:515–532.

Landsberg G, Hunthausen W, Ackerman L. 1997. *Handbook of behavior problems of the dog and cat*. Oxford, UK: Butterworth Heinemann.

Marder AR. 1991. Psychotropic drugs and behavioral therapy. *Vet Clin N Am-Small* 21:329–342.

Marder AR, Bergman L. 1999. Guidelines for the use of psychotropic drugs for behavior problems. In: Hetts S (ed), *Pet behavior protocols*. Lakewood, CO: American Animal Hospital Association Press:299-314.

Mills DS, Simpson BS. 2002. Psychotropic agents. In: Horwitz DF, Mills DS, Heath S (eds), *BSAVA manual of canine and feline behavioral medicine*. Gloucester, UK, BSAVA Press:237–248.

Novartis. 2000. Clomicalm®, Package Insert. Basel, Switzerland: Novartis International.

Overall KL. 1997. *Clinical behavioral medicine for small animals*. St. Louis: Mosby.

Overall KL. 2000. Behavioral pharmacology. Proceedings of the American Animal Hospital Association 67th Annual Meeting, Toronto.

Paget P, Gaultier E. 2003. Current research in canine and feline pheromones. *Vet Clin N Am-Small* 33:201–208.

Papich MG. 2002. *Saunders handbook of veterinary drugs*. Philadelphia: WB Saunders.

Pfizer. 2000. Anipryl®, Package Insert. New York: Pfizer.

Plumb DC. 1988. *Veterinary pharmacy formulary*, 2nd ed. St. Paul: Minnesota Veterinary Teaching Hospital.

Reisner I, Houpt K. 2000. Behavioral disorders. In: Ettinger S, Feldman E (eds), *Textbook of veterinary internal medicine: Diseases of the dog and cat*, 5th ed. Philadelphia, WB Saunders:156-162.

Sawyer LS, Moon-Fanelli AA, Dodman NH. 1999. Psychogenic alopecia in cats: 11 cases (1993–1996). *J Am Vet Med Assoc* 214:71–74.

Schwartz S. 1999. Use of cyproheptadine to control urine spraying and masturbation in a cat. *J Am Vet Med Assoc* 214:369–371.

Voith VL, Marder AR. 1998. Canine behavioral disorders. In: Morgan RV (ed), *Handbook of small animal practice*. New York: Churchill Livingstone: 1245-1267.

12
Emotional Maltreatment in Animals

Franklin D. McMillan

During the latter part of the twentieth century, society saw a growing appreciation of and respect for the welfare of animals (Lacroix & Wilson 1998). Animal maltreatment has received much attention in the popular press, fueled by a number of well-publicized incidents of deliberate cruelty that have provoked widespread public outrage (Patronek 1997). Unfortunately, the efforts at combating animal neglect and abuse have encountered the same problem well described in the field of child maltreatment: a disproportionate focus on physical neglect and abuse, with little attention devoted to emotional maltreatment. In children, emotional abuse is regarded as an elusive and nebulous phenomenon, and authorities have historically tended to view it as less serious than other forms of abuse (Iwaniec 1995, Kowal 1998, Kent & Waller 2000). Childhood emotional abuse does not generate the public interest or outrage that physical and sexual abuse do, in part because emotional maltreatment is harder to recognize, as it does not leave visible scars or overtly recognizable injury like that found in physical neglect and abuse (Iwaniec 1995, Kowal 1998). In animals, the disparity in reaction and response (legal and otherwise) to emotional, as opposed to physical, maltreatment closely resembles the early situation in the field of child abuse. The focus of maltreatment in animals has traditionally been on physical harm, also likely due in a large part to the fact that the outcome of physical trauma is graphic and shocking in nature as compared to that of emotional trauma (Jorgensen 1990, Kent & Waller 2000). Furthermore, it is well known that physical abuse can cause death, whereas emotional abuse would not be expected to have any such extreme outcome. Although efforts have been made to detail the signs of animal maltreatment (Leonard 2000, Sinclair 2000), these have addressed signs of physical abuse and neglect; no such standards have been proposed for emotional maltreatment. As a further example of this lopsided focus, of the animal cruelty statutes of the 50 states and the District of Columbia, none include language specifically acknowledging or addressing emotional neglect, abuse, or suffering in their definitions of cruelty. Furthermore, nine states specifically prohibit consideration of emotional suffering by specifying that any injury or suffering must be physical in nature (Animal Protection Institute 2001).

This deficiency in animal care and protection is especially important in light of the recent advancements in the study of the psychological components of animal well-being. In the past three decades, there has been a rapid proliferation of research in the fields of the cognitive sciences, ethology, comparative psychology, neuroscience, and clinical animal behavior, which collectively has led to a vastly increased understanding of emotions. This new knowledge has alerted scientists and nonscientists alike to the scope of animal suffering that is associated with mental states (Dodman 1997, Patronek 1998, McMillan 2002) and has expanded the scope of animal care to include the attendance to emotional needs, distress, and suffering. Because of the potential for emotions to inflict discomfort, anguish, and suffering (McMillan 2002, 2003), the goal of understanding and addressing emotional maltreatment in animals necessarily deserves a high priority in animal care.

In addition to the direct suffering caused by unpleasant emotional states, emotional maltreatment warrants full attention because of the relationship between mental and physical health. An extensive body of research that substantiates a strong association between unpleasant emotional states and adverse health effects has accumulated (for a review, see McMillan 1999). For the distress and suffering it causes, as well as the link to bodily health, the protection of animals against emotional maltreatment assumes a critically important aspect of comprehensive animal care.

All emotions appear to have an associated affective (feeling) component, and this affect has either a pleasant or unpleasant quality. The emotions relevant to the issue of emotional maltreatment are those with unpleasant affect. Unpleasant emotions for which substantial evidence exists in animals include fear (and phobias), anxiety, separation anxiety (or separation distress), loneliness (and isolation-related emotions), boredom, frustration, anger, grief, helplessness, hopelessness, and depression (Panksepp 1998). Additional unpleasant emotions present in human beings (Lazarus 1999) but currently lacking strong evidence supporting their existence in animals include jealousy, embarrassment, shame, and guilt.

PROBLEMS IN DEFINITION

A consensus on definitions and terminology in the study of emotional maltreatment in children—and its component parts, emotional neglect and emotional abuse—continues to elude researchers (Wolfe 1999, Kent & Waller 2000). Although all forms of childhood neglect and abuse have proved difficult to define, the very private, subjective, and nebulous qualities of emotional maltreatment present especially difficult definitional challenges (Iwaniec 1995, Kent & Waller 2000). In contrast to physical abuse, childhood emotional abuse is exceedingly hard to clearly recognize because no consensus exists about what constitutes emotional abuse, its harm is in the form of emotional rather than physical scars, no pathognomonic findings are recognizable on examination, and the harm can vary dramatically from one child to another (Owen & Coant 1992, Jellen et al. 2001).

The problems faced in the human field become even more difficult in our dealings with animals. As has been noted in regard to parenting methods with human infants, what some may consider in animal care to be abusive, others may consider acceptable, necessary, and even normal care. In children, formulating a clinical picture of the signs of physical abuse was an important starting point for addressing the problem of this form of abuse. Child abuse had existed for millennia, but only as recently as 1962, with the publication of the landmark paper "The Battered Child Syndrome" by Kempe *et al.*, were the clinical criteria for physical abuse established.

Kempe and colleagues proposed that distinct patterns of injury, such as multiple bone fractures at different stages of healing and unexplained hemorrhage of the brain or retinas, were evidence suggesting physical abuse—a "battered child."

In contrast to the rather precise descriptions in children, no clinical signs in animals are currently established as "highly suggestive" of non-accidental injury, and none are "virtually diagnostic" (Munro 1998). To date, no comprehensive and reliable description of the "battered pet" exists that is in any way comparable to the clinical picture in the physically abused child (Patronek 1997, Ascione & Barnard 1998). The little that has been written focuses almost exclusively on physical neglect rather than abuse. For example, a scoring tool has recently been developed for evaluating body condition with the goal of objectively quantifying physical neglect (Patronek 1998). As was the case in child maltreatment, the problems inherent in the seemingly straightforward task of describing the animal victim of physical maltreatment pale in comparison to the challenges of describing the victim of emotional maltreatment.

The difficulty of defining maltreatment—physical or emotional—is complicated further by the uncertainty as to whether the emphasis should be on the caregiver's actions (or inactions) or the effect on the animal victim. Is maltreatment based on the *act* of the caregiver, the *intent* of the caregiver, the *response* of the victim, the *harm* to the victim, or some combination of these? Certainly, the most appropriate focus would appear to be the harm—actual or potential—to the victim, because for an act to qualify as maltreatment, it would require at least the potential for harm to occur. However, because in animals we do not have direct access via self-reports to the victim's mind, it is not currently possible to determine the full extent of harm to an animal that has been emotionally maltreated.

Actual or potential harm is not the only factor relevant to defining maltreatment. The *intent* of the caregiver plays a role in maltreatment; however, this role is not at all straightforward. Consider three instances of an animal being deprived of water to the point of dehydration and severe thirst. In the first instance, the water deprivation is done intentionally by a researcher studying the effects of thirst on sodium regulation in the kidneys. In the second instance, the thirst is induced by a pet's owner in the context of a water deprivation test to diagnose a medical disorder afflicting that pet. The third instance involves a sociopathic teenager who deprives the family pet of water because he enjoys seeing the animal suffer. The act is the same in each of the three cases; what differs is the intent of the act. If we label the researcher's actions acceptable, even laudable; the owner's actions proper and admirable; and the teenager's actions abusive, intent is the only reason for the difference in the labels. For animals, as for human infants, harm to the victim exists *from the perspective of the victim* and does not factor in the intent of the perpetrator. Regardless of the differences in caregivers' intentions, the victim's perspective is that any harm, injury, pain, morbidity, or mortality is the same (Ludwig 1992). In the example above, all three dogs suffer thirst; they are not aware of the intent. It is for this reason that the prevailing view holds that intent should not be considered when defining maltreatment in children (Ludwig 1992, Glaser 2000) and animals (Vermeulen & Odendaal 1993), and current definitions of child abuse and neglect are not predicated on the intention to harm the child. Applying this principle to animal care, maltreatment would be defined at least partially by the animal's harm or risk of harm, independent of the caregiver's intent. Although the definition of maltreatment does not incorporate caregiver intent, as we will see, intent is important in categorizing the acts of maltreatment as neglect or abuse.

Defining maltreatment runs into even more difficulties when the issue of quantification is considered. At what point, or quantity, does an act that is aversive to the animal become maltreatment? For example, crate training is a currently popular method of raising and training a dog. In units of time, where is the point at which confining a dog to a crate turns from an acceptable action to emotional neglect or abuse? One hour? Twelve hours? Three days? Six months?

In children, these quantification questions have been approached by specifically avoiding the drawing of clear-cut lines between acceptable and unacceptable parental actions. Recent definitions of childhood emotional abuse have conceptualized it as that of a continuum with the repetitive, sustained nature of the acts being a crucial defining feature (Kent & Waller 2000). Because single acts may cause harm, however, the definition of child maltreatment must include single events as well as patterns of behavior (Glaser 2000).

MALTREATMENT, NEGLECT, AND ABUSE

Because the terminology of maltreatment has rarely appeared in the context of animal care, no common terminology for animal neglect or abuse currently exists (Kowal 1998). Because the concept of maltreatment in animals appears to have extensive parallels with that in children, however, it is useful to draw from the terminology used for child maltreatment when developing definitions for use in animals. *Maltreatment* may be defined as actions or inactions that are neglectful, abusive, or otherwise threatening to an individual's welfare (US Department of Health, Education, and Welfare 1992). *Maltreatment* is commonly used as a collective term for its two constituent parts: neglect and abuse (US Department of Health, Education, and Welfare 1992).

Neglect is widely considered to be a passive process, or an act of omission, in which the basic needs—physical and emotional—of a dependent individual are not adequately met by the caregivers (Owen & Coant 1992, Oates 1996, Munro 1998). In child care, parents are considered to have responsibilities to their children; they must provide food, clothing, shelter, health care, education, a safe environment, along with love, affection, and emotional support (Owen & Coant 1992, Munro 1998). Neglect is distinguished by its lack of intent to harm the child; rather, acts of neglect result from a poor understanding or ignorance of the child's needs, a lack of motivation, or poor judgment (Owen & Coant 1992). In animals, it has been estimated that neglect accounts for 80 percent or more of instances of maltreatment (Hubrecht 1995; Patronek 1997, 1998). Needs, which constitute the basis for neglect, can be physical or emotional; hence, two types of neglect—physical and emotional—exist.

In contrast to the passive nature of neglect, *abuse* is a form of maltreatment that is an active process consisting of acts of aggression with intent to harm the victim. Abuse may include acts of commission or omission, but in both cases, the caregiver is conscious of the fact that the result will inflict harm. Like neglect, harm may be physical or emotional; therefore, abuse also exists in both forms.

Cruelty is an extensively used term in reference to animals—frequently in a legal context such as in state and local anti-cruelty statutes—and is often used interchangeably with animal abuse (Munro 1998). Kellert and Felthous (1985) defined animal cruelty as "the willful infliction of harm, injury, and intended pain on a nonhuman animal." Although definitions of abuse and cruelty overlap and resemble one another, several writers have suggested that cruelty implies an action more serious and more malicious than abuse (Trowbridge 1998). The

American Humane Association regards cruelty as much like abuse and uses the definition "knowingly, willfully, or negligently inflicting physical or emotional suffering on another living creature" (Jakober 2003).

EMOTIONAL MALTREATMENT

The most widely accepted classification of maltreatment in children identifies four major types: physical abuse, sexual abuse, neglect, and emotional abuse (Wolfe 1999). Similar categories have been proposed for use in animals (Vermeulen & Odendaal 1993, Ascione & Barnard 1998). In categorizing maltreatment in animals, because both neglect and abuse may be subdivided into physical and emotional components (Oates 1996, Wolfe 1999), it would seem most correct to use a modification of the human classification and subdivide animal maltreatment into four categories: physical abuse, physical neglect, emotional abuse, and emotional neglect (Table 12.1).

Like all maltreatment classification schemes developed to date, these four classes of maltreatment are not mutually exclusive. Considerable gray areas and overlap occur within and between the classes.

For children, no method for defining and subdividing emotional maltreatment has yet gained universal acceptance (Hobbs et al. 1993). The most widely utilized classification scheme is that developed by Garbarino et al. (1986) and amended by Pearl (1994). In their landmark 1986 book *The Psychologically Battered Child*, Garbarino *et al.* (who preferred the term psychological maltreatment over emotional maltreatment because they believed it incorporates both affective and cognitive aspects of maltreatment [Jellen et al. 2001], whereas others [Hobbs et al. 1993, Iwaniec 1995, Monteleone 1996] prefer the term emotional maltreatment) identified five forms of childhood psychological maltreatment: rejecting, terrorizing, isolating, corrupting, and ignoring. Garbarino (1993) described the forms accordingly:

Table 12.1. Classification of forms of maltreatment in animals.

	Neglect (passive)	Abuse (active)
Emotional	Inadequate provision of • Security • Control • Social companionship, love, and affection • Mental stimulation • Freedom of movement	• Rejecting • Terrorizing • Taunting • Isolating • Abandoning • Overpressuring
Physical	Inadequate provision of • Clean water • Proper quantities (neither too much nor too little) of complete and balanced nutrition • Shelter and protection from aversive environmental conditions • Health care • Sanitation and hygiene • Rest and sleep	• Assault • Burning • Poisoning • Shooting • Mutilating • Drowning • Suffocating • Abandoning • Excessively restricting movement; inadequate exercise • Transporting (unprotected, overloaded) • Overworking (excessive labor) • Fighting intentionally • Committing bestiality • Inflicting sexual-genital trauma

Note: many of these actions may be due to either neglect or abuse, depending on the intent of the caregiver. For instance, insufficient clean water would be an example of neglect if it was forgotten or if the caregiver did not know how much water to provide, whereas it would be abuse if the caregiver intentionally withheld water. The same would be true for social companionship, confinement, sleep, and the like.

rejecting involves actions that send messages of rejection to the child; *ignoring* is being psychologically unavailable to the child; *terrorizing* refers to behavior that uses intense fear as a weapon against the child (creating a climate of fear or unpredictable threat, hostility, and anxiety, thus preventing the child from gaining feelings of safety and security [Monteleone 1996, Hamarman & Bernet 2000]); *isolating* involves cutting the child off from normal social relationships; and *corrupting* is missocializing the child into self-destructive and antisocial patterns of behavior (teaching and encouraging destructive antisocial behavior, reinforcing deviance, and making the child unfit for normal social experiences [Hamarman & Bernet 2000]). Garbarino (1993) classifies emotional neglect as one type of emotional abuse. Although other investigators have classified and defined terms of emotional maltreatment differently, general agreement now exists that emotional maltreatment consists of two major types: active abuse and passive neglect (Owen & Coant 1992, Iwaniec 1995).

EMOTIONAL NEGLECT

THE ROLE OF EMOTIONAL NEEDS

Needs, both physical and emotional (incorporating psychological, social, and behavioral needs), are those factors required for normal function. Basic needs must be satisfied for an animal to maintain a state of physical and psychological homeostasis (Clark et al. 1997). Examples of physical needs include oxygen, water, balanced nutrition, shelter, health care, exercise, optimal temperature, and excretion of waste products. Examples of emotional needs identified in animals include social companionship, mental stimulation, and others to be discussed in the next section. Serpell (1996) has suggested that emotional needs, such as the need for social companionship, have acquired many of the properties of a physical need such as hunger and that satisfying these needs is required for a state of happiness and fulfillment.

In the course of evolution, needs and affect appear to have forged a critically important relationship. Evidence suggests that the brains of higher animals are constructed such that the animal is signaled, through unpleasant feelings, when it *needs* something, whether it be a physical factor such as water, salt, or warmth or an emotional factor such as social companionship. An *emotional need* may thus be defined as *any need that is signaled by an emotional affect.*

When a need is insufficiently satisfied, unpleasant affect will persist until the need is fulfilled (or the need otherwise abates). When one is motivated to lessen unpleasant affect but is unable or unsuccessful in achieving this goal, distress may result (Dawkins 1990). For example, if a social animal such as a dog were motivated by unpleasant loneliness-like feelings to seek companionship (a need) but was prevented from meeting the need because of solitary confinement in a backyard, then the unpleasant affect would persistently exert its effects. For this reason, any caregiver actions (or inactions) that impede the meeting of emotional needs would be harmful to animals.

EMOTIONAL NEGLECT

Neglect is defined as the failure to provide for a dependent individual's needs. Accordingly, emotional neglect refers to a failure to meet the emotional needs of the individual (child or animal) (Owen & Coant 1992, Iwaniec 1995, Wolfe 1999). Owen and Coant (1992) have described emotional neglect in children to be a lack of nurturing and psychological support for the child by the parent or primary caregiver, which results in a failure to meet the child's emotional needs and a state of emotional deprivation. They point out that although emotional neglect reflects a passive attitude on the part of the parent, the child is hurt because of inadequate provision for the emotional needs necessary for mental health and well-being.

Emotional needs are the foundation for emotional neglect; therefore, knowledge of the emotional needs of the individual is necessary to recognize and prevent emotional neglect. This is often a challenge in infants and toddlers but is a much more complex problem in animals. Children have differing needs at different ages, but examples of emotional needs common to all children include attention, affection and love, security and protection, new experiences, social companionship, acceptance, belongingness, praise, recognition, personal identity, and a positive self-image and self-esteem (Hobbs et al. 1993, Iwaniec 1995). Deprivation of any of these needs by a parent or caregiver's inactions constitutes emotional neglect.

Emotional needs in animals vary widely according to such factors as species, sex, age, and individual traits. However, a number of emotional needs have been widely accepted as being shared by most sentient animals, and include

- control (ability to exert meaningful change to situations, especially those of an unpleasant nature, in one's life) (Seligman 1975)

- abilities and resources to cope with aversive ("stressful") events (Wechsler 1995, Koolhaus et al. 1999)
- sufficient living space (Fox 1984)
- mental stimulation (Wemelsfelder 1990, this volume; Sackett 1991)
- safety, security, and protection from danger, such as hiding places (Hubrecht 1995, Bracke et al. 1999)
- social companionship (for social animals) (Serpell 1996; Dettmer & Fragaszy 2000; Van Loo et al. 2001; Panksepp, this volume)
- adequate predictability and stability to life events (Seligman 1975, Bracke et al. 1999)

Human influences often directly contribute to the creation of emotional needs, which may result in emotional neglect. Confinement of animals in man-made environments—such as zoological parks, farms, research laboratories, and even private homes—places animals in environments that often differ greatly from the one to which the animal evolved to be adapted. The positive consequence of this is that these environments often provide improved physical safety and disease control. The negative consequences are due to the fact that such environments frequently create emotional needs that in the natural setting can be easily fulfilled, such as social companionship and stimulating activities. Man-made environments frequently prevent or otherwise lack the resources necessary for the animal to fulfill these needs.

Other human influences on emotional needs may be less obvious yet exert powerful effects. One specific factor by which human intervention has contributed to the emotional pain of social separation is domestication of the dog. In this species, the enhanced emotional attachment of dogs to humans at least partially brought about by domestication has thereby also intensified an emotional need that now appears to be intensely unpleasant when unfulfilled (Panksepp 1998). In contrast to the frequently espoused view that dogs exhibit unconditional love (Masson 1997), I believe it is probably more accurate to say that dogs exhibit unconditional *need*. Because any factor that creates or intensifies emotional needs will ultimately play a role in emotional maltreatment, it is important to identify and attend to all such factors.

EMOTIONAL ABUSE

Emotional abuse has been described in children to differ from emotional neglect in that it is an active

process in which some deliberate action on the part of the parent is taken against the child (Oates 1996). Emotional abuse includes acts or omissions by the parents or caregivers that have caused or could cause serious behavioral, cognitive, emotional, or mental disorders (Wolfe 1999). This basic concept of emotional abuse in children is appropriate for use in animal care, and emotional abuse can be defined similarly in all sentient species (including human) as the deliberate infliction of emotional distress on another individual.

Kowal (1998) has pointed out that emotional abuse may not seem relevant to animals, because much of the child protection literature focuses on the damaged self-image and self-esteem of children whose parents or caregivers berate them, belittle them, call them derogatory names, and deny them love and affection. However, several categories of emotional abuse identified in children (Monteleone 1996) have direct application to animal care. Categories that have the greatest usefulness include *rejecting, terrorizing, taunting, isolating, abandonment*, and *overpressuring*. Whereas ignoring is a passive inattention to the individual's emotional needs and involves no intent of harm, *rejecting* is an active, purposeful denial of a child's or animal's emotional needs for which the resulting emotional deprivation is intended by the abuser. An example in animals would be the dog that is excessively confined to a small crate as punishment for a minor incident of undesired behavior such as whimpering for attention or getting hair all over the couch. *Terrorizing* refers to the creation of a "climate of fear" or unpredictable threat or hostility, preventing the victim from ever enjoying feelings of safety and security. Included in this category are the use of discipline and punishment that is inconsistent and capricious, extreme, or bizarre. An example of this type of abuse would be the use of harsh punishment in training (breaking) circus elephants to achieve control, domination, intimidation, and rule by fear (PRNewswire 2001). *Taunting* includes any teasing, provoking, or harassing that causes frustration, anger, or mental anguish. Examples include taunting a dog at the end of a tether or from behind another barrier such as a fence or cage bars. *Isolating* involves the active prevention of social interactions and companionship and is a source of emotional distress for social animals. *Abandonment* is the desertion and termination of care by the caregiver. This category of abuse overlaps with neglect because of the failure to meet the victim's needs; however, it is an active rather than passive behavior on the part of the caregiver. Examples include discarding a litter of kittens in a garbage dumpster, tossing a pet dog onto the roadside in the country to fend for itself, or moving out of an apartment and leaving a pet animal behind. *Overpressuring* in humans involves excessive demands and pressure placed on the child to perform or achieve. Examples in animals might include situations in which performance animals—such as race horses, circus animals, carriage and other horses used for labor, sled dogs, and marine mammals used in shows—are driven to perform in excess of their physical or mental capabilities.

PROPOSED DEFINITION OF EMOTIONAL MALTREATMENT

A definition of maltreatment, whether referring to physical or emotional forms, must meet certain criteria. It must specify, to the greatest extent that current knowledge permits, the central role of affect in the harmful effects, the issue of intent, criteria for differentiating lesser actions that do not rise to the level of maltreatment from actions that do, and exemption criteria for those actions that cause emotional harm but are intended to benefit the animal (such as eliciting fear in a cat by taking it to the veterinarian's office for medical care).

The following is a proposed definition of emotional maltreatment: *Actions (or inactions) of the animal caregiver or other person(s) which, intentionally or unintentionally, cause, perpetuate, or intensify emotional distress. Emotional distress is here defined as unpleasant emotional affect at a level that exceeds coping capacity. Such actions (or inactions), when intentional, are not maltreatment when a reasonable expectation exists that the ultimate outcome will be a meaningful net increase in that animal's overall (psychological and physical) well-being. Emotional maltreatment consists of two types: passive neglect and active abuse.*

EMOTIONAL MALTREATMENT AS THE CORE OF ALL MALTREATMENT

According to the above definition, emotional maltreatment occurs whenever any human action or inaction—emotional or physical in nature—heightens emotional distress. Physical abuse or neglect can therefore also be regarded as emotional maltreatment if it causes the victim to experience emotional distress.

This notion has been widely accepted in childhood maltreatment. For children, many researchers have recognized that all physical abuse and neglect has a psychological component (Jorgensen 1990, Hobbs et al. 1993, Monteleone 1996, Oates 1996, Wolfe 1999, Hamarman & Bernet 2000, Kent & Waller 2000, Jellen et al. 2001). No form of childhood maltreatment is believed to occur without coexisting fear, terror, anxiety, loneliness, hopelessness, helplessness, or other negative emotional state. Emotional maltreatment is considered part of or an inevitable consequence of all other kinds of abuse and neglect, and all maltreated children are regarded to be victims of emotional harm, the impact of which may persist long after the physical injuries have healed (Jorgensen 1990, Hobbs et al. 1993, Hamarman & Bernet 2000). Emotional maltreatment is widely considered the common factor underlying all other forms of maltreatment, and for this reason, emotional maltreatment is regarded as the core issue and major destructive force in the broader topic of child maltreatment (Monteleone 1996, Oates 1996, Jellen et al. 2001).

Ascione and Barnard (1998) have made the same observation for maltreatment in animals. They stated that an abused animal may also be considered emotionally maltreated.

THE HARMS OF EMOTIONAL MALTREATMENT

Physical maltreatment attracts far more attention, concern, and outrage than emotional maltreatment in both animals and children. This emotional response, or "gut reaction," is not necessarily supported by scientific data. To the contrary, substantial evidence now exists to support the notion that in both animals (Agrawal et al. 1967; Wolfle 1987, 1990) and children (Garbarino et al. 1986, O'Hagan 1993, Iwaniec 1995, Monteleone 1996, Oates 1996, Wolfe 1999, Jellen et al. 2001), the harm caused by emotional maltreatment is frequently *worse* than that from physical neglect and abuse. A growing consensus exists among childcare professionals that emotional maltreatment has the potential to harm the child in ways over and beyond the effects of physical injuries and is more damaging in the long term than other forms of abuse (O'Hagan 1993, Iwaniec 1995). In animals, some unpleasant emotional states appear to have a greater impact on animal well-being than physical pain (Wolfle 1987, 1990; McMillan 2002). For example, it has been proposed that for social animals such as dogs, withdrawal of social interaction is far more punishing than is physical abuse (Agrawal et al. 1967).

At present, identifying the harm of emotional maltreatment in an animal is very problematic.

First, because emotional maltreatment exists, to some degree, in all forms of maltreatment, the specific consequences attributable to emotional maltreatment are often hard to identify (Garbarino et al. 1986, Wolfe 1999). Second, the harm of emotional maltreatment is dependent on the coping ability of the individual. Oates (1996) mentions that when children fail to have their needs met, there is a variation in how children respond to such deprivations, leading to some children faring better than others. This is readily observed in animals as well. When dogs are separated from their owners and confined to cages (such as in a boarding facility), some dogs clearly cope better than others. Those who cope poorly (vocalize continuously, run in circles, chew at the bars on the cage, refuse to eat) presumably experience greater emotional harm than those that cope well (have calm, friendly demeanor; eat well). This variability in coping abilities renders any measurement technique for emotional harm in animals very elusive and difficult.

The harms of emotional maltreatment in children appear to bear considerable similarities with those in animals; however, extreme caution must be exercised in drawing analogies between children and animals. Much of the harm in children involves disturbances in development of a positive self-concept and self-esteem (Monteleone 1996, Jellen et al. 2001), and such complex cognitive concepts have not been demonstrated in animals. Many other relatively complex effects identified in children, however, appear possible and even likely in animals. These include impaired ability to learn, inability to build or maintain satisfactory social relationships, inappropriate behavior and feelings under normal circumstances (e.g., separation anxiety), a pervasive mood of unhappiness or depression, and a tendency to develop physical symptoms (Jellen et al. 2001).

It is well-recognized in children that the consequences of emotional maltreatment can be immediate and long-term (Hobbs et al. 1993, Monteleone 1996). Hobbs *et al.* (1993) point out that maltreated infants and children will suffer not only at the time but will also carry the long-term consequences with them into the future.

IMMEDIATE HARM

The most obvious immediate harm of emotional maltreatment in any sentient species is the emotional pain and discomfort of the unpleasant emotional states elicited by the maltreatment. Unpleasant emotions such as fear, anxiety, isolation and social deprivation, boredom, frustration, anger, helplessness, grief, and depression appear to be capable of causing distress and suffering of great intensity in animals (Panksepp 1998). Even in instances of emotional maltreatment that have no long-term consequences, the immediate distress warrants the most vigorous efforts directed at prevention and relief.

Another important immediate harm of emotional maltreatment is the adverse effects of unpleasant emotions ("stress") on physical health. Research spanning much of the past century has demonstrated convincingly that the mental states of animals—emotional and cognitive—are inseparable from their somatic aspects (Riley 1981, McMillan 1999). Mental states interact continuously with bodily states, and emotions appear to have an influence on all disease processes (Ader 1980, Gallon 1982). Acute emotional events can be severe enough to cause death (Riley 1981).

LONG-TERM HARM

The evidence for the long-term consequences of emotional maltreatment in animals is less clear than that for the immediate consequences. Long-term harm has not been as well studied in animals as in people, not only because the effects are often difficult to recognize, but also because of the unknown history of many animals. Unlike the situation in people, one cannot ask a mature animal with an unknown background what happened to it at an earlier age. As a result, it has become common for pet owners, as well as veterinarians and clinical behaviorists (Dodman 1997, Overall 1997), to assume earlier abuse when an animal shows certain signs such as an inordinate fear of humans.

When emotional maltreatment occurs during the individual's formative stages of life, healthy brain development is impaired, which leads to numerous emotional problems throughout life. Research has consistently shown that children who are emotionally neglected experience persistent feelings of resentment and emotional distress and may be psychologically scarred for life (Bremner et al. 1995, Bugental et al. 2003). Agrawal *et al.* (1967) found that when puppies are socially isolated from 3 days to 20 weeks of age, regardless of having their physiologic needs met, they are emotionally disturbed for life. In rodent and nonhuman primates, maternal deprivation during infancy is associated with increased stress reactivity, greater vulnerability to stress-induced illness, and more-intense fear and startle responses in novelty tests (Charmandari et al. 2003). Dozens of studies examining the effects of social deprivation in chimpanzees indicate that the resulting damage can be permanent.

Serpell and Jagoe (1995) noted that long periods of daily social isolation or abandonment by the owner appear to intensify some dogs' attachments for their owners and may lead to separation-related emotional distress problems in adulthood. These findings in dogs coincide with a well-recognized effect of emotional maltreatment in young children. Iwaniec (1995) has noted that a rejected child is likely to be more dependent; more clinging; more intensely possessive; and more seeking of parental nurturance, attention, and physical contact than the accepted child. She goes further to state that if a child's caregivers are rejecting and if the child's needs for warmth and affection are unfulfilled, the child will increase its efforts to attract love and attention, becoming hyperdependent. It is striking how nearly exact language has been used to describe shelter and abandoned dogs. For example, several investigators have noted that rescued, shelter-obtained, re-homed, and abandoned dogs have a significantly higher risk for separation anxiety than dogs coming from more stable environments (e.g., breeders, family or friends) or living in stable homes (Flannigan & Dodman 2001, Overall et al. 2001).

It is not only during infancy when emotional maltreatment may inflict long-term harm. Several investigators have reported that psychological trauma in dogs of any age may cause manifestations of severe mental disorders and maladaptive behavior that endure for a lifetime (Serpell & Jagoe 1995, Overall 1997, Thompson 1998). Animals have demonstrated many of the signs of post-traumatic stress syndrome, a well-studied consequence of severe emotional trauma in humans (Thompson 1998).

PREVENTING EMOTIONAL MALTREATMENT

Addressing maltreatment after it has occurred is quite obviously not the optimal strategy for protecting animals. Clearly, the ideal goal is prevention. After several decades of research, parental education, and criminal prosecution of abusers, emotional maltreatment in children still occurs in extremely high numbers. It is therefore very naïve to believe that emotional maltreatment of animals will be eliminated any time soon. However, some important first steps will help us get started.

The first and most important step is research in the field of animal emotions. Without a thorough understanding of the unpleasant emotions and emotional needs of animals, we can make little progress in identifying and preventing emotional maltreatment. Much study is also needed in identifying the signs of emotional maltreatment, which would, at the minimum, entail study of the behavior of animals with documented histories of emotional neglect and abuse.

Education of the public is a critical step in the prevention of emotional maltreatment. Aware that most of the emotional neglect in children is a result not of malice but of an inadequate understanding of the child's emotional needs, child protection workers have focused on educating the well-meaning parents to make the home more nurturing and emotionally fulfilling for the child. In animal care, several writers (Vermeulen & Odendaal 1993, Patronek 1997, Kowal 1998) have expressed similar ideas with regard to physical maltreatment. For example, Patronek (1997) has written that there is ample anecdotal evidence that the overwhelming majority of animal maltreatment involves neglect rather than an intent to harm. Butler et al. (1998) stated that animal control officers have reported that although some harmful actions are done intentionally, most maltreatment stems from high levels of frustration, a lack of resources, and insufficient knowledge about the animals' needs and about responsible ways to care for animals.

For public education to be effective, it is first essential that veterinarians, animal control officers, and humane workers be well educated about emotional maltreatment. Counseling on proper animal care is only possible if the animal care professional is knowledgeable in all aspects of care, including emotional needs and sufferings. The training of humane workers and animal shelter personnel would then be used in the screening process for prospective animal adopters. During the screening, questions regarding a potential adopter's ability to meet the animal's emotional needs should carry equal weight as the standard questions about meeting the animal's physical needs of nutrition, water, shelter, and health care.

An effective prevention program must include enactment and strong enforcement of humane laws that recognize and clearly define emotional maltreatment. Current state cruelty statutes need to be amended to include *emotional* injury, pain, suffering, and trauma. In addition, progress in child protective services demonstrates the benefits of mandated reporting of all forms of maltreatment. Ascione and Barnard (1998) have pointed out that the advent of definitions and mandated reporting statutes for child neglect and abuse resulted in substantial strengthening of the response to cases of child maltreatment. They proposed that taking the same steps in the recognition and reporting of animal maltreatment would similarly strengthen the response to animal maltreatment. Cappucci and Gbadamosi (1998) suggested the possibility that someday, mandated training of veterinary medical students and graduate veterinarians on identification and reporting of animal abuse and cruelty may be required as a prerequisite for licensure, just as the state of New York mandates training on recognizing and reporting child abuse for licensure of physicians, psychologists, psychiatrists, nurses, teachers, and other professionals (Cappucci & Gbadamosi 1998).

FINAL COMMENTS

From an ethical and scientific standpoint, the rationale and principles for managing pain are essentially the same for physical and emotional pain. Unpleasant emotions harm the animal by way of the distress and suffering they cause and by the adverse health effects with which they are associated. It is reasonable to believe that the animal experiencing unpleasant feelings does not care about the source of the discomfort—whether it has an emotional or physical origin—that the animal only desires to be rid of the unpleasantness. This applies to all aspects of the animal's life, but particularly to the distress and suffering caused by neglect and abuse.

It is probable that many of the behavioral problems presented to veterinarians, behaviorists, and trainers are caused, at least in part, by emotional maltreatment. It is also possible that many somatic health disorders seen in veterinary medical practice are associated with emotional maltreatment (McMillan 1999, Buffington 2002). If this proves to be the case, then emotional maltreatment will assume a heretofore unrecognized prominence in veterinary care.

Animal abuse and undesirable behavior may have an especially detrimental relationship. It has been said that undesirable pet behavior is the most likely cause of animal abuse (Tripp 2001). Conversely, emotional neglect and abuse can cause abnormal and undesired behaviors such as fear aggression, anxiety-induced inappropriate urination, excessive vocalizing, and self-injurious behaviors (Dodman 1997, Overall 1997). This sets up a highly destructive vicious cycle in which undesired behaviors may lead to rejection, resentment, and loss of affection by the pet owner (i.e., emotional neglect), which then exacerbates the undesired behavior, which then causes more resentment and rejection, and on and on. More tragic is when abnormal behavior cycles with abuse. In these cases, the undesired behavior elicits yelling, social deprivation through banishment to outdoors, or the threat of abuse as punishment for the behavior, which then may perpetuate or worsen the behavior. One example is the cat with anxiety-induced inappropriate urination in a multi-cat household to which the owners respond with yelling and threatening, which creates a heightened climate of fear, causing the cat to urinate even more around the house, which leads to more yelling, and so on. In such cases, the animal may ultimately be relinquished to the local animal shelter or face euthanasia. Only an understanding of the emotional needs of animals and the motivations for the undesired behaviors can avert these heartbreaking situations.

Certainly one of the largest impediments to moving forward in our efforts to tend to emotional maltreatment is the difficulties inherent in recognizing emotional maltreatment when it occurs and discerning the signs of emotional harm; however, the same problem plagued the early efforts in the field of childhood emotional maltreatment. Ludwig (1992) commented that the difficulties in defining maltreatment are not a reason to shrink from the duty to protect children. He further noted that definitions may vary between individuals and change over time, commenting that, "Child abuse as a concept has evolved over time and will continue to evolve. What was considered to be normal child care practice 50 years ago may now seem abusive. The way our children are treated today may be viewed as abusive by future generations" (Ludwig 1992). The same can be said about animal maltreatment. Disciplinary practices viewed as acceptable in the past, such as beating horses and shoving dogs' faces in feces, have changed over time and are now widely considered to be unacceptable.

With his colleagues, Cornell University's James Garbarino (1986), perhaps the most widely recognized researcher on childhood emotional maltreatment, aptly stated, "rather than casting psychological maltreatment as an ancillary issue, subordinate to other forms of abuse and neglect, we should place it as the centerpiece of efforts to understand family functioning and to protect children." Protecting animals would involve nothing less.

REFERENCES

Ader R. 1980. Psychosomatic and psychoimmuno-logic research. *Psychosom Med* 42:307–321.

Agrawal HC, Fox MW, Himwich WA. 1967. Neurochemical and behavioral effects of isolation-rearing in the dog. *Life Sci* 6:71–78.

Animal Protection Institute. 2001. State animal cruelty laws. Accessed 8/24/01 from http://www.api4animals.org

Ascione FR, Barnard S. 1998. The link between animal abuse and violence to humans: Why veterinarians should care. In: *Recognizing and reporting animal abuse: A veterinarian's guide*. Denver, CO, American Humane Association:4–10.

Bracke MBM, Spruijt BM, Metz JHM. 1999. Overall animal welfare reviewed. Part 3: Welfare assessment based on needs and supported by expert opinion. *Neth J Agr Sci* 47:307–322.

Bremner JD, Randall P, Scott TM, et al. 1995. Deficits in short-term memory in adult survivors of childhood abuse. *Psychiat Res* 59:97–107.

Buffington CAT. 2002. External and internal influences on disease risk in cats. *J Am Vet Med Assoc* 220:994–1002.

Bugental DB, Martorell GA, Barraza V. 2003. The hormonal costs of subtle forms of infant maltreatment. *Horm Behav* 43:237–244.

Butler C, Lagoni L, Olson P. 1998. Reporting animal cruelty. In: *Recognizing and reporting animal abuse: A veterinarian's guide*. Denver, CO, American Humane Association:50–54.

Cappucci DT, Gbadamosi SG. 1998. Prevention of animal abuse: Reflections on a public health malady. In: *Recognizing and reporting animal abuse: A veterinarian's guide*. Denver, CO, American Humane Association:11–19.

Charmandari E, Kino T, Souvatzoglou E, et al. 2003. Pediatric stress: Hormonal mediators and human development. *Horm Res* 59:161–179.

Clark JD, Rager DR, Calpin JP. 1997. Animal well-being I. General considerations. *Lab Anim Sci* 47:564–570.

Dawkins MS. 1990. From an animal's point of view: Motivation, fitness, and animal welfare. *Behav Brain Sci* 13:1–61.

Dettmer E, Fragaszy D. 2000. Determining the value of social companionship to captive tufted capuchin monkeys (*Cebus apella*). *J Appl Anim Welf Sci* 3:293–304.

Dodman N. 1997. *The cat who cried for help: Attitudes, emotions, and the psychology of cats*. New York: Bantam Books.

Flannigan G, Dodman NH. 2001. Risk factors and behaviors associated with separation anxiety in dogs. *J Am Vet Med Assoc* 219:460–466.

Fox MW. 1984. *Farm animals: Husbandry, behavior, and veterinary practice*. Baltimore: University Park Press.

Gallon RL. 1982. *The psychosomatic approach to illness*. New York: Elsevier Biomedical.

Garbarino J. 1993. Psychological child maltreatment. A developmental view. *Primary Care* 20:307–315.

Garbarino J, Guttman E, Seeley JW. 1986. *The psychologically battered child: Strategies for identification, assessment, and intervention*. San Francisco: Jossey-Bass.

Glaser D. 2000. Child abuse and neglect and the brain—a review. *J Child Psychol Psyc* 41:97–116.

Hamarman S, Bernet W. 2000. Evaluating and reporting emotional abuse in children: Parent-based, action-based focus aids in clinical decision-making. *J Am Acad Child Psy* 39:928–930.

Hobbs CJ, Hanks HGI, Wynne JM. 1993. *Child abuse and neglect—A clinician's handbook*. Edinburgh: Churchill Livingstone.

Hubrecht R. 1995. The welfare of dogs in human care. In: Serpell J (ed), *The domestic dog: Its evolution, behaviour and interactions with people*. Cambridge, UK, Cambridge University Press:179–198.

Iwaniec D. 1995. *The emotionally abused and neglected child—Identification, assessment and intervention*. Chichester, UK: John Wiley & Sons.

Jakober A. 2003. Personal communication. American Humane Association.

Jellen LK, McCarroll JE, Thayer LE. 2001. Child emotional maltreatment: A 2-year study of US Army cases. *Child Abuse Neglect* 25:623–639.

Jorgensen EC. 1990. Child abuse—A practical guide for those who help others. New York: Continuum.

Kellert S, Felthous A. 1985. Childhood cruelty towards animals among criminals and noncriminals. Hum Relat 38:1113–1129.

Kempe CH, Silverman FN, Steele BF, et al. 1962. The battered child syndrome. J Amer Med Assoc 181:17–24.

Kent A, Waller G. 2000. Childhood emotional abuse and eating psychopathology. Clin Psychol Rev 20:887–903.

Koolhaus JM, Korte SM, DeBoer SF, et al. 1999. Coping styles in animals: Current status in behavior and stress-physiology. Neurosci Biobehav R 23:925–935.

Kowal LW. 1998. Recognizing animal abuse: What veterinarians can learn from the field of child abuse and neglect. In: Recognizing and reporting animal abuse: A veterinarian's guide. Denver, CO, American Humane Association:40–49.

Lacroix CA, Wilson JF. 1998. State animal anti-cruelty laws. In: Recognizing and reporting animal abuse: A veterinarian's guide. Denver, CO, American Humane Association:20–24.

Lazarus RS. 1999. Stress and emotion. New York: Springer.

Leonard EA. 2000. Signs and symptoms of animal abuse. Proceedings of the American Veterinary Medical Association Annual Convention, Salt Lake City.

Ludwig S. 1992. Defining child abuse: Clinical mandate—evolving concepts. In: Ludwig S, Kornberg AE (eds), *Child abuse: A medical reference*, 2nd ed. New York, Churchill Livingstone:1–12.

Masson JM. 1997. *Dogs never lie about love*. New York: Crown.

McMillan FD. 1999. Influence of mental states on somatic health in animals. *J Am Vet Med Assoc* 214:1221–1225.

McMillan FD. 2002. Emotional pain management. *Vet Med* 97:822–834.

McMillan FD. 2003. A world of hurts—Is pain special? *J Am Vet Med Assoc* 223:183–186.

Monteleone JA. 1996. *Recognition of child abuse for the mandated reporter*, 2nd ed. St. Louis, MO: G.W. Medical Publishing.

Munro HMC. 1998. The battered pet syndrome. In: *Recognizing and reporting animal abuse: A veterinarian's guide*. Denver, CO, American Humane Association:76–81.

Oates RK. 1996. The spectrum of child abuse—Assessment, treatment, and prevention. New York: Brunner/Mazel.

O'Hagan KP. 1993. Emotional and psychological abuse of children. Buckingham, UK: Open University Press.

Overall KL. 1997. Clinical behavioral medicine for small animals. St. Louis, MO: Mosby.

Overall KL, Dunham AE, Frank D. 2001. Frequency of nonspecific clinical signs in dogs with separation anxiety, thunderstorm phobia, and noise phobia, alone or in combination. J Am Vet Med Assoc 219:467–473.

Owen M, Coant P. 1992. Other forms of neglect. In: Ludwig S, Kornberg AE (eds), Child abuse: A medical reference, 2nd ed. New York, Churchill Livingstone:349–355.

Panksepp J. 1998. Affective neuroscience: The foundations of human and animal emotions. New York: Oxford University Press.

Patronek GJ. 1997. Animal cruelty, abuse and neglect: Issues for veterinarians. Proceedings of the American Animal Hospital Association Annual Meeting, San Diego, CA:375–379.

Patronek GJ. 1998. Issues and guidelines for veterinarians in recognizing, reporting, and assessing

animal neglect and abuse. In: *Recognizing and reporting animal abuse: A veterinarian's guide*. Denver, CO, American Humane Association:25–39.

Pearl P. 1994. Emotional abuse. In: Brodeur AE, Monteleone JA (eds), *Child maltreatment: A clinical guide and reference*. St. Louis, MO: GW Medical Publishing:37–51.

PRNewswire. 2001. ASPCA learns Mark Oliver Gebel cited for elephant abuse. Accessed 9/19/01 from www.prnewswire.com

Riley V. 1981. Psychoneuroendocrine influences on immunocompetence and neoplasia. *Science* 212:1100–1109.

Sackett GP. 1991. The human model of psychological well-being in primates. In: Novak MA, Petto AJ (eds), *Through the looking glass: Issues of psychological well-being in captive nonhuman primates*. Washington, DC, American Psychological Association:35–42.

Seligman ME. 1975. *Helplessness: On depression, development, and death*. San Francisco: W.H. Freeman.

Serpell J. 1996. *In the company of animals*. Cambridge, UK: Cambridge University Press.

Serpell J, Jagoe JA. 1995. Early experience and the development of behaviour. In: Serpell J (ed), *The domestic dog: Its evolution, behaviour and interactions with people*. Cambridge, UK, Cambridge University Press:79–102.

Sinclair LR. 2000. Signs and symptoms of animal neglect. Proceedings of the American Veterinary Medical Association Annual Convention. Salt Lake City, UT.

Thompson SB. 1998. Pharmacologic treatment of phobias. In: Dodman NH, Shuster L (eds), *Psychopharmacology of animal behavior disorders*. Malden, MA, Blackwell Science:141–182.

Tripp R. 2001. Behavior techniques can prevent canine death, abuse. *DVM Newsmagazine Practice Builder* Sept:28–31.

Trowbridge D. 1998. Definitions for animal cruelty laws. In: *Recognizing and reporting animal abuse: A veterinarian's guide*. Denver, CO, American Humane Association:1–3.

US Department of Health, Education, and Welfare. 1992. Interdisciplinary glossary on child and neglect. In: Ludwig S, Kornberg AE (eds), *Child abuse: A medical reference*, 2nd ed. New York, Churchill Livingstone:479–484

Van Loo PLP, de Groot AC, Van Zutphen BFM, et al. 2001. Do male mice prefer or avoid each other's company? Influence of hierarchy, kinship, and familiarity. *J Appl Anim Welf Sci* 4:91–103.

Vermeulen H, Odendaal JSJ. 1993. Proposed typology of companion animal abuse. *Anthrozoos* 6:248–257.

Wechsler B. 1995. Coping and coping strategies: A behavioural view. *Appl Anim Behav Sci* 43:123–134.

Wemelsfelder F. 1990. Boredom and laboratory animal welfare. In: Rollin BE, Kesel ML (eds), *The experimental animal in biomedical research*. Boca Raton, FL, CRC Press:243–272.

Wolfe DA. 1999. *Child abuse—Implications for child development and psychopathology*. Thousand Oaks, CA: SAGE.

Wolfe TL. 1987. Control of stress using non-drug approaches. *J Am Vet Med Assoc* 191:1219–1221.

Wolfe TL. 1990. Policy, program, and people: The three P's to well-being. In: Mench JA, Krulisch L (eds), *Canine research environment*. Bethesda, MD, Scientists' Center for Animal Welfare:41–47.

Part III
Mental Wellness

13
The Concept of Quality of Life in Animals

Franklin D. McMillan

THE CHALLENGES OF QUALITY OF LIFE

Everyone knows what quality of life is. If one asks a pet owner to evaluate their animal's quality of life, he or she will invariably undertake the task with no question as to what they are supposed to be evaluating. They just *know*. Ask any veterinarian to evaluate a patient's quality of life, and he or she feels no need to ponder what he or she is looking for. They, too, just know. When we see a photo of Elizabeth Taylor petting the immaculately groomed silver Persian cat on her lap while the cat is eating caviar out of a crystal goblet, our thinking is automatic—this kitty has the consummate quality of life. When we read of the sad death of the majestic 550-pound silverback gorilla that had been captured and taken from the wild at two years of age and spent the remaining 38 years of his life alone in a small, barren cement-and-bar enclosure in a decrepit zoo in Afghanistan, we do not question that the gorilla had a very poor quality of life. When a drug company claims that its new drug improves the quality of life of dogs with heart failure, we know exactly what it means. And if you were visiting a friend's house and her dog said to you, "You've got to help me—I've got a terrible quality of life," you'd know exactly what he meant.

Or would you? He looks very healthy, so it couldn't have the same meaning as the quality of life that the drug company is referring to regarding their new product. He's got a great house and yard, so it couldn't have the same meaning as the gorilla's quality of life. Would his terrible quality of life mean that his life is the *opposite* of that of Liz Taylor's cat? And what would *that* mean? And if he couldn't talk, how would you even know that his quality of life was so poor? Is it possible, you ask yourself, that you, along with every other visitor your friend has had over, have been walking into and out of her house without ever knowing that her dog was living in misery?

There is a strong intuitive sense as to what quality of life (QOL) means as well as the feeling that it carries immense importance in the care of animals. Yet our sense of familiarity with the term belies its true elusive nature. Quality of life, like happiness, currently defies precise description (see McMillan, this volume, Chapter 16). This is not a problem confined to animals; QOL in humans, even when people can provide detailed self-evaluations, remains confounding and controversial. This is because QOL is a personal, private, subjective experience that has no "normal," "average," or any other frame of reference, lacks any units of measurement, and means different things to different people. Even so much as one contributing factor to QOL—such as anxiety or physical pain—is extremely hard to measure, making the much more complex mental experience of QOL seem almost incomprehensibly difficult to quantify. Quality of life is incredibly simple yet profoundly complex, constantly changing and adapting throughout life yet very consistent and seemingly fixed and nearly immutable, and lends itself to one word assessments (e.g., "excellent," or "poor") yet escapes accurate measurement with even the most exhaustively comprehensive questionnaires and interviews. It is little wonder why QOL presents such a challenge to understand. Yet, in spite of these obstacles, the extreme importance of QOL in the lives of all sentient animals makes it imperative that we work to move beyond "gut-level" and intuitive assessments of QOL.

Although QOL has become strongly associated with health care, the term had its origins as a descriptor for the conditions for a good life in human society (Musschenga 1997). With the diagnostic and therapeutic advances in modern medicine, it became clear that health and disease played a prominent role in individual and societal QOL. The term therefore became useful in examining the quality and delivery of health care, and over the past three decades of the twentieth century, QOL made a gradual transition from its collective economic and societal meaning to represent the individual's view of his or her life. Its heavy usage in medical care often made QOL seem to be a synonym for health status, but a broad consensus now exists that QOL is influenced by a multitude of factors including, but not at all limited to, health status. In its applications to animal care, this means that QOL involves all facets of an animal's life and that efforts to maximize QOL must attend to all relevant life events and circumstances.

Interestingly, the successes of modern medicine are the main reasons why the medical profession has embraced and extensively utilized the concept of QOL. The remarkable medical advances of the past half century have steadily improved the ability of medicine to increase the patients' *quantity* of life. Unfortunately, this led to the emergence of a steadily growing gap between what *can* be achieved and what *should* be achieved from the patient's perspective. With the advancing technology, the promise of medicine to protect and preserve life came to acquire the more negative connotation of *prolonging* life. With these remarkable new abilities to keep people alive, it became increasingly clear that doing everything science had to offer to prevent death was not always in the individual's best interest (Treurniet et al. 1997) and that a new measure for success of health care was needed. Quality of life came to fill that need. Quality of life was adopted to serve as the more appropriate objective for health care decisions (Pal 1996). Quality of life has become a useful means of assuring that the perspective of the patient—rather than the cold statistics of morbidity and mortality—remains the focus of modern medicine.

Over the past 30 years, a robust study and analysis has been made of the concept of QOL in the fields of human medicine and psychology. In contrast, QOL received no attention in animals until 2000 (McMillan 2000). Promisingly, in the past four years, a budding interest in animal QOL has emerged, as evidenced by an abstract on QOL in heart patients presented by Freeman et al. (2003) at the 2003 Forum of the American College of Veterinary Internal Medicine, a one-day seminar organized by the British Veterinary Association (BVA) Animal Welfare Foundation and the BVA Ethics Committee held in London in June 2003 (Anonymous 2003), a series of one-day seminars on QOL throughout 2004 sponsored by Boehringer Ingelheim and Hill's Canada, and a recent journal report (Yazbek & Fantoni 2004). This relative dearth of interest in animal QOL does not mean that the related concepts of psychological well-being and welfare have been ignored. On the contrary, the past two decades have seen a rapidly growing body of literature on these issues of mental well-being in animals. Because all of these concepts are not clearly distinguishable from one another, it may turn out that animal QOL has actually been receiving a great deal of attention but under a different name.

Many difficulties impede the understanding of QOL. Consider, for example, the situation in children with severe mental disabilities. Many health professionals who work with these children have approached their work with a presumption that these children have a diminished QOL and that an important focus of the care of these children should be on increasing their QOL (Hatton 1998). Other investigators, however, have challenged this basic premise, questioning the presumption of a diminished QOL. How would we know? Does raising their QOL mean trying to give them what "normal" people have? How do we know they would want this? And how do we know that giving them this would increase their QOL?

We must ask similar questions about animals. For obvious reasons, much of what an animal thinks, feels, and desires is unknowable to us. We have to be very careful not to bring a possibly misguided presumption to the table when we explore QOL in animals. We must not, in other words, presume that animals want to be human beings or that making them more human or giving them more of what humans want is sure to elevate their QOL.

To set the stage for our look at QOL in animals, I must make two points at the outset:

- QOL is, as the name implies, about *life*. It is not restricted to what kind of housing the animal has, the type of food he gets, the luxuriousness of her bed, the number of walks he gets per day, what size of yard she has to play in, whether he goes to doggie day care or stays home alone all day, or whether she has animal companions to play with. And most important, it is not restricted to—or equivalent to—his health status. QOL is a compilation of all of these factors and more, *and* of the animal's reaction to and feelings about them.

- The goal of improving an animal's QOL involves attention to all aspects of life that can lessen QOL. For many animals—specifically those that are in good physical health—such efforts may not involve health issues at all.

WHAT IS QUALITY OF LIFE?

Quality of life in humans refers to how an individual feels about how his or her life is faring. In a simplified, though accurate, view, QOL may be regarded as one's general enjoyment of life overall. The potential benefits of QOL assessments are well accepted, yet no consensus has been achieved as to its definition or influential factors (Glaser & Walker 1995). Like "happiness," it is a concept that feels understood but is exceptionally difficult to describe in precise terms (Slevin 1992). In the human field, numerous models of QOL have been proposed, most approaching QOL in terms of its component parts rather than as a single, unified concept (Hunt 1997). Quality of life is closely related, and may be equivalent, to a number of other concepts of subjective life experience such as *well-being* (often specified as subjective, emotional, psychological, or mental well-being), *welfare, happiness, life satisfaction,* and *contentment* (Novak & Suomi 1988; DeGrazia 1996; Clark et al. 1997a; Hetts et al., this volume; McMillan, this volume, Chapter 16). In everyday discourse, *emotional fulfillment* and *peace of mind* refer to similar phenomena as QOL.

It is well accepted that QOL, as currently understood, refers to a state of mind: It is a conscious subjective mental experience. Hence, QOL requires a state of consciousness. Beings that are not conscious, such as (presumably) animals with no central nervous systems, may have a quality *to* their lives (such as being healthy or diseased, living where food is plentiful or scarce, or being comforted or "picked on" by conspecifics) but would lack the capacity for the *experience* we are calling QOL. In addition, individuals that are in a comatose state, in some forms of deep sleep, or under general anesthesia, would not have the experience of QOL

while unconscious (although what occurs to and around them during the unconscious state certainly could impact their QOL if and when they regain consciousness).

In humans, QOL is considered strictly a view from within; it is not an external evaluation of how others judge a person's life but how that person feels about the circumstances and events making up his or her own life and what they mean to that person, and that person alone. This quality of QOL has led to the general consensus that QOL should be assessed from the perspective of the individual, with that individual utilizing his or her own values (Osoba 1994).

Another feature of QOL is that it is very individualized, based on each person's or animal's unique genetic make-up, personality, and learned experiences. In people, one's QOL is largely determined by the individual's past experiences and by the values and meaning that the person attaches to those experiences (Stewart et al. 1999). Individual preferences, desires, and needs lead each individual—animal or human—to assign different values to the vast array of events and conditions in his or her life. For example, one person may value family relationships over his career, whereas another person may value the same things oppositely. A good illustration in animals is the value of human companionship in dogs. If deprived of human interaction and companionship, one dog may be unaffected, whereas another dog may be emotionally debilitated. Pain tolerance, fear of strangers, enjoyment of certain toys or games, interest in exercise, desire to be outside, preferences in foods and treats, propensity to anxiety in strange places, and social affiliations with other animals are just a few of the qualities and traits of animals that, by differing among individuals, cause each animal to assign different values to various facets of life. Accordingly, the components of QOL will carry different weights for each animal. The experience of QOL is dependent on what *matters* to the individual animal, and what matters varies greatly among individuals.

All interpretations view QOL as a continuum, ranging from very high (good) to very low (bad). Because such determinations are subjective and vary not only between individuals but also in the same individual over time and under different circumstances, there are no clear-cut demarcations or recognizable cutoff points on the continuum, for example, above which QOL is "satisfactory," "acceptable," "reasonable," or "good," or below which QOL is "unacceptable."

An important point that must be kept in mind whenever we apply any of the concepts developed for human QOL to animals is that human QOL and animal QOL may differ, possibly substantially. Although it appears that the foundational structure of QOL—a general sense of how one's overall life is faring—is very similar between humans and animals, animal QOL is not likely as complex and may not involve as many contributing factors as human QOL. For example, a dog doesn't appear to set and pursue life goals that can be achieved or denied, fret about how his loved ones will support themselves if he were to die, worry about the fate of humankind and the world in the face of global terrorism, or find fulfillment in religion. Utilizing these ideas and the following discussion, I will offer a proposal for the definition of QOL later in the chapter.

THE PRIMACY OF AFFECT

If we accept that QOL involves all aspects of the individual's life, we still face the questions of *which* aspects, and *how* do these aspects of life manifest their influences on QOL? Most importantly, what raises QOL, and what lowers it? What specific factors affect QOL, and what factors do not?

Consider the latter question. How does one decide whether something affects an animal's QOL? Imagine that you are given a list of factors in your pet dog's life and you are asked to place each factor in one of two columns: Has an effect on QOL and Does not have an effect on QOL. You are given such factors as: painted toenails, very tasty food and treats, a loving and caring human family, a scar on his face, diamond studs in her collar, lots of play and trips to the dog park, partial loss of vision in one eye, being left at home alone for 14 hours every day and all weekends, having her white doghouse painted light blue, having been born with the outside toe missing on his left front foot, having prosthetic testicles implanted after being neutered, being physically abused, living in a city that doesn't have a Starbucks, being shuffled from one foster home to another every few months, having severe osteoarthritis, having a small lipoma on her abdomen, having epilepsy, living her entire life in a tiny dirty cage having litter after litter in a puppy mill, being a quadriplegic, and being the descendant of a line of best-in-show grand champions. As you place each factor into one column or the other, you are obviously using some criterion to decide into which column to place each one. Some distinguishing factor clearly separates the items in the "Has an

effect" column from those in the "Does not have an effect" column. What *is* that factor?

For all the complexity of QOL and the myriad factors that contribute to it, the answer is surprisingly simple: It *matters* to the animal. The items you placed on the "Has an effect on QOL" list all have that factor in common. The "Has an effect" list could be retitled "Matters to the animal." Likewise, the "Does not have an effect on QOL" could be retitled "Does not matter to the animal." If we accept the reasoning that QOL can only be affected by things that matter to the individual, we then must ask: What matters, and how can we tell?

Animals—human and, presumably, nonhuman—seem to feel some affect (feelings) during virtually all of their waking lives. All affect appears to have a hedonic valence; that is, a pleasant or unpleasant experiential quality is associated with each feeling. Hence it appears that affect contributes pleasantness or unpleasantness continually to personal experience (Diener & Larsen 1993). It follows, then, that a definition of quality of life will include emotional pleasantness, specifically, the intensities of the affect and the relative times experiencing pleasant and unpleasant affect in one's life over time.

Feelings have physical or emotional origins. *Pleasant affect* includes the positive emotions of social interaction and companionship, joy (such as experienced during play), mental stimulation, and the physical origin pleasures such as tasty foods, physical touch, and sexual activity. *Unpleasant affect* of physical origin includes hypercapnea, thirst, hunger, nausea, full urinary bladder, bloatedness, extremely bright lights, pruritus, temperature extremes, pain, and many others. Emotional origins of unpleasant affect include fear, anxiety, isolation distress, separation anxiety, grief, frustration, boredom, helplessness, and anger.

Feelings appear to have evolved to serve as a mechanism that equips the brain to encode value to the vast array of external and internal stimuli constantly inundating the nervous system. Stimuli that have value, or are relevant, for survival and reproduction elicit feelings. In general, stimuli that are beneficial to well-being elicit pleasurable affect, while those that are threatening or detrimental to well-being elicit unpleasant affect (Panksepp 1998). In general, the intensity of the affect appears to be proportional to the degree of importance and urgency of the stimulus. In this view, feelings evolved to represent those things that *matter* to the animal. The *way* these things matter is related to their effects on success in natural selection: reproductive fitness (i.e., survival and reproduction). Feelings, then, signal to the animal that certain stimuli or events—external, such as an approaching predator, or internal, such as a full bladder—are important to pay attention to in order to increase one's chances for successful survival and reproduction. The *intensity* of the feeling appears to represent how *much* those things matter to the animal. In this sense, feelings are the rough units, or currency, of what matters to the animal. Because QOL would presumably involve only those things that matter to the animal, and feelings are elicited by and represent those things that matter, we can reasonably conclude that feelings are the central, and possibly *only*, constituent of QOL in animals. In support of this contention, studies in people have shown that the quality of emotional pleasantness is one of the strongest predictors of life satisfaction (Diener & Larsen 1993). Similarly, QOL in animals appears to be represented by the pleasant and unpleasant feelings in the individual's life over time.

Affect appears to play such a central role in QOL in animals that it is not unreasonable for us to suggest that it is through feelings that anything influences QOL. Any factor that does not elicit a feeling—which is to say, anything that does not matter to the animal—does not appear to have any influence on an animal's QOL. Examples of factors that elicit feelings include painful glaucoma or osteoarthritis, vestibular disease or azotemia causing nausea, deprivation of social companionship causing loneliness, and tasty foods causing pleasant feelings. All of these factors elicit some type of feeling that would influence QOL. Conversely, painted toenails, prosthetic testicles, and fancy collars do not (presumably) elicit feelings, and hence appear to have no effect on the animal's QOL—likewise for certain medical disorders such as a small patch of hair loss, a benign heart murmur, or partial vision loss in one eye. If, however, a condition progresses or otherwise changes, it will affect QOL *at the point where it elicits a feeling*. Current research and observations suggest this axiom: Unaffected feelings means unaffected quality of life.

If we look again at the scenario of placing various life events and factors into the two columns of those factors that have an effect on QOL and those factors that do not, we now clearly see what the distinguishing feature was in deciding which column to put the item in. Those factors that elicit affect—a feeling of any kind—have an effect on QOL. Those that elicit no feelings do not have an effect on QOL. As mentioned above, if QOL is influenced by those things that matter—and "mattering" is identified and measured by feelings—then feelings would appear to be *the* distinguishing feature for factors influential to QOL.

Needs constitute a fundamental component of the evaluation of the subjective quality of a person's life. In some human models of QOL, needs play such a prominent role that they are proposed to be the primary determinant of QOL. In general, these "needs models" posit that QOL is at its best when all, or most, of a person's needs are met and becomes worse as fewer needs are met (Hunt 1997). In animals, needs have been proposed to be an important aspect of well-being (Dresser 1988). Odendaal (1994) has defined needs in terms of their effects on QOL. In his view, basic needs are those things necessary for an animal to have an acceptable QOL.

Fulfillment of needs appears to be an important function of affect. Feelings signal many and probably most needs to the animal and motivate the animal to fulfill those needs. For example, thirst alerts the animal to the need for water, and the unpleasantness motivates the animal to seek and consume water. Separation distress in infant mammals when separated from their mother appears to be the signal for unmet needs—security, warmth, and nutrition—and motivates the infant to vocalize loudly to reestablish contact with its mother. Many more examples can be identified, such as hunger, loneliness and isolation distress, feelings of ambient temperature, salt cravings, and boredom from unmet needs of stimulation. Because of the strong association between affect and needs, needs clearly play an important role in QOL.

DIFFERENTIAL CONTRIBUTIONS OF FEELINGS

Of all the situations, conditions, and stimuli an animal faces moment by moment throughout its life, many matter to the animal and many do not. The ones that matter do so in different degrees (and these degrees can vary under different circumstances; for example, water matters much more in hot weather than in temperate weather).

Because they are protective against threats and critical to survival, unpleasant feelings command more attention, priority, and urgency than the pleasant feelings of life. They do this by inflicting feelings that *hurt*, which ensures that the animal pays attention to and acts to rectify the threat. In addition, the consequences of a malfunction or failure differ dramatically between unpleasant and pleasant feelings. If an unpleasant feeling fails or is ignored, it could result in death, whereas the same happening for a pleasant feeling would do little more than cause the animal to miss out on an opportunity, such as a meal.

Consequently, unpleasant feelings appear to have been constructed to contribute disproportionately more to one's subjective life experiences than do pleasant feelings. Recent sensory and neurophysiologic studies support this notion. Zuker (2004) notes that the human tongue has 30 different types of receptors for bitter flavors but only two for sweet flavors. Oya et al. (2002) found that when recordings are made directly from single neurons in the human amygdala, a larger proportion of neurons are tuned to unpleasant stimuli than to pleasant. Kawasaki et al. (2001), in studies of human neurological patients being assessed for the surgical treatment of seizures, evaluated the responses of neurons of the ventromedial prefrontal region to pleasant and unpleasant stimuli (photographs). They found that neurons responded faster, more intensely, and more frequently to unpleasant stimuli than to pleasant stimuli.

In addition to the greater experiential weight of unpleasant affect, as a threat increases (e.g., as the urinary bladder continues to fill, oxygen intake diminishes, or the predator continues to approach), the unpleasant feeling correspondingly increases in intensity, steadily narrowing the animal's focus of attention on the threat and lessening the mental focus on all other (less urgent) matters. If the threat remains uncorrected, the mental focus ultimately becomes solely on the discomfort, with little to no attention directed toward anything else. Every person has experienced this him- or herself; a common situation is that of the filling bladder. While the discomfort intensifies, the mind is increasingly unable to focus on virtually anything other than obtaining relief. An ideal illustration of this mental process is the motto of the American Lung Association, which reads: When you can't breathe nothing else matters. These seven words ideally encapsulate the evolutionary history of feelings. When facing a severe and urgent threat, feelings are extremely effective in focusing the animal's attention on correcting the dangerous situation and removing the threat while also taking focus off other matters. Accordingly, when experiencing hypercapnea, pain, fear, or any number of other unpleasant feelings at high intensity, one finds it virtually impossible to enjoy any pleasurable activities. The overall effect of unpleasant affect on QOL is therefore twofold: the unpleasant experience itself, and the inability to focus on or experience pleasures. As a consequence, the contribution of unpleasant feelings to QOL has the potential to be extremely aversive.

The greater weight of unpleasant affect as compared to pleasant affect is not the only variance in value of affect. If we limit ourselves to looking at only the unpleasant feelings and calculating their impact on QOL, it is readily evident that the distress potential is not the same for all unpleasant feelings. The survival value of unpleasant feelings differs, and their contributions to QOL correspondingly differ. This development would seem to be an obvious evolutionary necessity, in order that in situations where more than one unpleasant affect was motivating the animal to perform a specific behavior, the priorities would be clear. For example, consider an impala on the African savannah. While approaching a water hole to alleviate its thirst, the impala feels the sun too uncomfortably hot to stand in for too long. The impala must weigh the urgency and importance of drinking with that of seeking shade. The presence and intensity (i.e., magnitude of unpleasantness) of the feelings "tell" the impala which to tend to first. If the thirst is severe, seeking the water becomes the animal's priority at that moment. But now picture this thirsty, hot impala approaching the water hole, and a lion leaps out of the bush and charges. Now the impala has three competing feelings—fear, thirst, and excessive heat. If the feelings didn't prioritize the importance of the various stimuli (and fast!), this impala would see (or, more precisely, *feel*) all three necessary actions as equally important, and thus would have no reason to act on its fear before its thirst.

As evolutionary logic would predict, situations and stimuli that are most urgently threatening to life have apparently come to be associated with the most intensely unpleasant feelings and include the extreme threat to life of deficient oxygen intake (detected indirectly via increased carbon dioxide levels and attributable to such causes as airway obstruction, pleural effusion, pulmonary edema, and being trapped underwater), which elicits not only the unpleasant feeling of hypercapnea but also feelings of terror and panic (Panksepp 1998). Most people can recall a time in their lives when they were swimming underwater and running out of breath. The feelings that arose were not simply the unpleasant affect of hypercapnea and acid-base imbalance but also feelings of extreme terror and urgency—all figuratively screaming at you, "Get to the surface fast!" These feelings were hard-wired into our brains by natural selection—all to protect us and animals to get ourselves out of danger. Without such powerful motivation, you might linger around, looking at the colorful underwater coral reef until it's too late to survive. With such punishing feelings as an enforcement tool, you won't be inclined to ignore their message. Tissue damage, especially major trauma such as fractured bones, is another major threat to well-being and life, and hence elicits the intense feelings of discomfort that we call pain. A third prominent threat to life elicits the emotion of fear. Many things pose grave dangers to one's life— such as the approach of a large predator, standing near a cliff edge, a violent shaking of the ground under one's feet, and an approaching fire—and fear represents the signal of imminent danger, which alerts, motivates, and prepares the animal to take self-protective actions.

THE AFFECT-BALANCE MODEL OF QUALITY OF LIFE

Quality of life appears to comprise the pleasant and unpleasant feeling states and, more specifically, the balance between these feelings (Bradburn 1969,

Spruijt et al. 2001). In this way, QOL may be viewed as a set of scales with pleasant feelings on one side and unpleasant on the other (Figure 13.1). The direction of tipping of the scales represents the QOL. Quality of life increases when the balance tips toward the pleasant feelings and declines when the balance tips toward unpleasant feelings. This model provides a clear view as to which factors contribute to QOL. Anything that tips the QOL scales in either direction is an influence on QOL; anything that does not tip the scales is not relevant to QOL. For example, the reason dying your carpet a darker color would not affect your dog's QOL whereas replacing your current carpet with one that your dog is allergic to would is because the former would not tip the QOL scales (no feelings elicited), and the latter would (unpleasant feelings of the allergy). Likewise for a cat that has a wall painting of a mountain range added to its household (no tipping of the scales) or the addition of an aggressive, bullying male cat (tipping of the scales). On the QOL scales, the intensity of the feelings dictates the *degree* to which the scales are tipped, and hence defines the *magnitude* of influence that factor has on QOL.

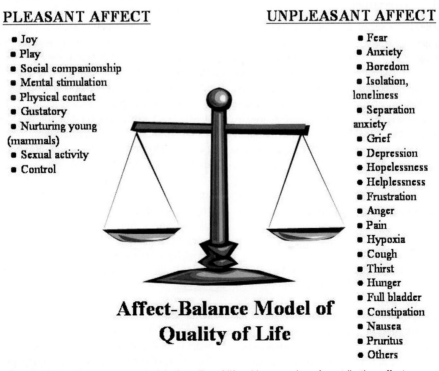

PLEASANT AFFECT

- Joy
- Play
- Social companionship
- Mental stimulation
- Physical contact
- Gustatory
- Nurturing young (mammals)
- Sexual activity
- Control

UNPLEASANT AFFECT

- Fear
- Anxiety
- Boredom
- Isolation, loneliness
- Separation anxiety
- Grief
- Depression
- Hopelessness
- Helplessness
- Frustration
- Anger
- Pain
- Hypoxia
- Cough
- Thirst
- Hunger
- Full bladder
- Constipation
- Nausea
- Pruritus
- Others

Affect-Balance Model of Quality of Life

Figure 13.1. Affect-balance model of quality of life with examples of contributing affect.

This affect-balance model of QOL explains the reason for the intuitive sense that an animal's QOL is compromised when a painful condition exists (the unpleasant feeling of pain tips the scales negatively), when a pet is abused (the unpleasant feelings of fear, pain, loneliness, hunger, etc., strongly tip the scales), and when a pet is paralyzed (the inability to experience normally enjoyable activities lessens the pleasant feelings in life, thereby tipping the scales toward the unpleasant feelings).

If we once again look back at the initial exercise of placing life factors into the two columns of having or not having an effect on QOL, using the balance model described here, we can see that all factors placed in the "has an effect" column are those that tip the QOL scales (in either direction) and that those in the other column do not tip.

MAJOR CONTRIBUTING FACTORS TO QUALITY OF LIFE

A number of factors contribute to an animal's QOL, which I believe all exert their influence through their associated affect. Due to variation in personal preferences, needs, and desires, factors influential to QOL vary in their importance between individuals. Discussions of these factors have been presented in greater depth elsewhere (McMillan 2000, 2003).

SOCIAL RELATIONSHIPS

In social animals, a set of pleasant and unpleasant emotions appears to have evolved for the purpose of promoting and enforcing social relationships (Panksepp 1998). Evidence suggests that positive social affiliations and companionship elicit pleasant emotions, whereas separation and isolation elicit unpleasant emotions (e.g., isolation distress, loneliness). Together, these feelings form and maintain social bonds and affiliations (Panksepp 1998). Wolfle (2000) has suggested that for some social species such as dogs, non-human primates, and some rodents, social companionship is often considered *the* most important element in achieving well-being.

MENTAL STIMULATION

When monotonous, unchanging, and unchallenging environments provide insufficient mental stimulation, animals show signs of boredom. Studies in the behavior and physiology of animals suggest that boredom acts similarly through unpleasant feelings in human and many nonhuman species, often manifesting as abnormal behavior patterns (e.g., stereotypies and depression) (Wemelsfelder 1990, this

volume). Conversely, mental stimulation is very rewarding to animals, appearing to elicit highly pleasurable feelings (Panksepp 1982). Stimulation can be in the form of play, exploration, and many other forms of mental engagement and challenges.

HEALTH

Health factors are associated with a wide array of pleasant and unpleasant feelings and have been long regarded as a strong influence on QOL. The discomfort of disease states (e.g., nausea, pain, hypercapnea, equilibrium disturbances, pruritus, constipation, and the like) can contribute strong negative affect to one's overall subjective experience. Relief of these discomforts is a primary reason people seek health care (Gropper 1992). In addition, infirmity and physical disabilities (e.g., heart disease, blindness, osteoarthritis, and paralysis) limit one's opportunities for experiencing pleasurable events and activities (such as, for animals, playing catch and chasing balls, going on walks, and frolicking in pastures and parks). Some medical conditions may cause no feelings of discomfort to the animal but lead to unpleasant feelings indirectly—for example, malodorous skin or urinary incontinence, which may result in social rejection or banishment to outdoors by the pet owner. In such cases, the health disorder may have no direct influence on QOL but affects it indirectly by the resultant isolation and loneliness.

Some recent research in human and nonhuman primates suggests that health may not be as important to QOL as traditionally believed. It has been found in humans, for example, that QOL is only weakly linked to health factors and that health is not a necessary condition for happiness (Musschenga 1997). In interviews conducted with human asthma patients, Drummond (1997) found that when these individuals took pleasure in life, experienced the giving and receiving of love, and had a positive approach to everyday events, life had a high quality, regardless of the medical condition or the severity of the illness. Sackett (1991) has commented that work by Diener (1984) suggests that health indices should not be used as the sole, or perhaps even a major, indicator of psychological well-being in primates.

"STRESS"

"Stress" is commonly used as a catch-all term when what is really involved is a specific unpleasant emotional experience such as fear, anxiety, pain, loneliness, frustration, boredom, or anger (Burchfield

1979; McMillan, this volume, Chapter 7). In the affect-balance model of QOL, the classic physiologic stress response consisting of sympathetic and hypothalamic-pituitary-adrenal axis activation would be expected to contribute to QOL only through its influence on affect (Noble 2002; McMillan, this volume, Chapter 7). Any stress reaction that operates below consciousness and does not directly or indirectly influence the animal's affect is therefore not relevant to QOL.

The relationship between stressful events and QOL is not a simple inverse relationship. Much evidence supports the contention that some degree of stress is necessary and beneficial to animal well-being and that too little stress can be unpleasant to the animal and detrimental to well-being (Novak & Suomi 1988, Wemelsfelder 1990). The most important aspect of stress as it pertains to QOL appears to be the animal's ability to respond to the demands of its environment—that is, to cope effectively with stressors. The ability to cope, rather than the amount of stress encountered, appears to be the factor most correlated with the impact of stress on emotional well-being (Novak & Suomi 1988) and physical health (Seligman 1975).

CONTROL

A large body of research in animals and humans has demonstrated that a sense of control over one's life and circumstances, especially the unpleasant feelings and events, is one of the most reliable predictors of positive feelings of well-being and health (Seligman 1975, Myers 1992). As it is used in animals, control is the perceived ability to influence one's environment or one's relationship with the environment—that is, to affect outcomes. Control permits the animal to influence the psychological impact of stimuli by giving the animal the ability to increase the intensity of pleasant feeling states and decrease the intensity of unpleasant states. For animals, a sense of control over adverse conditions, specifically the ability to minimize the intensity and distress potential of unpleasant feelings, appears to be one of the most critical components of mental well-being (Weiss 1972, Seligman 1975). In people, and presumably in animals, the perception of control, even if the perceived control is not utilized, provides positive expectations about one's circumstances and creates a sense of hope that unpleasant life events will not endure. Animals deprived of any control over their own circumstances, especially under persistent or repetitive aversive conditions, may develop severe

emotional distress in the form of helplessness and hopelessness (Seligman 1975). Helplessness in animals is a debilitating emotional state that has been equated to and is used as a model for clinical depression in humans (Seligman 1975).

Many situations of animal care are structured such that nothing in the animal's environment is within the animal's power to change. As Lay (2000) has observed in farm animals, the one major factor that would allow livestock to cope better with stressful stimuli and situations is forbidden: control.

THE IMPORTANCE OF ADAPTATION

A major force affecting the experiential properties of QOL and all related concepts of subjective well-being—happiness, psychological well-being, life satisfaction, and the like—is the psychological mechanism of *adaptation* (for a more in-depth discussion, see McMillan, this volume, Chapter 16). It has been well-recognized that given enough time, people adapt to adverse events and, throughout life, continuously revise the personal value and meaning they assign to those events and their outcomes (Stewart et al. 1999). Ample evidence exists that as an individual comes to terms with the conditions of long-term illness or disability, psychological adjustments occur that preserve one's life satisfaction, and individuals can judge their QOL as good even when severe limitations exist on their physical abilities (Leplege & Hunt 1997). Argyle (2001) has suggested that adaptation may explain the finding that although the elderly are in poorer health, more likely to be socially isolated, and less well-off financially, they are not, on average, less satisfied with life than young people, and in fact may be more satisfied.

Although it is widely agreed that the capacity for adaptation evolved as a useful psychological tool for coping with adversity (as well as extremely pleasant events [Suh et al. 1996, Lykken 1999]), the precise mental mechanism behind adaptation is not understood. It is currently unclear whether adaptation represents a diminished emotional response to events, an adjustment in strategies for coping with the event, changes in one's own standards as to what defines a satisfying life, or some combination of these factors (Diener & Lucas 2000).

In animals, studies (Bauer et al. 1992) and anecdotal observations (Dodman 1997; McMillan, this volume, Chapter 16) suggest that adaptation works similarly in animals as in humans. It is therefore important to consider that conditions such as gradually acquired blindness and slowly progressive age-related disorders and disabilities may not be, from the perspective of that animal, as much of an adverse influence on QOL as may be assumed by an outside evaluator who is not afflicted with these conditions.

Another factor responsible for the dynamic nature of self-assessed QOL is the changing personal values that are a part of every individual's life. Stewart et al. (1999) point out that values change at various stages in life and that what was once important may at a later point in life seem insignificant, while things once ignored may acquire greater weight. They noted that terminally ill patients, during different phases of the dying process, may attach more importance to one aspect such as the cognitive ability to recognize family and friends than to other, formerly vital, matters such as walking or even bodily functions. Cohen and Mount (1992) studied human patients with terminal illnesses and noted that because of the changing view of oneself as disease progresses, QOL can remain stable *or even improve* as physical suffering and disability increase.

We can easily conceive of a scenario in an animal that would suggest a similar process. Consider a dog whose life has consisted of confinement in a small enclosure with little or no social companionship (e.g., a racing dog, a dog used as a blood donor, or a dog used in medical research). During this time, social companionship may be the most important matter, and hence the most influential factor, affecting the dog's QOL. Then the dog is placed in a loving home with abundant human and canine companionship. Now having all of its social needs fulfilled, social factors are no longer the most important concern for the dog, and hence no longer a major influential factor on its QOL. Now the greatest value is attached to other things such as exploring new places and chasing squirrels.

In a very real way, changing values and the process of adaptation, which imparts frequent and continual changes to one's self-assessment of QOL throughout one's lifetime, make QOL a "moving target." The clear lesson is that it is essential that we judge QOL from the perspective of the individual, using his or her personal values and meanings of events—which are subject to adaptational changes—rather than judging in terms of the meaning others attribute to the experiences of the individual (Stewart et al. 1999).

A PROPOSED DEFINITION OF QUALITY OF LIFE

In humans, QOL is a subjective experience consisting of a cognitive and affective component. Whereas both components are present in humans and it is widely accepted that many animals have a comparable affective component, the contribution of a cognitive component in animal QOL is unclear. That is, in nonhuman species a cognitive evaluation of how one's life is faring may be minimal and possibly nonexistent. The affective component appears to consist of a general mood state reflecting the goodness or badness of one's life. In humans, this affective component is generally conceived to be a mood state over time and represent, or is otherwise linked to, the cognitive component of the individual's degree of satisfaction with and enjoyment of his or her life. Human QOL is not considered to be, or represent, the current transient affective state. It is reasonable to suggest that nonhuman animals have a more limited cognitive evaluation of life overall, and, accordingly, experience QOL on the basis of the current affective state(s) to a greater degree than occurs in humans. That is, whereas a person currently experiencing severe pain may still report his or her QOL as good (because the person can see his or her life as incorporating much more than the pain, know that the pain is only transient, or both), a dog with the same degree of pain may use that unpleasant affect as the primary (or sole) basis for its QOL. Hence, regardless of the animal's life circumstances and affects over time, during the pain experience the dog may assess its QOL as poor.

In this sense, when humans self-assess their QOL they are able to report a cognitive assessment, that is, how they *think* about their lives, in such terms as "I've got a good family, career, health, etc.," and "I've achieved most of my life's goals." The affective component, in contrast, is how the person *feels about* his or her life, on a good-to-bad continuum, in such terms as "I *feel* fulfilled," and "I *feel* good about how things are going." It is the cognitive component that psychotherapists work to change in order to influence the affective component of QOL. Due to cognitive limitations, language limitations, or both, animal QOL may be exclusively the affective (i.e., feeling, mood) component. The animal experience of QOL may be purely a *feeling* of how their life is faring, no more complex than an affective experience expressable as "life is good."

Based on the affect-balance model of quality of life and modified from definitions for human QOL (Jenney & Campbell 1997) and my earlier definition of animal QOL (McMillan 2000), the following definition for QOL in animals is proposed: *Quality of life is the affective and cognitive (to the degree that the animal can form such a cognitive construct) assessment that an animal makes of its life overall, of how its life is faring, experienced on a continuum of good to bad. This assessment is derived from the balance between the various pleasant and unpleasant affects experienced by the animal at and recently preceding the QOL assessment. In general, the further the affect balance tips toward the pleasant side, the higher the QOL. The contributory weights of the specific affects vary between individuals and are determined by the psychological impact of the affects to that individual.*

MEASURING QUALITY OF LIFE

Measurement of QOL continues to be a source of great controversy, debate, and difficulty in the human field, and to date, no consensus exists as to the best method for assessment. Because of its highly subjective nature, QOL continues to defy efforts at quantification (Leplege & Hunt 1997). Much greater agreement exists about *why* we should measure QOL than *how* to do it (Eiser 1997).

The usual method of collecting QOL information in people is through patient self-assessment questionnaires (Stephens et al. 1997). An *instrument* (or *index*) is the collection of items used for obtaining the desired data (Gill & Feinstein 1994) and may be comprised of a single question, such as "How do you rate your quality of life?" or a series of questions in a lengthy questionnaire format (Gill & Feinstein 1994). A number of standard instruments have been developed to measure QOL in human beings. Most instruments are designed to generate a single aggregate score (Bender 1996, Hunt 1997); however, as logical as these scores appear, their inherent meanings in terms of QOL remain unclear (Bender 1996, Hunt 1997).

QUANTIFYING SUBJECTIVE PHENOMENA

Measurement of QOL requires quantification of a subjective phenomenon. Because of the extreme difficulties this entails, many studies of QOL in humans are designed to use objective criteria to reflect the individual's subjective status. Measuring objective criteria has an appeal because of the ease of quantifying such items as compared to subjective criteria. Furthermore, objective measures permit standardization and provide an established anchor point that can be compared across studies. Examples of objective criteria commonly measured have

included physical functioning and activity level, disease and physiologic measures, appetite, and social support. Subjective criteria—considered the truest reflection of QOL—involve the way an individual *feels about* aspects of life (e.g., health, companionship) and life overall.

PROXY MEASUREMENT

It is now well accepted that the individual should be the primary source of information regarding his or her QOL (Sprangers & Aaronson 1992, Bradlyn et al. 1996). Individuals have unique interests, values, needs, and desires—all contributing to an individual mental disposition that uniquely characterizes the QOL experience.

Measuring QOL from the individual's own perspective is a problem when the individual is incapable of providing first-hand information regarding his or her subjective experiences. In humans, such individuals include neonates, infants, the mentally disabled, and the severely ill. To avoid excluding such individuals from QOL analyses, researchers have devised instruments to acquire QOL information from closely associated alternative sources such as parents, spouses, partners, caregivers, siblings, friends, and health care providers. Such individuals are termed "proxy" informants. Because of communication barriers, subjective information concerning QOL of nonhuman animals must, with rare exceptions (Dawkins 1990, Rushen 1996), come from sources other than the animals themselves. The issue of the accuracy of proxy measurements is therefore crucial to QOL assessment in animals.

The accuracy of proxy ratings has been studied extensively in adolescent humans by comparing data from proxy informants with data from pediatric patients themselves. Poor agreement between children and parents on measures of private experiences such as emotions and subjective states, regardless of whether the child is healthy or sick, is well documented. The importance for animal care is that if parent-child proxy QOL assessment is inaccurate, then person-animal assessment is likely to be even more so.

UNITS, STANDARDS, AND STATISTICAL ANALYSES

A central problem with quantifying QOL is the same problem identified by Robertson (2002) in reference to pain: "We can measure many things, including blood pressure, weight, temperature, the number of white cells in the blood, and the amount of oxygen or acid in the blood. All of these have a unit attached to them and are completely objective measures. What is the unit of pain? There is none." This problem exists for all subjective experiential matters, particularly the highly complex concept of QOL.

Another statistical barrier associated with the measurement of QOL is the absence of any "gold standard" for comparison—no external criterion of QOL against which measures can be tested exists (Hunt 1997, Jenney & Campbell 1997). Unlike physiological data, QOL has no normal range, and as Hunt (1997) has noted, the notion of an "average" QOL is meaningless.

The practical problems in QOL measurement have led researchers to concede that the demand that measures have robust statistical properties is very difficult to meet and that it is perhaps unrealistic to demand that a QOL scale should attain the same level of statistical rigor as can be achieved in the physical sciences (Eiser 1997). Even so, researchers have insisted that any measures proposed to assess QOL must meet standards for reliability and validity and conform to scientific standards for instrument development (Reaman & Haase 1996, Eiser 1997).

STATISTICAL VERSUS CLINICAL SIGNIFICANCE

Bradlyn et al. (1996) observed that in assessing QOL, the relationship between statistical significance and clinical significance is unclear. It has yet to be conclusively demonstrated that a statistically significant difference in any type of QOL measurement corresponds to a clinically meaningful difference to the individual (Bender 1996). With the metric associated with QOL being so poorly understood at this time (e.g., what do five QOL units of difference between treatments actually reflect?), the translation of QOL findings into clinical applications is not currently reliable (Bradlyn et al. 1996).

POTENTIAL FOR BIAS

All of the aforementioned difficulties making QOL assessment a very inexact science open the door to influences such as personal bias. Many, if not most, animal caregivers and those with animal care interests—pet owners, zookeepers, livestock producers, marine aquariums, animal refuges, research scientists, as well as animal welfare and animal rights organizations—have some degree of personal stake in the QOL assessment made for the animals in their care or area of concern. In situations where bias is influencing QOL assessments and multiple assessors disagree—such as when an animal rights group

claims that sows in farrowing crates have a miserable QOL but swine producers claim just the opposite—the absence of an accurate, objective method for measuring QOL makes it difficult and often impossible to conclusively determine who is most correct.

QUALITY OF LIFE MEASUREMENT IN ANIMALS

Although only a single method of measurement of QOL in animals has, to my knowledge, appeared in the literature (Yazbek & Fantoni 2004), much has been written about measurement of closely related concepts, particularly welfare and psychological well-being. Because of the similarities (and possible equality) of these concepts and QOL, much of what has been proposed regarding their measurement appears relevant and applicable to the concept of QOL. Specific assessment criteria have been categorized by authors in various ways, and include behavior (normal, abnormal, and preference studies), neurochemical and endocrine factors (e.g., catecholamines, glucocorticoids, and other indices), health status, physical functioning (i.e., degree of disability), immune function, morphologic changes, and brain imaging (Novak & Suomi 1988; Dawkins 1990; Rushen 1996; Clark et al. 1997b, 1997c).

The affect-balance view of psychological well-being led Bradburn (1969) to develop the Affect-Balance Scale (ABS) for use in humans. In Bradburn's view, happiness is the degree to which a person's positive feelings in life outweigh the negative feelings. The ABS consists of 10 questions, half devoted to pleasant affect and half to unpleasant affect. Because Bradburn's subjects had the ability to provide self-reports, Bradburn could design his ABS to collect a large amount of information about affect with very broad questions. One question, for example, asked whether the person felt "on top of the world," and another asked if the person felt like "things were going your way." This allowed Bradburn to get maximal information using a minimal number of questions.

In my view, the affect-balance model of animal QOL and its measurement is necessarily more complex than Bradburn's ABS. The specific manner in which I propose that affect be utilized in the affect-balance model can be viewed as a set of four steps. The first step in measuring an animal's QOL is to inventory all feelings in the animal's life—pleasant and unpleasant, emotional and physical in origin, health-related and non-health related. The second step is to attempt to adjust contributory weight of each feeling for the level of biological, or survival, value and urgency. Among the unpleasant feelings, proportionately more weight should be assigned to those feelings that are evolutionarily associated with the most serious and immediate threats to survival such as hypercapnea, pain, fear, and separation distress in infant mammals separated from their mothers. Step three is to individualize the weights of feelings. For example, loneliness-type feelings would be assigned much more weight in a dog with separation anxiety than in a dog that is relaxed when left alone at home. The final step is to construct a scale weighing the adjusted-importance feelings. At present, this step lacks any precision and in many instances may be simply a best guess.

The overriding goal in measurement is to assess QOL from the perspective of the animal. Interests, needs, and desires are meaningful only as they are perceived by and in that animal's mind. This goal is not currently attainable due to language barriers and vast differences among species, sexes, breeds, age groups, and individuals regarding values and sources of unpleasant and pleasant affect. When this goal cannot be achieved, proxy assessment should serve in its stead, preferably conducted by the person who has the greatest knowledge of the individual animal's personality and nature. Fortunately, innovative behavioral research techniques are providing a window to the subjective worlds of animals (e.g., preference testing [Clark et al. 1997b], aversion learning [Rushen 1996], and demand curve analysis [Dawkins 1990]), offering great promise that the private feelings of animals will become increasingly accessible.

MAXIMIZING QUALITY OF LIFE

THE GUIDING PRINCIPLE FOR MAXIMIZING QUALITY OF LIFE

Despite the difficulties in measuring QOL, quantification problems, fortunately, do not seriously hamper our ability to maximize QOL, as the basic approach is effective at all levels of QOL. Maximizing QOL can be summarized by a single principle: Tip the QOL scales as far toward the pleasant side as possible. Based on the affect-balance model of QOL, this goal is accomplished by the dual effort of minimizing unpleasant affect and promoting pleasant affect. This basic principle applies to all animals, healthy and ill. For animals with an illness, the main effort is to restore QOL by alleviating the unpleasant feelings associated with the disease. For healthy animals, the main emphasis

is promoting pleasures. In all cases, QOL should be expected to rise as the scales tip increasingly toward the positive side.

Each of the major contributing factors to QOL discussed in the earlier section (e.g., social companionships, mental stimulation, health, etc.) should be individually addressed. Each factor has its associated feelings, pleasant and unpleasant, and these deserve individual attention when we attempt to tip the balance of the QOL scales. Table 13.1 presents each major contributing factor and the specific approaches to QOL enhancement for each.

Probably the single most important element of any QOL enhancement program—for all animals, healthy and ill—is to provide the animal with a degree of *control* (Weiss 1972, Seligman 1975). Having the power to alter conditions of the environment, and especially to alleviate unpleasant affect, is most likely the best protection against distress (for a discussion of a proposed relationship between control and distress, see McMillan, this volume, Chapter 7). Control can be provided by offering the animal meaningful opportunities to make choices (e.g., going outside or staying inside, which direction to go on a walk, which toy to play with) and giving the animal some say-so in its life by allowing the animal to make requests (e.g., for play, walks outside). Control entails ensuring that the animal has or perceives some ability to lessen the intensity of unpleasant feelings or to improve an unpleasant situation such as boredom, loneliness, frustration, or fear, which is at least partially accomplished by providing the animal with a secure place to escape or hide and the means to obtain mental stimulation.

MAXIMIZING QUALITY OF LIFE IN THE ILL ANIMAL

In the ill or disabled animal, the QOL balance is expected to be tipped toward the unpleasant side because of three factors: (1) the increase in unpleasant feelings associated with the disease state, (2) loss of some opportunities to experience pleasurable events and activities, and (3) the tendency of unpleasant feelings to focus attention progressively more on the discomfort and progressively less on pleasant feelings. Restoration of health is the most effective means to regain the pre-illness QOL, but when cure is not attainable, other methods (such as oxygen supplementation; analgesic, anti-nausea, and antiinflammatory medications; psychotropic medications such as antianxiety and antidepressant drugs; laxatives; chemotherapy drugs; and gentle and soothing human contact such as stroking, petting, and talking to the

Table 13.1. Major contributing factors to quality of life and methods for counteracting any adverse effects caused by each factor.

Contributing Factor to QOL	How QOL is Affected	Methods for Maximization of QOL
Social relationships	• Social interaction and companionship are associated with pleasant feelings • Separation and isolation are associated with unpleasant feelings	• Provide abundant social interaction and companionship—human, other animals
Mental stimulation	• Insufficient stimulation results in boredom, a potentially devastating emotional distress • When the animal receives stimulation, pleasant feelings are elicited	• Stimulation can be in the form of novelty, variety, activities, play, fun, recreation, challenges, exploration, and other forms of mental stimulation and engagement. Specific examples include treasure hunts with food snacks, interactive toys, continual supply of novel objects to investigate and explore, outings (e.g., dog parks, camping trips), games, chase and pounce, working for food.
Health	• Discomforts of illness (e.g., hypercapnea, nausea, pain, pruritus). Certain medical conditions may impair QOL by indirectly eliciting unpleasant feelings—for example, bad skin odor or urinary incontinence may lead to social rejection or banishment to outdoors, resulting in loneliness • Physical impairments and disabilities (e.g., paralysis, blindness, deafness) can limit one's opportunities for experiencing pleasurable events and activities	• Provide high-quality health care • Alleviate all discomforts associated with disease—ideally with elimination of disease, but if cure is not possible, then alleviation of all discomforts to the greatest degree possible • Restore lost functions of disabilities to promote pleasures • Mental health disorders: pharmacologic and nonpharmacologic (e.g., behavioral modification, counterconditioning, desensitization) interventions to lessen the intensity of unpleasant feelings
Stress	• Stress contributes to QOL through specific emotional states such as fear, anxiety, pain, loneliness, boredom, anger, and frustration.	• Alleviate the specific emotion involved. • Reduce the stimuli eliciting the unpleasant emotions. • Enhance the animal's opportunities to adapt to the stressor by providing the means for coping—e.g., controllability (see below), social support, predictability.
Control	• Control over stressors lessens the impact of stressors. • A perception of no control leads to feelings of helplessness,	• Offer meaningful opportunities to make choices (e.g., going outside or staying inside, which food to eat today, which toy to play with, etc.).

Contributing Factor to QOL	How QOL is Affected	Methods for Maximization of QOL
	which can be a severe emotional distress and extremely detrimental to QOL. Lack of control over stressors makes the negative impact of stressors greater.	• Give animal say-so in its life by allowing animal to make requests (signaling to the owner when the pet would like to go outside or on a walk, when it would like the owner to play, etc.) • Ensure that the pet has a meaningful ability to lessen the intensity of unpleasant feelings or to improve an unpleasant situation such as boredom, loneliness, frustration, fear, or pain (e.g., by having a secure place to escape or hide, seeking out stimulation or better conditions, or actively easing any discomforts).

Adapted from McMillan FD. 2003. Maximizing quality of life in ill animals. *J Am Anim Hosp Assoc* 39:227–235. The Journal of the American Animal Hospital Association by Frucci, Jill E. Copyright (c) 2003 by Am Animal Hosp Assn/AAHA. Reproduced and modified with permission of Am Animal Hosp Assn/AAHA in the format Textbook via Copyright Clearance Center.

animal, which can attenuate feelings of pain, anxiety, fear, and loneliness [for a review, see McMillan 1999]) are used to alleviate unpleasant feelings. Attention should be prioritized according to the distress potential of the specific unpleasant feelings.

As the totality of this book makes clear, when considering illness in animals, it is essential that we include mental health in the spectrum of health disorders. An animal could be in perfect physical health and yet have an extremely poor QOL. Emotional illnesses such as phobias and separation anxiety elicit unpleasant feelings that appear to be every bit as, and in some cases more, distressing than physical illness. The intense fear experienced in phobic disorders, especially when the condition is unrelenting, may elicit profound suffering. Alleviating discomforts of mental illnesses is of equal importance as those of physical illness for elevating a diminished QOL. Methods to alleviate the unpleasant feelings of emotional illness include pharmacological and nonpharmacological interventions and have been recently described (McMillan 2002; Marder & Posage, this volume; Wright et al., this volume).

Although the primary focus for QOL enhancement in ill animals is the alleviation of unpleasant feelings, it is also important to promote pleasant affect. In human patients with serious illnesses, social support, fun activities, and humor are often used to increase pleasant affect, induce positive moods and increase happiness levels (Argyle 2001, Hassed 2001). It has been found in animals that vocal pain responses to nociceptive stimulation are diminished when animals have abundant social companionship (Panksepp 1980). Providing the ill animal with more pleasurable experiences would be expected to elevate QOL. Because of the individual nature of QOL, the type and quantity of pleasure-eliciting stimuli must be individualized for each animal. Accordingly, the person who is most familiar with the animal's unique personality and nature is best suited to compile the list of pleasures to be used in the QOL maximization program.

For patients with disabilities such as paralysis, blindness, and generalized weakness, no increase in unpleasant feelings may occur. In these cases, the restoration of a diminished QOL involves replacing any losses in the ability to experience pleasures such as chasing, running, and playing. These losses can be at least partially restored through such measures as carts and sling-walks for paraparalysis patients and hand signals for communication with deaf animals.

Care must be taken that pleasant activities are suitable for the specific disease or disability. Chasing a ball, for example, may be inappropriate for a patient with severe heart disease or a slipped disc. Any pleasurable feelings that can be increased without risking additional unpleasant feelings should be fully promoted. Even activities that elicit unpleasant feelings may be ultimately beneficial to QOL, as long as the net effect is to tip the QOL scales toward the pleasant side. For example, if going on walks leads a dog to feel some discomfort of arthritis, but the walks are highly pleasurable and desired, then continuing the walks could be expected to result in a net improvement to QOL.

As disease states progress, the QOL scales will tip increasingly toward unpleasant feelings. This is due to an increasing magnitude of the unpleasant feelings and lessening of pleasurable feelings. Eventually, efforts to increase QOL will be insufficient to counteract the progressively negative tipping of the scales.

ENHANCING QUALITY OF LIFE IN THE HEALTHY ANIMAL

Because the healthy animal is not obviously suffering any malady, it is often presumed that life is good. This may not be true, as the animal could still be experiencing any of a wide array of unpleasant feelings that are not health-related. Examples include isolation distress, loneliness, boredom, frustration, hunger, thirst, and unpleasant temperature extremes. Many of these are the results of unmet physical and emotional needs.

A useful and important method of enhancing the QOL of healthy animals is the concept of *environmental enrichment*. Already accepted as an important aspect of care for animals in captivity, such as those in zoos, in laboratories, and on farms, environmental enrichment has recently been proposed as an important aspect of pet animal care (Neville 1997). Environmental enrichment has been defined as "an animal husbandry principle that seeks to enhance quality of captive animal care by identifying and providing the environmental stimuli necessary for optimal psychological and physiological well-being" (Shepherdson 1998) and entails the modification of the animal's environment by adding structural, social, temporal, climatic, or dietary diversity to the animal's housing (Burghardt 1999). Environmental enrichment provides an excellent illustration for how QOL is enhanced by tipping the scales toward the pleasant side. When novel and interesting objects, events, and social companions are added to the animal's environment, the unpleasant feelings of boredom and loneliness are alleviated, and the pleasant feelings of mental stimulation and social companionship are promoted. A specific example of environmental enrichment in pet animals is providing indoor cats with a continuous supply of novel objects to investigate and explore (such as cardboard boxes, tree branches, toys), "treasure

hunt" games in which food treats are hidden around the house, chase-and-pounce games with toys and people, a fish tank, and leash walks outside on a harness (Neville 1997, Delzio & Ribarich 1999).

Once emotional and physical needs are met (thereby eliminating the unpleasant feelings associated with unmet needs), the animal may be said to have a comfortable life. At this point—when physical and mental health are good—efforts to further elevate QOL can turn a comfortable life into an enjoyable, happy, fun, and emotionally-fulfilled life. With little or no unpleasant affect, the emphasis in enhancing QOL in the healthy animal is the promotion of pleasurable feelings and experiences. Known sources of pleasurable feelings include social interaction and companionship (with humans and other animals), mentally stimulating and engaging activities (variety, novelty, play, chases, games, hunting for hidden objects, exploring, outings, interactive toys, leash walks outside), taste pleasures (palatable foods, snacks), human touch (petting, massage, laying in lap), climbing, digging up things, and lounging in sunlight.

The true nature of quality of life in animals is not understood. No question exists that affect plays an important role, but does the affect-balance model of QOL—in which affect is the sole determinant of QOL—fully explain QOL in nonhuman animals? In their overview of subjective well-being, Kahneman et al. (1999) assert that in humans, "quality of life cannot be reduced to the balance of pleasure and pain." Studies in humans tend to confirm this; a special quality to QOL exists in people that seems to transcend affect, involving factors such as purpose and meaning in life, which does not always correlate with reported affect. Various studies have shown that as people age, positive affect rises in some but not others, negative affect decreases in some but not others (Mroczek & Kolarz 1998), but that overall life satisfaction is consistently found to increase with age (Cantril 1965). This suggests that in humans, the amounts of positive and negative affect are not the whole story—other factors also influence people's self-assessments of their subjective well-being. Whether such a transcendent quality is part of animal QOL remains to be determined. For now, however, research in animal behavior, neuroscience, physiology, and evolutionary psychology point overwhelmingly in the same direction: Sentient animals make behavioral choices in life—a highly likely indication of the way they want their lives to run—by the pleasure principle, that is, maximize pleasure and minimize displeasure. It makes sense that a system of animal care committed to helping animals achieve this basic goal will be the type of care that is most effective, most compassionate, most appreciated, and, at the present time with our present knowledge, the most likely to give them the highest quality of life.

REFERENCES

Anonymous. 2003. How do you measure quality of life? *Vet Rec* 12:37–38.

Argyle M. 2001. *The psychology of happiness*, 2nd ed. New York: Taylor & Francis.

Bauer M, Glickman N, Glickman L, et al. 1992. Follow-up study of owner attitudes toward home care of paraplegic dogs. *J Am Vet Med Assoc* 200:1809–1816.

Bender BG. 1996. Measurement of quality of life in pediatric asthma clinical trials. *Ann Allerg Asthma Im* 77:438–445.

Bradburn NM. 1969. *The structure of psychological well-being*. Chicago: Aldine Publishing Company.

Bradlyn AS, Ritchey AK, Harris CV, et al. 1996. Quality of life research in pediatric oncology. *Cancer* 78:1333–1339.

Burchfield SR. 1979. The stress response: A new perspective. *Psychosom Med* 41:661–672.

Burghardt GM. 1999. Deprivation and enrichment in laboratory animal environments. *J Appl Anim Wel Sci* 2:263–266.

Cantril H. 1965. *The pattern of human concerns*. New Brunswick, NJ: Rutgers University Press.

Clark JD, Rager DR, Calpin JP. 1997a. Animal well-being I. General considerations. *Lab Anim Sci* 47:564–570.

Clark JD, Rager DR, Calpin JP. 1997b. Animal well-being III. An overview of assessment. *Lab Anim Sci* 47:580–585.

Clark JD, Rager DR, Calpin JP. 1997c. Animal well-being IV. Specific assessment criteria. *Lab Anim Sci* 47:586–597.

Cohen SR, Mount BM. 1992. Quality of life in terminal illness: Defining and measuring subjective well-being in the dying. *J Palliative Care* 8:40–45.

Dawkins MS. 1990. From an animal's point of view: Motivation, fitness, and animal welfare. *Behav Brain Sci* 13:1–61.

DeGrazia D. 1996. *Taking animals seriously*. Cambridge, UK: Cambridge University Press.

Delzio S, Ribarich C. 1999. *Felinestein: Pampering the genius in your cat*. New York: HarperPerennial.

Diener E. 1984. Subjective well-being. *Psychol Bull* 95:542–575.

Diener E, Larsen RJ. 1993. The experience of emotional well-being. In: Lewis M, Haviland JM (eds), *Handbook of emotions*. New York, The Guilford Press:405–415.

Diener E, Lucas RE. 2000. Subjective emotional well-being. In: Lewis M, Haviland-Jones JM (eds), *Handbook of emotions*, 2nd ed. New York, The Guilford Press:325–337.

Dodman N. 1997. *The cat who cried for help: Attitudes, emotions, and the psychology of cats*. New York: Bantam Books.

Dresser R. 1988. Assessing harm and justification in animal research: Federal policy opens the laboratory door. *Rutgers Law Rev* 4:723–729.

Drummond N. 1997. The quality of life in patients with asthma. Aberdeen, Scotland: University of Aberdeen. Thesis.

Eiser C. 1997. Children's quality of life measures. *Arch Dis Child* 77:350–354.

Freeman LM, Rush JE, Farabaugh AE, et al. 2003. Development and validation of the functional evaluation of cardiac health (FETCH) questionnaire for dogs. ACVIM Forum, Charlotte, NC (Abstract).

Gill TM, Feinstein AR. 1994. A critical appraisal of the quality of quality-of-life measurements. *J Amer Med Assoc* 272:619–626.

Glaser A, Walker D. 1995. Letter to the editor. *Lancet* 346:444.

Gropper EI. 1992. Promoting health by promoting comfort. *Nurs Forum* 27:5–8.

Hassed C. 2001. How humour keeps you well. *Aust Fam Physician* 30:25–28.

Hatton C. 1998. Whose quality of life is it anyway? Some problems with the emerging quality of life consensus. *Ment Retard* 36:104–115.

Hunt SM. 1997. The problem of quality of life. *Qual Life Res* 6:205–212.

Jenney MEM, Campbell S. 1997. Measuring quality of life. *Arch Dis Child* 77:347–350.

Kahneman D, Diener E, Schwarz N (eds). 1999. *Well-being: The foundations of hedonic psychology* (Preface). New York, Russell Sage Foundation:ix–xii.

Kawasaki H, Adolphs R, Kaufman O, et al. 2001. Single-unit responses to emotional visual stimuli recorded in human ventral prefrontal cortex. *Nat Neurosci* 4:15–16.

Lay DC. 2000. Consequences of stress during development. In: Moberg G, Mench JA (eds), *The biology of animal stress: Basic principles and implications for animal welfare*. Wallingford, UK, CABI:249–268.

Leplege A, Hunt S. 1997. The problem of quality of life in medicine. *J Amer Med Assoc* 278:47–50.

Lykken D. 1999. *Happiness*. New York: Golden Books.

McMillan FD. 1999. Effects of human contact on animal health and well-being. *J Am Vet Med Assoc* 215:1592–1598.

McMillan FD. 2000. Quality of life in animals. *J Am Vet Med Assoc* 216:1904–1910.

McMillan FD. 2002. Emotional pain management. *Vet Med* 97:822–834.

McMillan FD. 2003. Maximizing quality of life in ill animals. *J Am Anim Hosp Assoc* 39:227–235.

Mroczek DK, Kolarz CM. 1998. The effect of age on positive and negative affect: A developmental perspective on happiness. *J Pers Soc Psychol* 75:1333–1349.

Musschenga AW. 1997. The relation between concepts of quality-of-life, health and happiness. *J Med Philos* 22:11–28.

Myers DG. 1992. *The pursuit of happiness*. New York: Avon Books.

Neville PF. 1997. Preventing problems via social and environmental enrichment. Proceedings of the The North American Veterinary Conference, Orlando, FL:31–32.

Noble RE. 2002. Diagnosis of stress. *Metabolism* 51 Suppl 1:37–39.

Novak MA, Suomi SJ. 1988. Psychological well-being of primates in captivity. *Am Psychol* 43:765–773.

Odendaal JSJ. 1994. Veterinary ethology and animal welfare. *Rev Sci Tech Off Int Epiz* 13:291–302.

Osoba D. 1994. Lessons learned from measuring health-related quality of life in oncology. *J Clin Oncol* 12:608–616.

Oya H, Kawasaki H, Howard MA, et al. 2002. Electrophysiological responses recorded in the human amygdale discriminate emotion categories of visual stimuli. *J Neurosci* 22:9502–9512.

Pal DK. 1996. Quality of life assessment in children: A review of conceptual and methodological issues in multidimensional health status measures. *J Epidemiol Commun H* 50:391–396.

Panksepp J. 1980. Brief social isolation, pain responsivity, and morphine analgesia in young rats. *Psychopharmacology* 72:111–112.

Panksepp J. 1982. Toward a general psychobiological theory of emotions. *Behav Brain Sci* 5:407–467.

Panksepp J. 1998. *Affective neuroscience: The foundations of human and animal emotions*. New York: Oxford University Press.

Reaman GH, Haase GM. 1996. Quality of life research in childhood cancer. *Cancer* 78:1330–1332.

Robertson SA. 2002. What is pain? *J Am Vet Med Assoc* 221:202–204.

Rushen J. 1996. Using aversion learning techniques to assess the mental state, suffering, and welfare of farm animals. *J Anim Sci* 74:1990–1995.

Sackett GP. 1991. The human model of psychological well-being in primates. In: Novak MA, Petto AJ (eds), *Through the looking glass: Issues of psychological well-being in captive nonhuman primates*.

Washington, DC, American Psychological Association:35–42.

Seligman ME. 1975. *Helplessness: On depression, development, and death*. San Francisco: W.H. Freeman.

Shepherdson DJ. 1998. Introduction: Tracing the path of environmental enrichment in zoos. In: Shepherdson DJ (ed), *Second nature: Environmental enrichment for captive animals*. Washington, DC, Smithsonian Institute Press:114.

Slevin ML. 1992. Quality of life: Philosophical question or clinical reality? *Brit Med J* 305:466–469.

Sprangers MAG, Aaronson NK. 1992. The role of health care providers and significant others in evaluating the quality of life of patients with chronic disease: A review. *J Clin Epidemiol* 45:743–760.

Spruijt BM, van den Bos R, Pijlman FTA. 2001. A concept of welfare based on reward evaluating mechanisms in the brain: Anticipatory behaviour as an indicator for the state of reward systems. *Appl Anim Behav Sci* 72:145–171.

Stephens RJ, Hopwood P, Girling DJ, et al. 1997. Randomized trials with quality of life endpoints: Are doctors' ratings of patients' physical symptoms interchangeable with patients' self-ratings? *Qual Life Res* 6:225–236.

Stewart AL, Teno J, Patrick DL, et al. 1999. The concept of quality of life of dying persons in the context of health care. *J Pain Symptom Manag* 17:93–108.

Suh EM, Diener E, Fujita F. 1996. Events and subjective well-being: Only recent events matter. *J Pers Soc Psychol* 70:1091–1102.

Treurniet HF, Essink-Bot ML, Mackenbach JP, et al. 1997. Health-related quality of life: An indicator of quality of care? *Qual Life Res* 6:363–369.

Weiss JM. 1972. Psychological factors in stress and disease. *Sci Am* 226:104–113.

Wemelsfelder F. 1990. Boredom and laboratory animal welfare. In: Rollin BE, Kesel ML (eds), *The experimental animal in biomedical research*. Boca Raton, FL, CRC Press:243–272.

Wolfle TL. 2000. Understanding the role of stress in animal welfare: Practical considerations. In: Moberg G, Mench JA (eds), *The biology of animal stress: Basic principles and implications for animal welfare*. Wallingford, UK, CABI:355–368.

Yazbek KVB, Fantoni DT. 2004. Validity of a health-related quality-of-life scale for dogs with cancer pain. *J Am Vet Med Assoc*: in press.

Zuker C. 2004. Personal communication. University of California San Deigo School of Medicine.

14
Giving Power to Animals

Hal Markowitz and Katherine Eckert

MENTAL HEALTH OF ANIMALS

How does one accurately assess the mental health of another animal, whether human or nonhuman? Inevitably, the answer for scientists is that one can only accomplish this task by careful observation of behavior and eventual ability to predict successive behavior of the animal in question. In humans, this task becomes extremely complicated by the fact that verbal behavior has been a major focus of mental health practitioners and is often surprisingly unreliable. Although assessing human mental health is not the focus of the current text, we should note that when human mental health is being assessed verbally, the patient's report is frequently more related to what he or she thinks is the expectation of the therapist than it is to his or her own actual past or present behavior (Quay 1959). We begin our chapter in this odd manner to point out that in assessing the apparent mental health of *any* animal, we are ultimately dependent on the careful analysis of behavior to decide about its well-being.

Whether the other animal is human or not, we make our judgments based on how the individual functions in his or her environment. When we are talking about nonverbal animals, especially those maintained in captivity for human companionship, amusement, research purposes, work, or exhibition, the task becomes very complex in its own way. For example, when a dog performs tricks at its "master's" command, bringing great glee to the one controlling its behavior, and does it repeatedly and reliably with a wagging tail, we are inclined to think that this is a happy creature. Of course we have no way to really know whether the dog in question is happy or whether it is laughing at the human for being entertained by this foolish unnatural stunt. When it comes to other animals for which we have less readily available knowledge of signs such as tail

wagging from which to infer contentedness or well-being, the task may be apparently insurmountable. For example, unless one believes in magic or has a great deal more information than your authors do about crocodiles, it is very difficult to decide whether a crocodile is *mentally* healthy, even after spending many weeks observing one in captivity.

If we have made our point adequately and expressed our personal convictions clearly, you may be asking yourself why we agreed to write a chapter on the mental health of animals. The answer is that we believe that modern scientists and good mental health practitioners make their assessments and predictions very tentatively and based on experience with the species in question as well as the individual of focus. This is the way of all good science, with history illustrating that today's most firmly held "truths" are often laughable tomorrow and best spelled with small t's.

Throughout this chapter, we will provide a review of some of the work that we believe indicates that the well-being of animals is enhanced by the animals' abilities to control aspects of their environments. The concept of controllability is complex, but we focus on research that gives animals the ability to learn control of novel situations or devices and to then use them to seek both predictable and new or innovative outcomes. We will also describe some data suggesting that inability to control one's environment greatly exposes animals (including humans) to the negative affects of stressful conditions.

METHODS FOR INFERRING WELL-BEING

With the increasing emphasis on institutional assessment of well-being in animals in the institution's care (see Markowitz & Timmel, this volume), more focus has been placed on ways to assess animals' apparent behavioral health. Most often, the criteria employed are based on one of two kinds of inferences. The first kind utilizes information about the "natural" behavior of conspecifics and assumes that if animals show characteristic behavior of their species, they are "well." Thus, for example, if a captive animal eats in a normal fashion, engages in species-typical sexual behavior, and generally does not exhibit quantitative or qualitative abnormalities in behavior as compared with wild counterparts, we deem them to be well off (see, for example, Erwin & Deni 1979).

The second category is used primarily to assess whether attempts to enrich environments have been successful in improving the well-being of the animals. The use of this kind of criterion is based on the assumption that if animals utilize the "improvements," they are better off. (One can see the analogy to our earlier example of the pet owner who assumes that his or her pet is happy to use the toys that the owner is happy to show the pet's willingness to use.)

Much confusion exists when it comes to animals with which we feel a closer kinship. It seems to those of us who have worked with great apes that we can tell when they are happy, mischievous, "sorry" for their misbehavior, or sad. For example, the first author remembers a day when, in preparation for trying to convince a zoo administration to provide a more natural habitat for young orangutans, he was trying to persuade a young captive-born orang to join him in climbing trees (Figure 14.1). At first, the youngster was quite trepidacious, having grown up in an almost totally concrete environment with limited place to climb and no large open vistas to explore. Then he joined Markowitz in the tree, climbing into Markowitz's arms for apparent reassurance. Soon, the human was rewarded for his efforts as the now-excited orang gleefully bit through the author's tennis shoe. Hearing the cry of pain, the orang "apologized" by lifting Markowitz's tee shirt and licking his naval.

Empathetically, it certainly seemed that much of the young orang's behavior was understandable. As he became more comfortable with regular sojourns to this forested area, he seemed more at home and happy to have this new opportunity, as measured by his increased usage of the trees and decreased ability of humans to retrieve him from the forest. Although behavioral ecologists have provided ample evidence that the notion of a *scala natura* in the Aristotelian sense is outmoded (Zuk 2002), it still seems apparent that we can empathize with some animals more so than with others. Consequently, throughout the remainder of this chapter, we will make the very tentative assumption that our familiarity with the individual animals

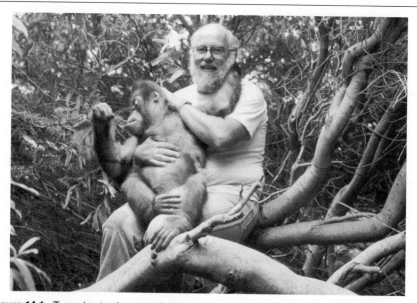

Figure 14.1. Two primates hang out in the trees.

about which we are writing and our knowledge of the species in general allow us to make useful inferences about their well-beings.

CONTROL OF THE ENVIRONMENT

When we look at animals in many captive circumstances such as zoos and laboratory quarters, we are inclined to think that they are "dying of boredom." The frequent absurdity of this assumption becomes apparent on hearing some of the most common complaints from visitors to these facilities. For example, wolves are reported to be "bored because they are pacing." Careful observation may reveal that the species-typical behavior of pacing is actually reduced in captive wolves when compared with their wild conspecifics. In the wild, humans often track wolves by looking for the repetitive evidence of where the wolves have redundantly paced. Lions and tigers that spend much of their days sleeping in nature are presumed to be sleeping in captivity because they are bored. But are we suggesting that life in captivity is wonderful? Most certainly not.

In the course of their evolutionary history, animals have become specialized in their abilities to hunt and gather food. When we deprive them of the opportunity to exercise these abilities, we essentially rob them of their natural existence, their source of pride, their sense of well-being. Of course we provide them with nutrition and shelter from the elements and predators, but this very provision and protection may contribute to the powerlessness which we believe is at the heart of the problem for captive animals. How can we expect animals in our charge to be "mentally healthy" if nothing that they do matters? How can we expect them to be healthy members of their species if we limit our praise and rewards to those circumstances in which they do exactly what we desire?

EARLY EXAMPLES OF EMPOWERING ANIMALS AND APPARENT CHANGES IN THEIR MENTAL HEALTH

Work begun more than 30 years ago in zoos and aquariums provides evidence that animals will actively use new opportunities to control some of their own environmental schedules and that this can have salutary effects on their well-beings (Markowitz & Stevens 1978). The first of these projects involved providing white handed gibbons the opportunity to obtain food regularly throughout the day by brachiating or leaping between widely spaced stations midway up the wall in a traditional barren zoo environment. Not only did these apes learn to effectively utilize the opportunity, but a young gibbon learned to effectively forage this way by watching his elders. Everyone marveled at the gymnastics of Harvey Wallbanger, the most proficient of the gibbons at food earning (Figure 14.2). This included another gibbon, Venus, who had brutalized a previous male that had been introduced to her in the hopes that they would mate. Now introduced into Harvey's captive home, instead of aggressing, Venus stayed quiet and watched him show off his abilities to fly through the air, rapidly "magically" producing a variety of attractive foodstuffs automatically delivered to him for his efforts (Markowitz 1982).

The first eight hours of this introduction were recorded on videotape and show Venus allowing Harvey to approach her and "peck" her on the cheek within the first hour. Venus watched Harvey intently for a long time and seemed content to share his food offerings. Within days, Venus learned to earn much of her own food, and these gibbons remained paired for years until they were sent to another zoo.

An apparatus that detected polar bear vocalizations was installed and tuned so that only non-aggressive sounds were rewarded by catapulting fish treats into or near a pond in the bears' exhibit home. Not only did the bears learn to use it, but a previously aggressive but otherwise indolent male began to actively dive into the pool when the fish flew in (Figure 14.3). This male had never before been able to put on the species-typical physiologic reserve of fat but now became heavier and more active (Schmidt & Markowitz 1977, Markowitz et al. 1978).

The dynamics in a family of Diana monkeys given an opportunity to earn tokens that could be exchanged in an "automat" for food astonished even the most jaded observer (Markowitz 1976)(Figure 14.4). These monkeys learned to move so quickly in foraging for food in this unusual manner that when filmed presentations were made at meetings, audience members asked if the film had been shown in fast motion. These monkeys displayed amazing abilities to ensure that they got an early share of the food earned in this manner each day. The most remarkable example was from a juvenile who learned to fool his mother so that she would not steal the food he had ordered from the automat. He would pretend to deposit the token but "palm" it

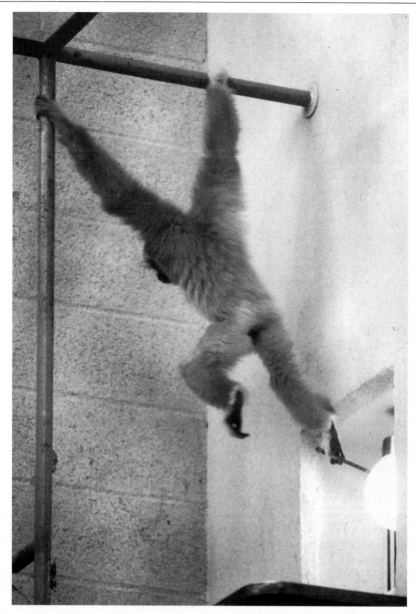

Figure 14.2. Gibbon earning food and showing natural abilities in an unnatural setting.

instead. When his mother eventually moved away from the food delivery device in apparent bewilderment, the youngster would then actually deposit the token and take the food for himself.

It seems important to note here that this not only increased healthful activity high in the environment, as opposed to previous feeding on the ground for these arboreal monkeys, but also gained the monkeys new admiration from many visitors. Instead of cowering from the occasional foolish behavior of visitors, these monkeys largely ignored the people and entertained themselves by earning food whenever they wished. They certainly appeared more mentally healthy than they had when waiting all day for keepers to deliver their food.

In another, nearby, large concrete-and-fencing cage lived a group of mandrills with unhealthy behavioral dynamics. The male frequently aggressed against his mates, and careful systematic observation revealed that the other mandrills were

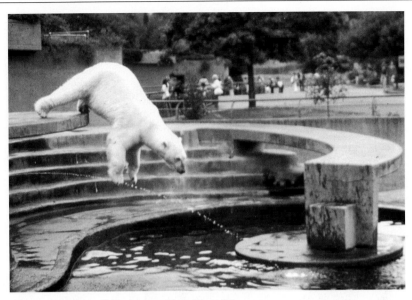

Figure 14.3. Polar bear diving into pool to retrieve fish.

restricted to a very limited portion of their environment (Yanofsky & Markowitz 1978). A game was installed, which allowed active competition between the mandrills and the public (or an electronic "adversary" when the public was not there to play)(Figure 14.5).

The male now dominated the game instead of aggressing against his cage-mates. The other mandrills were able to use most of the cage other than this small area occupied by the male and the game console. Although the only time the male relented and let others play was when he was courting a female, the apparent comfort and well-being of all in the cage was improved. The male's behavior clearly gave evidence that he gained pride from his regular success in defeating humans who competed with him on "his" speed game (Markowitz 1982).

Although small-clawed Asian river otters in an aquatic park had a rather limited captive environment, their caretakers were able to provide them some active hunting opportunities. Given the chance to listen for the sound of crickets and hunt for them when they were randomly delivered to various places in the otters' home structure, these otters developed active hunting strategies of various sorts and were very responsive to this new opportunity (Foster-Turley & Markowitz 1982).

One of the otters "outsmarted" the electronic device's requirement for active hunting in the exhibit to find the prey. He watched the three places where prey were actively delivered. Then he waited when the cricket sounds began until his exhibit-mates eliminated a place or two, thus greatly reducing his required activity for success in foraging for crickets. This is yet another example that suggests to us that providing power to animals for even limited control of delivery of their own food may stimulate active thinking and strategy building, which seem indicative of better mental health.

LABORATORY RESEARCH EXAMPLES

Bruno Prielowski, who conducted laboratory research in southern Germany, decided to adopt some of these techniques for research in his work on brain mechanisms in macaques. He designed a system that essentially allowed the monkeys to be trained to "run the experiment themselves," rather than being forced to perform on the researchers' schedules. Some of Prielowski's lab workers objected to the fact that they had lost control of the schedule and had to observe the monkeys when these nonhuman primates *chose* to work, but Prielowski reported that his research results were more significant than when he used traditional forced "trials" on the monkeys (Prielowski et al. 1988).

This result should not be surprising. A small but increasing body of experimental work is demon-

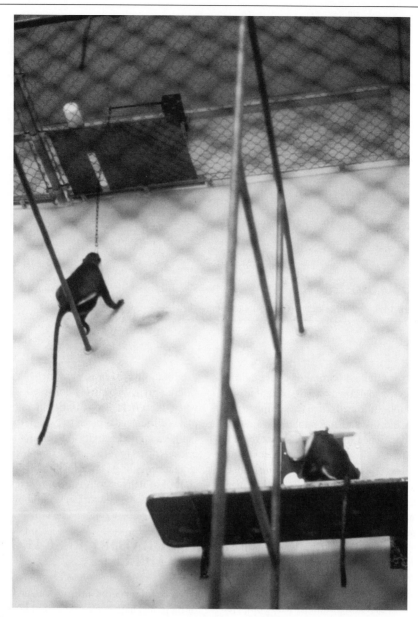

Figure 14.4. Diana monkeys exercising high in the cage to earn tokens for food at the automat.

strating the importance of control in the well-being of captive primates. For example, a study of a number of primate species in a zoo setting demonstrated that when the animals were given novel objects, they significantly preferred objects that could be controlled or changed over objects that could not, and controllability was shown to be of greater interest than object complexity to the individuals

(Sambrook & Buchanan-Smith 1996, 1997). In laboratory experiments, Mineka et al. (1986) showed that infant rhesus macaques develop increased exploratory behavior and lowered fear responses in novel situations when raised in conditions in which they were exposed to controllable stimulation. Our research group at the California Regional Primate Research Center (see Markowitz & Timmel, this

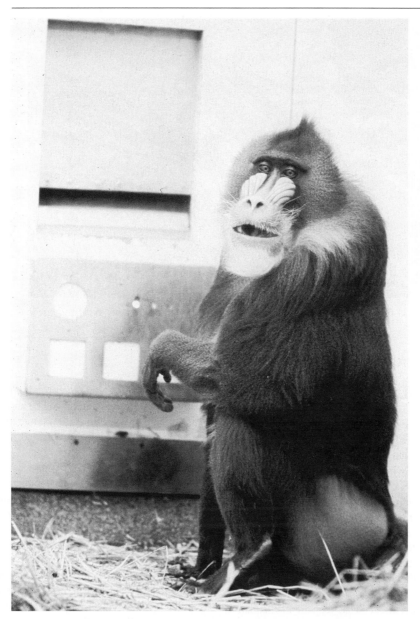

Figure 14.5. Mandrill inviting zoo visitors to compete with him in speed game.

volume) carried out research that indicated that providing primates even very limited control of their environments measurably reduced negative stress responses (Markowitz & Line 1989, Line et al. 1991). The ability to feed themselves food treats or to play music by touching a panel in their cage led to much shorter time in the primates returning to normal levels of heart rate and general activity following stresses such as being "squeezed" in their cages for medical procedures. More recently, laboratory studies of groups of chimpanzees (*Pan troglodytes*) challenged with stressful situations showed lower levels of visible tension (scratching) in the chimpanzees given control over videos and joystick-operated games than in chimpanzees that could see the screens but did not have control (Bloomsmith et al. 2000, Baker et al. 2001, Lambeth et al. 2001).

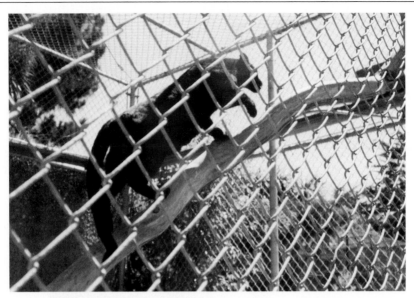

Figure 14.6. Black leopard pursuing acoustic prey in naturalistic manner in old zoo environment.

SOME THOUGHTS ABOUT THE FUTURE

Although the recent advent of powerful and inexpensive computers has greatly increased the chance for allowing animals truly active control of some aspects of their environments, we have been disappointed that only a few people and organizations responsible for animal care have responded to this opportunity. We recognize the limitations of budgets (cf., Markowitz & Timmel, this volume) and offer this last, more recent, example in the hope that it may stimulate others to use readily available technology to provide greater power to captive animals in their care.

Sabrina, a 16-year-old black leopard in the San Francisco Zoo, was provided with a way to actively forage for artificial prey in her home cage (Figure 14.6). She learned to actively pursue digitally recorded bird sounds controlled by a computer as they moved through her cage. After Sabrina chased the bird sounds up a large tree segment, bird parts (chicken) were delivered for her efforts at the end of the chase. Sabrina made very active use of this new opportunity, which resulted in an enhancement of her general activity and apparent well-being while reducing stereotypic behavior (Markowitz et al. 1995).

Thirty years ago, producing stimuli with this complexity and reliability might have cost at least ten thousand dollars for equipment and construction. Today, the major programming can be accomplished by simple computers costing a few hundred dollars at most. The use of acoustic stimuli and inexpensive motion detectors in work such as that described for Sabrina means that the cost of peripheral devices can also be kept within a reasonable range. Watching Sabrina's new behavior was wonderful and even inspiring to those of us who had the privilege to observe her. Like all cats, she chose to work when she wished, and if she felt like snoozing, she ignored the bird calls. Yet she was soon "capturing" all the prey offered in a day. Seeing her vigor in this hunt was amazing to us, considering her age, and her apparent joy in the hunt was a great reward for those who participated in providing her this opportunity.

We believe that we can do nothing more important for other animals than providing them active opportunity to control some parts of their existence.

REFERENCES

Baker K, Bloomsmith ML, Ross S, et al. 2001. Control vs. passive exposure to joystick-controlled computer tasks intended as enrichment for chimpanzees (*Pan troglodytes*). *Am J Primatol* 54(S1):64 (Abstract).

Bloomsmith MA, Lambeth SP, Perlman JE, et al. 2000. Control over videotape enrichment for socially housed chimpanzees. *Am J Primatol* 51(S1):44–45 (Abstract).

Erwin J, Deni R. 1979. Strangers in a strange land: Abnormal behaviors or abnormal environments? In: Erwin J, Maples TL, Mitchell G (eds), *Captivity and behavior: Primates in breeding colonies, laboratories, and zoos*. New York, Van Nostrand Reinhold:1–28.

Foster-Turley P, Markowitz H. 1982. Behavioral enrichment study: Small-clawed river otters. *Zoo Biol* 1:29–43.

Lambeth S, Bloomsmith M, Baker K, et al. 2001. Control over videotape enrichment for socially housed chimpanzees: Subsequent challenge tests. *Am J Primatol* 54(S1):62–63 (Abstract).

Line SW, Markowitz H, Morgan KN, et al. 1991. Effect of cage size and environmental enrichment on behavioral and physiological responses of rhesus macaques to the stress of daily events. In: Novak MA, Petto AJ (eds), *Through the looking glass. Issues of psychological well-being in captive nonhuman primates*. Washington, DC, American Psychological Association:160–179.

Markowitz H. 1976. New methods for increasing activity in zoo animals: Some results and proposals for the future. In: *Centennial Symposium of Science and Research,* Penrose Institute, Philadelphia Zoological Gardens. Topeka, KS, Hills Division Riviana Foods:151–162.

Markowitz H. 1982. *Behavioral enrichment in the zoo*. New York: Van Nostrand Reinhold.

Markowitz H, Aday C, Gavazzi A. 1995. Effectiveness of acoustic prey: Environmental enrichment for a captive African leopard (*Panthera pardus*). *Zoo Biol* 14:371–379.

Markowitz H, Line S. 1989. Primate research models and environmental enrichment. In: Segal EF (ed), *Housing, care and psychological well-being of captive and laboratory primates*. Park Ridge, NJ, Noyes Publications:202–212.

Markowitz H, Schmidt MJ, Moody A. 1978. Behavioural engineering and animal health in the zoo. *International Zoo Yearbook* 18:190–194.

Markowitz H, Stevens VJ (eds). 1978. *Behavior of captive wild animals*. Chicago: Nelson Hall.

Mineka S, Gunnar M, Champoux M. 1986. Control and early socioemotional development: Infant rhesus monkeys reared in controllable versus uncontrollable environments. *Child Dev* 57:1241–1256.

Preilowski B, Reger M, Engele H. 1988. Combining scientific experimentation with conventional housing, a pilot study with rhesus monkeys. *Am J Primatol* 14:223–234.

Quay H. 1959. The effect of verbal reinforcement on the recall of early memories. *J Abnorm Soc Psych* 59:254–257.

Sambrook TD, Buchanan-Smith HM. 1996. What makes novel objects enriching? A comparison of the qualities of control and complexity. *Laboratory Primate Newsletter* 35:1–3.

Sambrook TD, Buchanan-Smith HM. 1997. Control and complexity in novel object enrichment. *Anim Welfare* 6:207–216.

Schmidt MJ, Markowitz H. 1977. Behavioral engineering as an aid in the maintenance of healthy zoo animals. *J Am Vet Med Assoc* 171:966–969.

Yanofsky R, Markowitz H. 1978. Communication among captive talapoin monkeys (*Miopithecus talapoin*). *Folia Primatol* 18:244–255.

Zuk M. 2002. *Sexual selections: What we can and can't learn about sex from animals,* 1st ed. Berkeley: University of California Press.

15
Psychological Well-Being in Animals

Suzanne Hetts, Dan Estep, Amy R. Marder

PURPOSE OF THE CHAPTER

This chapter presents the concept of psychological well-being—what it is, what affects it, and how animal caregivers and veterinary professionals can help maximize well-being for the animals in their care. Psychological well-being and related concepts such as comfort, mental health, and behavioral welfare have been frequently used but not always clearly defined in the literature. Discrepancies among definitions are common and have led to confused thinking about these complex concepts. This chapter will discuss this confusion, present an overview of these issues, and offer a conceptual view of psychological well-being that animal caregivers can use to maximize the mental health of the animals in their care.

CONCEPTUAL ISSUES

As has been stressed in other chapters of this book, concern for the well-being of animals has mainly focused on the alleviation of suffering. Farmed animals, laboratory animals, and captive wild animals have been the major subjects of this concern, although the welfare of companion animals that might suffer as a result of neglect or cruelty has also been important. Only in the past few years has interest in the welfare of animals gone beyond suffering to consider the psychological wellness of animals, which includes positive concepts such as happiness, contentment, and comfort.

As animal behaviorists have learned more about the behavior and cognitive abilities of animals (see, for example, Griffin 1992 and Ristau 1991), they have found that many animals are psychologically more complex than previously believed. This complexity is reflected in an animal's psychological, behavioral, emotional, or cognitive needs. It is commonly assumed that if these needs are *not* met, well-

being is diminished and that if these needs *are* met, well-being is improved (Broom & Johnson 1993).

This chapter is concerned with these psychological needs and with the psychological wellness of animals, particularly companion animals. Our focus will be on how animal care providers can encourage and promote the positive aspects of well-being to increase the happiness, comfort, and contentment of companion animals and improve the human-animal relationship.

DEFINITIONS

Defining well-being, happiness, and comfort is difficult. Although most of us believe we have an intuitive understanding of these concepts, no consensus has yet been made on objective definitions that will allow their quantitative measurement. For many people, welfare and well-being are synonymous. Among the general public, welfare often means well-being, happiness, health, prosperity, comfort, or a state of faring well.

Duncan and Fraser (1997) provide one definition of welfare: "The 'welfare' of animals refers to their quality of life, and this involves many different elements such as health, happiness and longevity, to which different people attach different degrees of importance." Duncan and Fraser go on to point out the difficulties in defining the term: "One problem is that scientists have often tried to 'define' animal welfare as if it were a purely scientific concept. However, because our conception of animal welfare involves values as well as information, a conventional definition does little more than establish the general area of discourse."

Clark *et al.* (1997) echo these sentiments, saying, "Arriving at a universally acceptable definition of animal well-being is probably impossible because the way people define quality of nonhuman animal life depends on their personal experiences, views and values." Clark et al. (1997) and McMillan (2000) also see quality of life as equivalent to or very close to well-being.

Most scholars see well-being as existing on a continuum, varying from poor to very good. Well-being is not something an animal has or doesn't have, and it is not something that can be given to an animal. Most scholars also believe that the multiple factors influencing well-being are interactive and interrelated. A problem that is not often addressed in these definitions is the time frame for which well-being is specified. Is it over the entire life span of the animal, over a month, a day, or an hour? Clearly, well-being is a dynamic state and will vary over time, being better at some times than at others. Confusion arises when the time frame is not specified.

McMillan (2000) argues that quality of life is a direct function of affect; how the animal feels is the only relevant aspect of quality of life or well-being. This definition has limitations. For example, a dog with tapeworms may not show behavioral signs of not feeling well, but the parasite infestation is compromising his physical well-being.

Others scholars such as Broom and Johnson (1993) acknowledge that subjective feelings are important, but they argue that subjective feelings are not the only relevant aspects of welfare—health and behavior are also important independently. For purposes of this chapter, we will adopt the definition of Duncan and Fraser for welfare and consider quality of life and welfare as synonyms. We also recognize that the definitions we use in this chapter are influenced by our own experiences, views, and values, which are obviously different from others'.

Distinguishing between psychological and physical well-being is arbitrary in that all psychological events have a physical basis reflecting changes in the nervous system, hormones, and other bodily functions and structures. The psyche does not exist independently of the body.

Not all scholars make the distinction between psychological and physical well-being. However, by using the qualifier "psychological," we intend to emphasize the more cognitive and emotional aspects of welfare such as happiness, fear, thinking, and problem solving and to de-emphasize the more basic aspects concerned with survival, such as hunger, thirst, pain, and the provision of shelter.

McMillan (2002) states that "the central element in most descriptions of mental well-being is emotional pleasantness, or a balance between pleasant and unpleasant feelings (affect) over time in one's life." Poole (1992) expands on this, arguing that "psychological well-being is more than the absence of distress, it is a positive state of mental satisfaction resulting from the animal's psychological needs having been met." We see psychological and mental well-being as referring to the same thing.

NEEDS AND WELL-BEING

The idea of needs is central to notions of well-being. Needs are things that are required for normal functioning. When needs are not fulfilled to a significant degree, well-being declines. Needs are generally identified by examining the results of deprivation. If an animal is deprived of a necessity such as food, welfare is reduced.

Psychological needs are those that affect cognitive and emotional functioning. Needs are not the same as wants or desires. Wants and desires are things an animal would prefer to have but that are not necessary for normal functioning. A dog may want to sleep in the bed with his owners, but no evidence exists that this is necessary for normal functioning and that the dog's welfare is reduced by not fulfilling this desire.

Only in recent years has the notion of psychological needs of nonhuman animals been discussed. The literature includes references to both behavioral needs and psychological needs, but these appear to be similar if not identical to each other. Presently, no agreement exists about all of the psychological needs of any specific animal; too little is known about the behavior and psychology of most animals, and more research is needed to generate valid, reliable, and comprehensive lists of needs.

Serious attempts have been made to identify some needs in some animals. McMillan (2002) lists social companionship, mental stimulation, controllability and predictability in the environment, and skills for coping with stress and environmental challenges as emotional needs for animals. Poole's (1992) view of the behavioral needs of mammals includes stability and security in the environment, environmental complexity, some novelty and unpredictability, and opportunities to achieve goals and companionship. The list of behavioral needs of companion animals compiled by Hetts et al. (2004) includes provision of safe, comfortable places to sleep and rest; freedom from or ability to escape from unnecessary pain, fear, threats, or discomfort; ability to control some aspects of the environment; opportunities to express some species-typical behaviors such as chewing or scratching; opportunities for exercise and play; opportunities for mental stimulation; and opportunities for pleasant social contacts with conspecifics or people.

These lists overlap to a considerable degree. Some needs may be common to diverse groups of species, and others may be specific to individual species or even individuals within a species. These lists of needs are provisional and will undoubtedly change as behavior scientists learn more about the behavior and psychology of animals.

FACTORS THAT AFFECT PSYCHOLOGICAL WELL-BEING

Generally speaking, the factors that influence behavior are the same ones that influence mental or psychological states. This is because the major way psychological change is inferred is from behavioral change and because behavioral changes are assumed to be due, in part, to psychological changes.

GENETIC PREDISPOSITIONS

One important influence on psychological well-being is the genetic predisposition of the animal. Genetics influence all aspects of the animal from basic physiological processes such as production of hormones to cognitive and emotional states such as problem solving and fear.

A good example of the way that genetic predispositions can influence well-being is illustrated in the work of Murphree and colleagues (Murphree et al. 1967, Dykman et al. 1979). They selectively bred two lines of pointers, one for normal or stable behavior and the other for nervous or unstable behavior. In a very few generations, the dogs in the nervous line were much more fearful of people than those in the normal line.

From the descriptions of these animals when they were approached by people (e.g., freezing), it is likely that the fearful pointers had reduced well-being compared to their non-fearful counterparts. Mills et al. (1997) point out that genetic selection for traits that influence welfare, such as lack of fearfulness and adaptability to changing environments, may be a powerful way to improve the well-being of some animals. The disadvantages are that such changes will come slowly over many generations and that our ability and commitment to selectively breed based on these criteria on a wide scale don't yet exist (see also Rollin, this volume, Chapter 17).

ENVIRONMENTAL INFLUENCES

The environment is the other major influence on psychological well-being. The environment can exert its influences through early experiences, learning in later life, and immediate environmental stimuli.

Early Experiences

Prenatal influences on behavior have been demonstrated. In rodent species, pregnant females subjected to stressful experiences are more likely to produce reactive or emotional offspring, independent of genetic influences (Denenberg & Morton 1962, DeFries et al. 1967). During the canine neonatal period (birth to three weeks), puppies given a variety of environmental stimulation were more confident, exploratory, and socially dominant than unstimulated controls when tested later in novel situations (Fox 1978).

In mammals and birds, a sensitive period for socialization occurs soon after birth or hatching, during which time it is easiest for animals to develop social attachments to others (see review in McCune et al. 1995, Serpell & Jagoe 1995). In dogs, the sensitive period is between 3 and 12 weeks of age, and in cats, it is between 2 and 7 weeks of age. During this time, the young animal learns its social identity as well as which individuals it should treat as social partners. Exposure to conspecifics, people, or other species during this time predisposes the animal to form rewarding attachments to similar individuals later in life and reduces the likelihood of fearful or aggressive reactions to those types of animals.

Also around this age are sensitive periods for the acclimatization of animals to novel stimuli and for environmental enrichment (see McCune et al. 1995). Exposure at this time to the places, things, sights, and sounds an animal is likely to encounter as an adult can reduce fear of novel things later in life. Clearly, reducing fearfulness and increasing an animal's network of social companions will improve well-being. Exposure to specific enrichment activities may also improve cognitive abilities and well-being later in life.

Later Learning

Learning in later life can also influence well-being. Aversive experiences such as unpredictable punishment by people can lead to a pattern of learned helplessness that affects health, emotional and cognitive processes, and behavior, making it more difficult for the animal to learn and adapt in similar circumstances (Seligman 1975). In a similar way, encouraging and rewarding friendly behavior toward unfamiliar people can lead to consistent patterns of tolerance and friendly behavior in which fear and aggression are reduced and enjoyment or comfortable tolerance are increased.

Immediate Effect of Environmental Factors

Environments that do a poor job of meeting an animal's behavioral needs are likely to reduce psychological well-being because they are likely to produce conflict, pain, fear, frustration, boredom, discomfort, or physical illness. Environments that promote the behavioral needs of animals will likely improve the psychological well-being of animals by enabling animals to better cope with their environments, to be more comfortable, and to be happier. Many of the chapters in Appleby and Hughes (1997) and in the second part of this book describe environmental events that can influence well-being.

THE PROMOTION OF PSYCHOLOGICAL WELL-BEING IN ANIMALS

The question of primary importance to animal care professionals is how can we promote the psychological well-being of animals? Many other chapters in this book discuss the primary goals of recognizing, preventing, and reducing suffering.

Animal caregivers must also be able to recognize and promote the positive aspects of well-being. For our purposes, animal caregivers are all individuals who deliver care to animals—owners; breeders; veterinarians and their staffs; animal behavior consultants; trainers; groomers; and animal shelter, day care, and kennel staff as well as zoo, farm, and laboratory caretakers.

Elements of behavior wellness care, defined as "the planned attention to a pet's conduct, and the active integration of behavior wellness programs into the delivery of pet related services, including routine veterinary medical supervision" (Hetts et al. 2004), can be delivered by most if not all animal caregivers. Heinke and Hetts (2002), Hetts et al. (2004), and McMillan (2002) have urged the creation of animal mental wellness and behavioral wellness programs for implementation by caregivers.

Behavior wellness programs are "protocols, procedures, services and systems that: educate pet-owners and professionals about what constitutes the behaviorally healthy/well pet; promote behavioral wellness through positive proaction, behavior assessments, early intervention, and timely referrals; and decrease unrealistic human expectations and interpretations of pet behavior that lead to

neglect, euthanasia or relinquishment" (Hetts et al. 2004). These programs take a proactive, preventive approach to well-being that goes beyond the alleviation of suffering to maximize well-being.

When caregivers are focused on suffering, discomfort, inappropriate behavior, and other negative aspects of well-being, they are unlikely to think about promoting the positive aspects. The thinking goes something like "As long as the animal isn't suffering, I don't need to worry about him." If caregivers don't think about how to promote appropriate behavior, cognitive activities, and emotions, the animal's well-being will never be maximized.

Hetts et al. (2004) have outlined steps that veterinarians and their staff can take to prevent and minimize negative aspects of well-being and promote the positive aspects of well-being in companion animals. With some modifications, these steps can be adapted for use by all animal caregivers for companion and non-companion animals. We describe these steps below.

DEVELOPMENT AND PROMOTION OF CRITERIA FOR RECOGNIZING A PSYCHOLOGICALLY HEALTHY ANIMAL

To improve the quality of life for animals, we need goals or criteria by which to evaluate their psychological health. When we have those goals, caregivers can be educated to recognize them and then to take steps to try to meet them.

Hetts et al. (2004) have taken a step in this direction by providing a set of criteria for behaviorally healthy companion dogs and cats. Those criteria are listed in Table 15.1. Each criterion is accompanied by a brief summary ditected to caregivers for how they can mold these behavior patterns and, in so doing, meet many of the pet's behavioral needs. That list of needs is described in an earlier section of this chapter.

Some criteria describe behaviors that make the animals "good citizens," such as not being a danger to the community, eliminating in acceptable areas, and not vocalizing to excess. Companion animals are an important part of the social environment of people, at least in most Western countries. As such, their behavior must be compatible with the needs of people and should improve, not diminish, the well-being of the people they live with.

In fact, a proposed definition of behavior wellness is the condition or state of normal and acceptable pet conduct that enhances the human-animal bond and the pet's quality of life (Hetts et al. 2004). It could be argued that behaviors that create problems for the community ultimately diminish the

Table 15.1. Characteristics of Behaviorally Healthy Dogs and Cats

✔ Are affectionate without being "needy" or annoying. Spend quality time with your pet and behave in a trustworthy and predictable fashion so a strong bond of companionship develops between the two of you. A behaviorally healthy dog or cat can also amuse him- or herself without constantly demanding attention. Avoid reinforcing annoying, pestering behaviors.

✔ Are friendly toward, or at least tolerant of, both people (including children) and other members of their own species. Socialize your pet by letting him or her have many pleasant experiences with different types of people, places, and things. The importance of socializing cats is often overlooked. Avoid physical or painful punishments that can result in aggressive behavior.

✔ Are at ease during normal, everyday handling and interactions such as having feet wiped, nails trimmed, mouth opened, or being petted and touched anywhere on the body. Gradually accustom your pet to these procedures by using gentle techniques and lots of "good things" such as tidbits and toys. The behaviorally healthy pet will enjoy being touched and petted and will permit everyday handling and restraint.

✔ Can be left alone for reasonable time periods in the house or yard without becoming anxious or panicked. Gradually accustom your dog or cat to being alone. Start with short time periods of 10 minutes or so. It is not a good idea to adopt a new pet one day and leave for an entire work-day the next. If you use a crate for your dog, you must take the time to gradually acclimate him or her to it over several days or a week.

✔ Eliminate only in desired areas—a yard, on leash walks, or in a litterbox, depending on your living arrangements. Use appropriate housetraining procedures, which do not involve discipline or punishment, and give your dog sufficient opportunities and appropriate locations for elimination. Provide at least as many litterboxes as you have cats, and be sure their characteristics (location, type of litter, cleanliness) meet your cat's behavioral preferences.

✔ Are not overly fearful of normal, everyday events or new things. When startled, excited, or frightened, behaviorally healthy dogs and cats can calm down easily. To help prevent fear-related problems, this requires socialization, as mentioned previously, ideally beginning in puppy- or kittenhood. Behaviorally healthy cats and dogs aren't easily startled or frightened and calm down easily when they are startled.

✔ Can adapt to change with minimal problems. Help your pet be resilient in times of change through training and socialization.

✔ Play well with others, by not becoming uncontrollable or rough. They also play with their own toys and are not often destructive. Both dogs and cats need adequate exercise and opportunities for play. Encourage acceptable play behaviors such as fetch for dogs or chasing and pouncing on cat-friendly toys for cats. Do not encourage your pet to use your body parts as play toys by batting your pet around his or her face, enticing him or her to chase or nip your fingers, or allowing him or her to grab your ankles.

✔ Are not nuisances or dangerous to the community. They do not run loose in the neighborhood or threaten innocent people who come into their territory. Securely contain your pet on your property using humane methods, and do not tie your dog out.

✔ Readily relinquishes control of food, toys, and other objects. Teach your pet that giving up control of these items is a good thing to do because a reward will follow.

✔ Vocalize (bark, meow, etc.) when appropriate, but not to excess. Barking, meowing, and other vocalizations are normal communication behaviors for dogs and cats. Provide a quality environment so excessive vocalizing due to boredom, fear, anxiety, or other reasons does not occur.

In addition, <u>behaviorally healthy dogs</u>:

✔ Reliably respond when told to sit, down, come, or stay. Teach your dog these behaviors using humane training techniques based on positive reinforcement. Practice in many different situations, including when your dog is distracted by other things such as wanting to chase a squirrel, so your dog will perform these behaviors no matter where you are.

In addition, <u>behaviorally healthy cats</u>:

✔ Scratch only items provided for this purpose. Provide a number of scratching objects whose location, texture, and size meet your cat's behavioral needs.

well-being of the animal as well because such problem animals are often abused, neglected, or euthanized.

The criteria for behaviorally healthy companion dogs and cats will likely change as we learn more about the cognitive and emotional needs of companion animals and their behavior. These criteria will not necessarily be applicable to dogs and cats living in other settings such as research laboratories, nor will they be applicable to other animals such as farmed cattle, wild animals in zoos, or working horses. Different criteria may be needed for each species and may be partially dependent on the environment in which the animal lives. Those concerned with the care and well-being of animals should generate such criteria.

PROMOTION OF HELPFUL ATTITUDES, REALISTIC EXPECTATIONS, AND AN UNDERSTANDING OF BEHAVIORAL NEEDS

Many companion animals have behavior problems and diminished well-being because their owners know very little about the psychological and behavioral needs of their animals. This lack of understanding of their animals leads to unrealistic expectations and poor attitudes.

For example, many owners of companion dogs don't realize, or at least don't accept, that most dogs have a need to chew on things. This need for chewing is especially true of puppies. If the owners aren't aware of this need and aren't trying to meet it, the dog will find other outlets for chewing, such as shoes and table legs.

Without knowledge of this need, the owner will have the unrealistic expectation that the dog should never chew on things. Finally, the owner may believe the dog is chewing shoes and table legs out of spite or revenge for some perceived misstep by the owner. This in turn may lead the owner into unnecessary and unproductive punishment of the dog. All of this ultimately leads to diminishment of the dog's well-being and a diminishment of the relationship between the dog and the owner.

All animal caregivers should become knowledgeable about the psychological needs and species-typical behavior of the animals under their care. Caregivers should also assume attitudes that allow them to better meet the needs of animals under their care. Uncritical anthropomorphism such as assigning spite, revenge, and guilt as motivations for behavior, as in the above example, can in turn lead to inappropriate treatment and diminished animal well-being.

This knowledge about animal behavior and psychological needs can be gained through books, lectures at professional meetings, special seminars, and even telecourses that present the information. For veterinarians, information about animal behavior is often presented at veterinary conferences. Books such as those by Hetts (1999) and Overall (1997) provide some information, as do the telecourses on canine ethology offered by private businesses.[1]

THE ASSESSMENT OF PSYCHOLOGICAL HEALTH

Determining criteria for behavioral health and identifying the psychological needs of animals provides the basis by which psychological well-being of animals can be measured and evaluated. We think it is possible to develop objective measures for each of the criteria for psychological health. Without objective criteria for psychological health and regular assessments, caregivers will only take steps to improve the well-being of their animals when they are suffering.

Certainly such measures have been generated to measure human mental health. These measures for nonhuman animals will be based on observable behaviors such as measures of friendliness to people, physiological measures such as immune system functioning, or both. Within the range for each measure, categories can be defined that identify low, normal, and high functioning, much as is done now for physical wellness by measuring blood levels of circulating hormones and other compounds such as cholesterol.

The assessment of the psychological wellness of the animal at any time will depend on measuring many of these criteria. Assessment must also take into account individual differences among animals within a given population. For example, a given cat may not need or want regular contact with other cats. In fact, such contact may make the cat anxious and fearful and diminish his or her well-being. For this cat, a low tolerance for other cats may be normal, and having no contact with other cats may lead to the best well-being.

All caregivers of managed animals should be familiar with assessments of psychological health and, at some level, should be able to monitor and assess well-being. Hetts et al. (2004) urge general practice veterinarians to provide such assessments for their patients during every nonemergency visit. Assessments at regular intervals can detect changes in well-being and warn of declines in wellness.

Veterinarians are already familiar with the promotion of physical wellness, so it is natural for them to also be involved in promoting psychological wellness (see Jevring & Catanzaro 1999). Additionally, the regular contact that veterinarians have with companion animals and their owners puts them in a good position to provide these assessments.

With assessments in hand, caregivers can identify areas of psychological health that can be improved and identify warning signs of potential problems. These assessments give caregivers positive goals to improve their animals' behavioral health. The caregivers can then learn what steps are needed to improve psychological health.

For example, if a dog is being crated for 18 hours a day to prevent normal destructive chewing, the owner can be advised how and when to transition the dog to being crated less, how to provide appropriate chew objects, and about other means of preventing damage to household items, all of which result in improved well-being of the dog.

POSITIVE PROACTION PLANS TO PREVENT PROBLEMS

Experienced caregivers recognize that certain conditions or environmental changes put their animals at increased risk of behavioral problems and diminished wellness. For example, companion cats can have serious problems with inappropriate elimination and aggression to people when new cats are introduced to the household. Owners can be educated about positive steps they can take to prevent such problems. Hetts et al. (2004) list five principles that should be addressed in these proaction plans:

1. Elicit and reinforce appropriate behavior.
2. Prevent or minimize inappropriate behavior.
3. Provide for the behavioral needs of the animal.
4. Use the "take-away" (negative punishment) method to discourage inappropriate behavior.
5. Minimize the use of "discipline" (positive punishment) and use it correctly when it is used.

For example, when a new cat is introduced to resident companion cats, owners should reward friendly, tolerant behavior between the animals; separate animals to prevent fights and conflicts from developing when the cats cannot be supervised; provide sufficient "resource stations" to minimize competition between cats; provide each cat with human contact and mental stimulation during the initial separation from each other; separate cats and withdraw rewards when conflicts arise; and avoid physical punishment of the cats if conflicts develop.

Table 15.2. Behaviors and situations for which positive proaction plans should be developed for companion dogs and cats

- ➤ Elimination behavior
- ➤ Play behaviors
- ➤ Normal destructive behaviors (due to play, investigation, chewing, or teething)
- ➤ Barking
- ➤ Introduction of new pets to family, especially for children and resident pets
- ➤ Introduction of new pets to resident family pets
- ➤ Acclimation of dogs to being left alone
- ➤ Acclimation of pets to being handled and examined

From (Hetts et al. 2004).

Table 15.2 lists behaviors and situations for which positive proaction plans have been developed for companion dogs and cats.

Positive proaction plans should be created for all animals under human care for situations that frequently result in problems. For example, laboratory animal and zoo animal caregivers will need to handle their charges regularly and sometimes perform complex procedures on them. By developing proaction plans to train the animals to tolerate and cooperate with the handling and implementing the plans as soon as the animals are acquired, caregivers can prevent, minimize, or prevent *and* minimize distressing interactions for the animals; improve the well-being of the animals; and increase the efficiency and safety of the handling for the caregivers.

Many zoos and laboratories have protocols for training animals to handling, and some follow the general principles described here. Few, however, have comprehensive proaction plans that attend to all the major problem areas. The systematic attention to potential problem areas and the development of comprehensive proaction plans can improve the well-being of all animals under human care.

SOLUTIONS FOR PSYCHOLOGICAL AND BEHAVIOR PROBLEMS AS THEY DEVELOP OR PROVISION OF TIMELY REFERRALS

When psychological or behavior problems are identified by routine assessments or when a crisis exists, solutions should be provided as soon as practical. Many of the chapters in the second part of this book discuss the identification and modification of psychological and behavioral conditions in animals. Many of these problems produce immediate suffering for the animal, and that suffering should be relieved as soon as possible.

Some problems can be alleviated by making simple changes to the environment. For example, fighting among horses around feeding troughs can be reduced by increasing the number of feeding troughs available at one time. Some cat elimination problems can be alleviated by making changes to the litterbox itself, such as changing the quality of the litter, the location of the box, or the number of boxes available.

Identifying the causes of other problems, knowing how to resolve problems, or both may require input from professionals from various fields. Some problems require complex changes to the environment, behavior modification plans, medications, or any combination thereof. Many companion animal owners and, indeed, many general practice veterinarians, are not equipped to deal with such complex problems. In these cases, the caregivers should be referred to specialized resources to provide this help. Taking haphazard, "try this, try that" approaches to the problem can create frustration with the problem, can make the problem worse, and can reduce the welfare of the animal.

Veterinarians routinely interact with many categories of animal caregivers and are in an excellent position to help caregivers find referrals to animal behavior consultants. Lists of certified animal behavior consultants are available in North America through the Animal Behavior Society and the American College of Veterinary Behaviorists.

MANAGEMENT OF ANIMAL ENVIRONMENTS TO MEET PSYCHOLOGICAL NEEDS

Some environments clearly do a better job of meeting the psychological needs of animals than others. In the past, animal facilities were designed primarily to reduce disease transmission, improve efficiency, and provide for the comfort of employees. Attention to the needs of the animals, particularly the psychological needs, was usually a secondary consideration.

More recently, those designing and managing animal facilities have paid more attention to the psychological needs of animals. Zoos were among the first to address the psychological needs of animals and provide enrichments that go beyond the alleviation of suffering (see, for example, Shepherdson et al. 1998). Laboratories and farm animal facilities have followed (see the chapters on special populations in this book).

Only recently have the psychological needs of companion animals been considered by those designing and managing their facilities. The provision of cognitive enrichment, social contact, training, and exercise is being tried in some animal shelters (see Sternberg 2003). Kennels and doggie day care facilities are beginning to provide various kinds of enrichment such as social play periods and interactive toys for their charges. These interests are even filtering down to veterinary hospitals, breeding facilities, and private homes.

Some veterinary hospitals, for example, provide separate entrances and reception areas for cats and dogs to reduce fear among the animals. Owners are beginning to provide environmental enrichments for their indoor-only cats using methods such as puzzle boxes, access to windows, and climbing platforms.

Anyone caring for animals, even if only for a short time, should consider the psychological needs of the animals in the design and management of the facility. Hetts et al. (2004) describe ways that veterinary hospitals can take the needs of the animals into account when designing the facilities or interacting with the animals.

PROVISION OF SOCIALIZATION EXPERIENCES FOR ANIMALS

As discussed earlier, experiences early in life can have profound and long-lasting effects on many animals. Exposing young animals to pleasant experiences with a variety of animals, people, places, and novel stimuli can minimize fearfulness and aggression and allow the animal to cope more effectively with a variety of social and physical challenges later in life (McCune et al. 1995). Providing these socialization experiences can be an important way to improve the psychological well-being of animals. Not providing these experiences or allowing fear-provoking or pain-inducing experiences can diminish the well-being of animals.

Animal behavior consultants, dog trainers, and veterinarians have urged companion animal owners to provide early socialization experiences for their animals and have promoted puppy classes and kitten kindergartens as ways to achieve this. These classes can also be an important way to educate owners about the behavioral needs of their animals, how to recognize psychological wellness, and ways to promote psychological well-being. Some veterinary hospitals are offering socialization classes for puppies and kittens as a way to provide these experiences and educate clients (Seksel 1997).

Caregivers of companion animals are not the only ones concerned with socialization experiences. Zoo workers have promoted early socialization experiences as a way to facilitate the breeding and welfare of their animals (Watts & Meder 1996).

Socialization does not end with the termination of the sensitive period for the animal. Animals continue to be influenced by their social experiences and experiences with other aspects of their environments throughout their lives. The promotion of socialization experiences and formal classes should not stop at adolescence. Owners and other caregivers should be encouraged to continue socializing their animals throughout the animals' lives.

Socialization may be especially important for animals acquired as adults. Their history may not be known, and they may not have had good socialization experiences when younger. Socialization of older animals is not impossible, but it does require more time and effort to effect change. The sooner animals are socialized, the better. Owners of newly acquired adult companion animals should be encouraged to attend socialization classes and do other things to socialize their animals.

SELECTION OF THE ANIMAL TO FIT THE ENVIRONMENT

Matching an animal's needs to the environmental characteristics is a way to improve well-being. Wild and domestic animals have evolved to be better-adapted to some environments than others. The genetic constitution and the prior experiences of animals may allow them to cope more effectively and to have better well-being in some environments than in others.

Among companion animals, dog breeds such as the Pekinese may be better off in an apartment and with little regular exercise than will breeds with a great need for exercise, such as the Dalmatian. Providing pet selection counseling to people wanting to acquire an animal can help prevent mismatches that can diminish the welfare of the animal. Some veterinary hospitals, as well as many animal shelters, provide this service in one form or another. A number of books also provide information that can aid in pet selection (Tortora 1980, Hart & Hart 1988).

Other types of caregivers can attempt to match the animal to his or her environment to improve well-being. In choosing research animals, laboratories often take the species, breed, or individual characteristics of the animal into account. Their primary consideration is usually the suitability of the animal for the particular research problem, but welfare of the animal should also be a consideration. Government research laboratories have created socialization criteria for animal vendors to follow for the vendor to be an eligible animal provider (Weed 2003).

Our contention is that if more attention were paid to the fit of the animal to his environment, well-being of the animal would be improved. For example, a retriever that had been used to a great deal of exercise and was subsequently acquired from a shelter for a research project may have lower well-being in a small laboratory cage than would a purpose-bred Beagle that was adapted to confinement in small cages.

SUMMARY

The psychological well-being of animals has become a consideration for many animal caregivers and for the public at large. Scientific studies are helping identify the factors that influence well-being and how they exert their influences. Those studies are also helping us identify the psychological needs of animals and develop criteria for psychological health.

We've presented a number of ways in which the psychological well-being of animals under human care can be improved. Caregivers should be encouraged to take steps to improve the psychological well-being of their animals. Veterinarians can play an important role in encouraging the improvement of psychological wellness because other animal caregivers, whether owners, breeders, laboratory caregivers, or shelter workers, are likely to come into regular contact with a veterinarian, who is in a position to educate and encourage others. Hetts et al. (2004) describe how general-practice veterinarians can promote these aspects of behavioral wellness as part of their practices and in such a way as to benefit the animal, the pet owners, and the veterinary hospital itself.

NOTE

1. Fundamentals of Canine Behavior. Animal Behavior Associates, Inc.; Phone: 303-932-9095; Website: www.AnimalBehaviorAssociates.com

REFERENCES

Appleby MC, Hughes BO (eds). 1997. *Animal welfare*. New York: CAB International.

Broom DM, Johnson KG. 1993. *Stress and animal welfare.* New York: Chapman and Hall.

Clark JD, Rager DR, Calpin JP. 1997. Animal well-being. I. General considerations. *Lab Anim Sci* 47:564–570.

DeFries JC, Weir MW, Hegmann JP. 1967. Differential effects of prenatal maternal stress on offspring behavior in mice as a function of genotype and stress. *J Comp Physiol Psych* 63:332–334.

Denenberg VH, Morton JRC. 1962. Effects of environmental complexity and social groupings upon modification of emotional behavior. *J Comp Physiol Psych* 55:242–246.

Duncan IJH, Fraser D. 1997. Understanding animal welfare. In: Appleby MC, Hughes BO (eds), *Animal welfare.* New York, CAB International:19–31.

Dykman RA, Murphree OD, Reese WG. 1979. Familial anthropophobia in pointer dogs? *Arch Gen Psychiat* 36:988–993.

Fox MW. 1978. The dog: Its domestication and behavior. New York: Garland STPM Press.

Griffin DR. 1992. Animal minds. Chicago: University of Chicago Press.

Hart BL, Hart LA. 1988. The perfect puppy: How to choose your dog by its behavior. New York: W.H. Freeman.

Heinke ML, Hetts S. 2002. Behavior wellness programs can create safe, compassionate environment. DVM Newsmagazine May:32–35.

Hetts S. 1999. Pet behavior protocols: What to say, what to do, when to refer. Lakewood, CO: American Animal Hospital Association Press.

Hetts S, Heinke ML, Estep DQ. 2004. Behavior wellness concepts for general veterinary practice. *J Am Vet Med Assoc* 255:506–513.

Jevring C, Catanzaro TE (eds). 1999. Healthcare of the well pet. Philadelphia: W. B. Saunders.

McCune S, McPherson JA, Bradshaw JWS. 1995. Avoiding problems: The importance of socialization. In: Robinson I (ed), The Waltham book of human-animal interaction. Tarrytown, NY, Elsevier Science:71–86.

McMillan FD. 2000. Quality of life in animals. *J Am Vet Med Assoc* 216:1904–1910.

McMillan FD. 2002. Development of a mental wellness program for animals. *J Am Vet Med Assoc* 220:965–972.

Mills AD, Beilharz RG, Hocking PM. 1997. Genetic selection. In: Appleby MC, Hughes BO (eds), *Animal welfare.* New York, CAB International:219–231.

Murphree OD, Dykman RA, Peters JE. 1967. Genetically-determined abnormal behavior in dogs: Results of behavioral tests. *Cond Reflex* 2:199–205.

Overall KL. 1997. *Clinical behavioral medicine for small animals.* St. Louis, MO: Mosby.

Poole TB. 1992. The nature and evolution of behavioural needs in mammals. *Anim Welfare* 1:203–220.

Ristau CA. 1991. *Cognitive ethology: The minds of other animals.* Hillsdale, NJ: Lawrence Erlbaum.

Seksel K. 1997. Puppy socialization classes. *Vet Clin N Am-Small* 27:465–477.

Seligman ME. 1975. *Helplessness: On depression, development, and death.* San Francisco: W.H. Freeman.

Serpell J, Jagoe JA. 1995. Early experience and development of behaviour. In: Serpell J (ed), *The domestic dog: Its evolution, behaviour and interactions with people.* New York, Cambridge University Press:79–102.

Shepherdson DJ, Mellen JD, Hutchins M (eds). 1998. *Second nature: Environmental enrichment for captive animals.* Washington, DC: Smithsonian Institution Press.

Sternberg S. 2003. *Great dog adoptions: A guide for shelters.* Alameda, CA: Latham Foundation Press.

Tortora DF. 1980. *The right dog for you.* New York: Simon and Schuster.

Watts E, Meder A. 1996. Introduction and socialization techniques for primates. In: Kleiman DG, Allen ME, Thompson KV, et al. (eds), *Wild animals in captivity: Principles and techniques.* Chicago, IL, University of Chicago Press:67–77.

Weed J. 2003. Personal communication. Veterinary Resources Program, Office of Research Services, NIH, Washington, DC.

16

Do Animals Experience True Happiness?

Franklin D. McMillan

Happiness is the most obvious of psychological concepts and at the same probably the most elusive. Studies have shown that people, when asked, claim to have an intuitive understanding of what happiness is (Argyle 2001). But when it comes to defining happiness with precision, the task for science has proven to be exceedingly difficult. One of the biggest problems is that happiness is not the same for everyone. When people conceptualize happiness, some describe it as being in a state of joy or other pleasurable emotion, while others think of it as being satisfied with one's life overall (Argyle 2001). For the first 75 years or so of the twentieth century, researchers in human psychology focused their studies nearly exclusively on the pains and sufferings of the mind and devoted little to no attention to the positive emotions and feelings of life. This is not surprising in light of the fact that unpleasant feelings command more attention and urgency and that the individual under their influence wants to be rid of them. Probably as a result of this personal sense of urgency commanded by unpleasant feelings, the relief of distress and suffering was the priority for scientific study. Happiness was presumed to be a result of the successful alleviation of unpleasant emotions and feelings and hence did not warrant specific study. Research specifically designed to examine happiness and its contributing factors began in earnest in only the past quarter century.

For something of such monumental importance to human existence, it seems remarkable that happiness was not an object of serious study until so recently. Fortunately, despite its very belated start, this new field in human psychology has achieved rapid progress in just the past few years (Diener & Larson 1993), including numerous books (Myers 1992, Lykken 1999, Argyle 2001) and, at the tail end of the twentieth century, the first textbook devoted to the science of happiness: *Well-being: The Foundations of Hedonic Psychology* (Kahneman et al. 1999). But if we regard the study of human happiness to be in its infancy, we can safely say that the understanding of happiness in animals is at the blastula stage. Although positive influences on well-being have been discussed by animal scientists, the interest they have received is dwarfed by the attention directed at the unpleasant experiences such as fear, frustration, and "stress" (Mench 1998). Encouragingly, in recent years, discussions of welfare in animals have increasingly mentioned "pleasure" (Mench 1998). Among the problems of understanding happiness in all animals—human and nonhuman—is the question of how happiness can be measured. The very essence of the enterprise of science is measurement; if something cannot be quantified in some way, it eludes study, at least by the standard scientific method. For this reason, many researchers claim that scientifically studying consciousness is not possible—in any living being—for how can one measure consciousness? How can *any* mental state be measured in animals? Happiness presents such difficulties in this respect that it has caused psychologist David G. Myers (1992) to lament, "Oh, for a happiness thermometer."

THE TERMINOLOGY OF HAPPINESS

What is happiness? To answer this question, we must first address one of the main points of confusion inherent in terminology. Two common uses exist for the terms happy and happiness. The expression "I am happy" may refer to one's current mood or to one's assessment of life overall. As Davis (1981) has noted, "happy" has the same ambiguous meaning as "warm" does. "It is warm in Florida" may refer to today's weather report *or* to Florida's general climate. This ambiguity leads to such confusing semantics as that of a person in the throes of sadness upon hearing that his mother just died being able to say he is happy. He is, of course, referring to being happy in his overall life. Currently, no consensus exists among scientists and philosophers on the meanings of happy and happiness; however, it is important to recognize the distinction between the two uses of the term—the short-term state of feeling good and the long-term mood state referring to one's evaluation of life overall.

In this chapter, I will use the term *happy* to refer to the short-term experience of pleasant feelings of the present moment, such as the emotional states of joy, pleasure, enthusiasm, contentment, emotional warmth, positive mood, and the like. In this sense, "the dog feels (or is) happy" will mean that the dog is currently enjoying a pleasurable emotional state. I will use the term *happiness*, and, more specifically, *true happiness* (as it is often termed in humans), to refer to the long-term mood state associated with one's evaluative overview of life. This form of happiness is the degree to which one perceives his or her own life to be fulfilling, meaningful, and pleasant—the pervasive sense that life is good (Myers 1992, DeGrazia 1996).[1]

Because happiness is regarded to necessarily involve the evaluation of one's own life as a whole and because it is generally believed that no nonhuman animal has the mental capacity to form evaluative judgments about their lives as a whole, happiness in animals has never received serious consideration. Whereas abundant evidence now exists that animals can feel pleasure and be happy (Cabanac 1979, 1992, this volume; Cabanac & Johnson 1983; Balasko & Cabanac 1998), the issue of happiness has not been explored. The purpose of this chapter is to examine the evidence supporting the existence of true happiness in animals.

THE HAPPY ANIMAL

Before presenting the case for happiness in nonhuman species, let us look briefly at the happy animal. That animals can be happy does not establish that they also experience the complex mental state of true happiness. It is certainly reasonable, however, to conclude that a prerequisite to experiencing happiness is the capacity to experience the transient pleasures and joys of feeling happy.

The presence of pleasure and joy in conscious animals is supported most strongly by the evolutionary value of such feeling states. As DeGrazia (1996) has argued,

> If they [animals] can have unpleasant or aversive mental states, they are, by definition, conscious. Such mental states in these creatures are motivational; pain, discomfort, distress, fear, anxiety, and suffering motivate doing things that tend to make the unpleasant experiences stop. It is difficult to see how evolution might have conferred consciousness on these animals, provided them aversive states, provided human beings both aversive states and pleasurable ones, yet not provided nonhuman animals any capacity for pleasure. For pleasure, too, is motivating; we seek it, other things being equal.

In fact, all of the foundational criteria associated with pleasurable feelings in humans—evolutionary value, motivational function, associated behavior, neuroanatomy, and neurophysiology—appear to be present in all mammal species (Cabanac 1992).

All mammals—and in all likelihood birds and probably other animals—appear to be equipped with brain circuits that motivate them to behave in ways that make them *feel* good (Lykken 1999; Cabanac, this volume). In this way, the mammalian brain is considered to be wired such that certain behavior triggers the delivery of an internal reward—in the form of a pleasurable feeling. Evidence suggests that the evolution of this mental circuitry forged an association between behavior beneficial to one's own fitness and pleasant feelings, which appears to be an important mechanism for keeping conscious animals motivated to do things that promote survival and reproduction. In comparing the association of human behavior and affective experiences—particularly that of nonverbal infants—with the behavior of animals, it appears highly likely that all conscious animals are programmed to seek and repeat doing those things that feel good and to avoid things that feel bad.

Supporting this contention is a substantial body of research that has demonstrated the remarkable similarities of affective experiences in humans and animals. Michel Cabanac (Cabanac 1979, 1992, this volume; Cabanac & Johnson 1983) has pioneered research revealing that the response patterns of humans and animals to various pleasure-eliciting stimuli—such as taste and ambient temperature—are essentially identical. Response frequencies, expressions of preferences among stimuli, the weighing of pleasant against unpleasant stimuli, and the relative and contextual nature of pleasure all show substantial consistency across human and many nonhuman species. Human ratings of pleasure or displeasure can be altered by physiological and environmental factors; for example, the pleasure associated with sugar is relative and varies according to one's blood glucose concentration, and the pleasure associated with a cold drink varies with the ambient temperature (Cabanac 1979). The affective reaction of rats to taste can be altered by the same sets of physiological and psychological factors. The changes in the animal behavior match the changes in human behavior when the humans report experiencing pleasurable affect (Grill & Berridge 1985, Berridge 1996). Furthermore, the *pain detection threshold*—the smallest intensity of a noxious stimulus that humans experience as painful 50% of the time—and the *pain tolerance threshold*—the level of pain that can no longer be borne or tolerated by a subject—are essentially the same in humans and a variety of nonhuman vertebrate species, as indicated by avoidance or escape behavior (Hardy et al. 1952, Vierck 1976, DeGrazia & Rowan 1991, Lascelles 1996). Many psychotropic drugs such as anxiolytics and antidepressants show very similar effects in humans and animals (Dodman 1997). In studies of self-administration of drugs such as opioids, barbiturates, alcohol, cocaine, and caffeine, animals show patterns of drug use strikingly similar to the patterns exhibited by human users of the same agents (Schuster & Thompson 1969, Colpaert et al. 1980). Rats with arthritis learn to self-administer or self-select food or water containing analgesic drugs (Colpaert et al. 1980, 2001).

Support for the emotional experience of pleasure and joy in animals is vast and derives from numerous methods of study: experimental evidence (as cited above), ethological study of animals in their natural environments, and anecdotal observations. This extensive body of evidence has convincingly demonstrated that many of the sources of joy in humans (Izard 1977) have been described in animals, including play (Poole 1997, Houpt 1998, Siviy 1998), competition (Brown 1993), discovery (Butler 1953, Montgomery 1954), creativity (Pryor et al. 1969), eating and drinking (Cabanac & Johnson 1983, Balasko & Cabanac 1998), companionship (Coren 1994, Panksepp 1998, Herzing 2000), and recognition of familiar persons or animals (Poole 2000).

To the extent that animals experience subjective pleasure, and joy in particular, it appears overwhelmingly likely that animals can be happy. The emotional capacity to experience pleasures of the moment is vastly different than the cognitive capacity to form an emotional appraisal of how one's overall life is faring, however. Do animals experience this much-more complex state of true happiness? And how could we distinguish *true happiness* in animals from merely being transiently *happy*?

ANIMAL HAPPINESS

For sentient animals, emotions are a relatively constant experience, their feelings giving either a pleasant or unpleasant quality to just about all of one's waking moments, but happiness is not the emotion one feels at any particular moment. Happiness is a pervasive sense *over time* that all is well (Myers 1992), an evaluation of life *as a whole* (Averill & More 1993, Argyle 2001). Happiness transcends the emotional ups and downs of day to day living; it has an enduring effect that outlasts temporary sufferings in such a way that one can possess happiness even while presently experiencing unpleasant feelings, such as the example given earlier of the man whose mother died. Happiness may include episodes of joy and other pleasant emotions, but happiness is not equated with these, and in fact may include episodes of struggle, turmoil, and suffering (Averill & More 1993). Research on happiness in people has led to the widely agreed conclusion that happiness consists of three main components: *life satisfaction*, *positive affect*, and *negative affect* (Argyle 2001). It has been proposed that as constituents of happiness, joy is the emotional component, whereas satisfaction is the cognitive component representing a reflective appraisal—a judgment—of how well things are going—and have been going—in one's life (Argyle 2001)

Animal happiness—in the sense that the term is being used here—has never been defined. In humans, *happiness* is often equated to *subjective well-being* (Averill & More 2000, Argyle 2001). In the animal literature, scientists who write about animal well-being characteristically avoid mention of the term happiness. A major reason for this appears to be attributable to the common belief that animals live only in the present and experience only emotions of the moment (Clark et al. 1997b) and hence presumably lack the capacity to cognitively evaluate their lives as a whole. In fact, to date, this central aspect of human happiness has not been demonstrated in animals. Therefore, the argument goes, although capable of being happy (experiencing joy and pleasure), animals have no capacity for true happiness as experienced by humans. In scrutinizing this long-held belief, we will consider some of the important qualities of happiness as it is conceived by psychologists.

Studies in humans and animals have identified a psychological trait shared by many species, and seemingly present in all mammals, that allows them to adapt to wide-ranging changes in their environments (Lykken 1999, Argyle 2001). The brains of these species are constructed in such a way that the animals habituate to changes in the input processed by the nervous system. By making the mental impact of events impermanent, this trait of *adaptation* equips the animal with the ability to rebound in a relatively short time from the emotional highs and lows of life's events. This psychological mechanism ensures that the animal is not incapacitated from psychological trauma, prevents complacency in the event of sudden good fortune, and, overall, appears to ensure that the individual is able to effectively respond to the next challenge it encounters in life. Numerous studies have shown that in humans, it is unusual for any single event—good or bad—to create a lasting alteration of the individual's sense of well-being, a phenomenon that holds true even for the greatest extremes of tragedy and triumph (Suh et al. 1996, Lykken 1999). The death of a cherished companion or spouse, severely disabling and permanent injuries and illnesses such as paralysis, loss of vision, or the diagnosis of a progressive fatal disease—or, conversely, receiving a major promotion, highly esteemed honor, or coveted award; winning a major professional competition or tournament championship; and even winning multimillion dollar prizes in gambling ventures—all lead to extreme emotional lows and highs that, in time, usually recover to the prior level of happiness (Myers 1992, Lykken 1999, Argyle 2001). Lottery winners interviewed a year later generally report that the "high" of winning has faded away (Lykken 1999). Likewise, studies of people seriously injured in car accidents have found that less than a month after victims suffered paralyzing spinal cord injuries, their pre-injury levels of happiness had often returned (Myers 1992, Lykken 1999). As psychologist David Myers (1992) has written, "The point cannot be overstated: Every desirable experience—passionate love, a spiritual high, the pleasure of a new possession, the exhilaration of success—is transitory."

In animals, evidence exists to suggest that the transitory nature of emotional ups and downs also occurs. A study of dogs that had become paralyzed in their hind legs showed that their mental attitudes,

as judged by their owners, was as good three months after as before the paralysis in 85 percent of the animals (Bauer et al. 1992). Anecdotal reports also attest to the resiliency of moods in animals that have experienced severe trauma. Two stray Jack Russell terriers were found roaming the streets of Essex, England, together (Anonymous 1998). When they were found, one of the dogs had a sharp stick protruding from each eye socket. Both eyes were too severely damaged to regain sight and were enucleated. The two dogs were then adopted out to live together in the home of a kind and loving woman, who named the blind dog Ben and his friend, Bill. A year after the adoption, this woman told me in a telephone conversation that the blind dog's life has been full of boundless energy, play, and fun (Becher 1999). She stated that this dog never acts as if he's disabled and that she could not imagine him showing a higher level of happiness. Although we cannot know the dog's happiness level before his tragedy, we can reasonably conclude that because his subsequent happiness appeared to be so high, he had made a complete emotional recovery after his trauma. Clinical observations suggest that the loss of a companion can induce signs of grief (Dodman 1997) and depression (Overall 2002) in animals. As in humans, these emotional lows appear to fade with time, and the animal recovers to its level of emotional well-being that existed prior to the emotional event (Dodman 1997).

Current evidence suggests that for humans and at least some nonhuman species, a stability in the average emotional life of individuals exists that transcends the momentary fluctuations in mood. Life events produce upward and downward shifts in momentary affect, but when moods are averaged over several weeks or months, these shifts average out to reveal one's mean level of emotion (Diener & Larson 1984). This stability and relative constancy of one's level of happiness represents a concept that has been termed the *happiness set point* (Lykken 1999). Base happiness levels appear analogous to a temperature thermostat, which always tends to return to the set point prior to the time when outside forces act to change it. Furthermore, the set point level has a strong genetic influence and differs substantially between individuals; some people have a high set point (persons reporting a high level of happiness), and others have a low set point (persons with self-reported unhappiness) (Lykken 1999). The transient nature of emotional fluctuations in animals suggests the presence of a set point not dissimilar from that in human happiness.

As previously mentioned, happiness in humans has three main components: life satisfaction, positive affect, and negative affect (Argyle 2001). A vast body of research has provided extensive evidence supporting the existence of two of these factors—positive and negative affect—in animals (Panksepp 1998). Therefore, it appears that animals possess two of the three main components of happiness in people. Let us now look at the third component—satisfaction.

The satisfaction component is the cognitive part of happiness—a reflective appraisal, a judgment, of how well things are going and have been going in one's life as a whole (Argyle 2001). A number of elements are extremely important contributors to life satisfaction in people. Among the most important elements are active and challenging engagement in the world (as opposed to passive observation), fulfilling one's needs and goals, a sense of accomplishment, and, of possibly the greatest importance, a sense of control (Averill & More 1993, Mench 1998). Although we cannot currently gain direct information about life satisfaction in animals, we can examine the role and importance in nonhuman species of these contributors to human life satisfaction.

Active engagement in the world is an important element in human happiness (Averill & More 1993). Being passively stimulated without active involvement is associated with diminished well-being, and engaging the environment is related to a higher sense of well-being. Research has shown that when white rats are provided with various forms of sensory stimulation but are prevented from interacting with the stimuli, they develop smaller brains than those rats that can freely interact with their environments (Wemelsfelder 1993). Even high levels of mental stimulation and changes in the animal's environment may be of no benefit to emotional well-being if the animal is prevented from interacting with that environment. In animals (Wemelsfelder 1993) as well as people (Averill & More 1993), interaction and active engagement with the environment appears to be a prerequisite to positive subjective well-being. As an example, the cat confined to indoors who has a window to watch the birds and other activity outside—but without the ability to interact—may be experiencing no greater emotional fulfillment than the cat who does not have a window from which to gaze out.

All animal species—human and nonhuman—have *needs*. For all sentient animals, well-being is strongly related to the meeting of the individual's basic needs. For people, evaluations of life's events as positive or negative will depend to a large degree on how much those events meet the person's needs. If persons interpret events as successfully meeting their needs, they will react with pleasant emotions (Diener & Larsen 1993). Animals have needs relevant to their mental as well as physical well-beings, and meeting these needs is essential for an animal to experience a comfortable and satisfactory life (Clark et al. 1997a). As in humans, a large proportion of an animal's needs—physical and mental—appear to be represented in the form of affect. A large body of evidence supports the notion that for a vast array of needs, unpleasant affect signals to the animal that the need has not been fulfilled. The unpleasant feelings also appear to serve as a highly effective motivational force compelling the animal to fulfill the need. Examples of unmet needs and their associated affects include insufficient food intake and hunger, inadequate social companionship and feelings of isolation or loneliness, deficiency in body fluid levels and thirst, inadequate cover and hiding places and fear, and inadequate body heat and feelings of cold.

Needs are generally interpreted as requirements for normal function; basic needs must be satisfied for an animal to maintain a state of physical and psychological balance (Clark et al. 1997a). Therefore, need satisfaction, by lessening unpleasant affect, also lessens threat to life or well-being. Conversely, unmet needs cause the brain to continually deliver unpleasant affect to the animal.

Needs vary widely between species, sexes, age groups, and individuals; however, some basic needs appear to be fundamental to all sentient animals. A partial list of specific examples includes oxygen, water, complete and balanced nutrition, social companionship (for social animals), mental stimulation, play, hiding places, population density compatible with available resources, and a structured, orderly, and relatively peaceful society. Although nonhuman animal needs are likely not as cognitively complex as those of humans, all evidence supports that in animals, like in humans, the successful meeting of needs—and possibly goals—is rewarded with heightened emotional pleasantness and hence is a positive influence on happiness.

Happiness in humans is associated with a sense of *accomplishment*, or achievement, of activities well-performed, and doing productive work (Averill & More 2000). In many studies involving many species of animals, it has been shown that, given a choice, animals most often prefer to work for their food even if the same food is freely available (Anderson & Chamove 1984, Wemelsfelder 1990). When given the choice between two sources of food—for one, they can obtain food without any effort, for the other, they have to do work or perform some task—many mammals and some birds, such as chickens and ostriches, exhibit a preference for the food for which they have to work to obtain. Because in both of these cases, the known reward is the same (i.e., food), this suggests that an unseen reward is guiding the choice for work. A reasonable conclusion is that the work itself is a meaningful reward to the animal; the animals are enjoying work for the sake of the work itself, not unlike humans who enjoy and take pride in their work. Numerous animal trainers have commented that they believe many of the working animals they have trained—such as rescue dogs, guide dogs, and racehorses—appear to enjoy the work that they do. An anecdotal report of a unique incident at a marine aquarium offers another example of animals appearing to enjoy the performance of their jobs, or taking pleasure in accomplishment. Marine mammal veterinarian James McBain (1999) recounts the time he was called to the aquarium because the curator had noticed that many of the performing seals had not been eating their food for nearly two weeks. Despite the apparent lack of food intake, all the seals appeared healthy, had lost no weight, and still performed well in the shows. Suspecting that small ocean fish had been getting in through a break in the single wall separating the seals' pen from the ocean, a diver went into the pen to check for fish. What he found instead was a large hole in the wall that allowed the seals to freely move in and out of their pen into the ocean any time they desired. The seals had been going out to the ocean to feed but had not missed a show in two weeks. Eschewing the freedom that was fully available, the seals were apparently getting considerable enjoyment out of their daily performances.

A critical element in the happiness equation in people is the sense of *control* one has over his own circumstances and fate. The individual who perceives that he has no control over his life circumstances—that whatever he does is ineffective in changing his situation—frequently develops the devastating emotional states of helplessness and hopelessness. A sense of control over one's life is one of the strongest and dependable predictors of positive feelings of well-being yet identified in people (Myers 1992). When people gain more control over events in their lives, they enjoy improved

health and morale. Studies of nursing home residents and prisoners—groups traditionally given little control over their lives—have shown that when control is given, such as allowing the residents to arrange furniture to their liking or schedule their own activities, the people become more active, alert, and happy (Myers 1992).

In nonhuman animals, control has been shown to have a powerful influence on well-being and health (Seligman 1975, Peterson 1999). Animals raised in situations where they were given control over such things as access to water, feeding, and the amount of light in their habitats grew up to be more exploratory, self-confident, and less anxious than animals that received the same water, food, and lighting but had no control over these factors (Fox 1986). Some experimental evidence supports the contention that control is desired for its own sake. When white-footed mice were given control over certain aspects of their captive environment, they appeared to engage in a battle for control with the experimenters (Kavanau 1967). If the experimenters made the lights bright, the mice would dim them to darkness. If the experimenters made the room dark, the mice would turn the lights up bright. Prior testing to determine the animals' preferences in lighting levels showed that when they controlled the lights, their selection of light levels in reversing the experimenters' manipulations would be beyond the levels they originally showed a preference for. If the mice were awakened from sleep and emerged from their nest boxes, they would soon go back inside on their own; however, if the experimenters picked the mice up and placed them in the nest box, the mice would immediately come back out, even if they were placed repeatedly back in the box. The mice chose to exert control, even if it meant more work or having the lights at levels they did not normally prefer.

Control is an important method for coping with threatening stimuli. When an individual perceives that he possesses the ability to control—and, more specifically, to lessen—the unpleasantness of an aversive situation, the negative psychological impact of the situation is diminished. Control may simply involve escaping the unpleasant stimulus; numerous experiments have shown that the psychological and physical damage of a stressor is low when the stressor is escapable and high when inescapable (Visintainer et al. 1982, Laudenslager et al. 1983, Shavit et al. 1983). For animals and humans, the perception of an ability to control the intensity of unpleasant affect (such as fear, anxiety, pain, and isolation distress), that is, a belief in one's own ability to influence outcomes, is a consistent correlate of well-being (Peterson 1999). The key to this sense of control seems to be the knowledge that the subject can *turn off* the unpleasantness at any time he or she chooses. The sense that one has control, even if it is not exerted, is highly effective in reducing the harmful effects of physiologic and emotional stress.

Animals in the research laboratory or in the wild, and humans in oppressive conditions, often develop the emotional states of helplessness and hopelessness when they experience repeated traumas over which they have no control (Myers 1992)—likewise for companion animals subjected to ongoing physical or emotional (such as loneliness) neglect and abuse, which show very close parallels to the emotional consequences of maltreatment in children (Hobbs et al. 1993; Bremner et al. 1995; McCobb et al. 2001; McMillan, this volume, Chapter 12). These individuals learn that anything they do to improve their trying circumstances is unsuccessful, and they suffer paralysis of the will, passive resignation, and motionless apathy. This condition, termed *learned helplessness*, may then generalize to all aspects of the animal's life. After exposure to uncontrollable stressors and developing learned helplessness, animals have great difficulty coping with a wide variety of life's tasks, even the most routine, such as competing for food or avoiding social aggression (Seligman 1975).

The importance of control and helplessness for our examination of happiness encompasses more than the generally pleasant and unpleasant affect experienced, respectively, with and without control. It seems clear that the affective unpleasantness associated with the lack of control, especially in intensively aversive circumstances, is a major detractor from an individual's level of happiness. However, the concept of control also involves a cognitive aspect that suggests an evaluative view of one's life. Helplessness appears to distort the animal's thinking processes such that it causes the animal to perceive the world very differently than the normal animal in terms of what their behavior can accomplish. Helpless animals do not evaluate each challenge individually as hopeful or not hopeful—they appear to evaluate their situations *overall* as hopeless. They lose motivation and hope across the board as the mood pervades all other aspects of life from simple challenges to the enjoyment of life's pleasures. The sense of helplessness often generalizes even to settings where the animal again has control over its situation (Peterson 1999). The animals seem to have a view of *life*, not just the task at hand, as hopeless. As Sapolsky (1994) has interpreted the situation, it is as if the animal looks at its situation in life as "there is nothing I can do. Ever." Helplessness from the perception of having no control appears to have profound consequences for the animal's entire behavior pattern in life.

The hopelessness and despair of helplessness show substantial similarities to clinical depression in humans. Both helplessness and depression appear to be a mental state resulting from a lack of control over long-term unpleasant and aversive circumstances (Wemelsfelder 1990). Like depressed persons, helpless animals lose interest in normal joys in life such as eating and sex (Sapolsky 1994). Moreover, the treatments used for depression—antidepressants and electroshock therapy—speed the animals' recovery from the state of learned helplessness (Sapolsky 1994).

Several theories of human happiness propose that a person's happiness level is in part determined by comparisons that he or she makes with him- or herself against some standard (Michalos 1985, Argyle 2001). Often, peoples' standards come from observing people around them or remembering what they themselves were like in the past. In this way, *social comparison theory* says that people judge their own happiness not simply by viewing their own situation but on a relative basis according to the discrepancies between their situations and those of other people or those of their own pasts (Michalos 1985, 1986). Because it is this discrepancy, or gap, that is proposed to be a key determinant of happiness, these views are also known as *gap theories* (Wills 1981, Michalos 1986, Smith et al. 1989). It is hypothesized that if the comparison is favorable, happiness is facilitated; if the comparison is unfavorable, happiness is impaired (Michalos 1985). For example, a man with a family and home may be quite content. Then he meets up with a group of old high school classmates and learns that they have all achieved far more than he has in life—in their careers, financial holdings, marriages, and raising successful children—*and* were able to retire at a young age when he knows it will be many years before he can retire. The contentedness quickly gives way to a sense of disappointment, disillusionment, and failure. Or consider the factory worker who is quite satisfied with his job but then learns that all of his coworkers are earning twice as much for the same work. The person is now bitter, angry, resentful, and unhappy. In both cases, the individual at first has happiness and then becomes less content when his situation compares unfavorably with those of others. In each case, nothing about the individual's circumstances has changed—the only change was the newfound awareness of a gap. Other examples abound: the teenage girl who compares her own body with those of all the current fashion models, the prison inmate who compares his current situation with his earlier situation when he was free, and so on. Social comparison theory says that knowledge of a gap in conditions is a major determining factor in the individual's happiness.

Like happiness itself, social comparison (gap) theory has not been a subject of interest in animals. Recent research, however, has offered some enlightening new insights into the use of comparisons in animals.

In a study from the Yerkes National Primate Research Center involving brown capuchin monkeys, Brosnan and de Waal (2003) found that the primates responded negatively to unequal reward distribution in exchanges with a human experimenter, an effect amplified when a fellow monkey received a reward with no effort at all. The monkeys were first trained to exchange a granite token for a food treat. Testing the monkeys in pairs, the researchers then offered rewards of varying value to the monkeys in exchange for a token. Choosing the rewards according to prior tests of food desirability, the experimenters selected a piece of cucumber to be the lower-value food and a grape for the higher-value food. When both monkeys were given a cucumber slice in exchange for a token, they made the trade 95 percent of the time, but when the subject monkey observed the other monkey being given a grape for an equal effort (1 token), the rate of cooperation from the subject monkey declined to 60 percent. In addition, the cheated monkey would sometimes throw the token or make the exchange but refuse to eat the cucumber, and when the fellow monkey did not have to do anything to get a grape, the subject monkey made the exchange for the cucumber only 20 percent of the time. The rate of refusal to exchange increased as the experiment proceeded. The researchers determined that it was not simply the sight of a better treat that made the monkeys dissatisfied with a normally accepted food treat, as control studies in which the monkeys receiving the low-value reward could see the high-value reward with no other monkey present resulted in fewer refusals of the cucumber. This suggested to the researchers that the change in satisfaction was based on seeing a partner receive a more prized reward rather than on the mere sight of the reward.

The scientists concluded that capuchin monkeys, like humans (Andreoni & Brown 2002), apparently measure reward in relative terms, comparing their own rewards and efforts with those of others. They appear less satisfied with normally acceptable rewards if another individual receives a better reward.

The monkeys in this study showed behavior highly consistent with basic elements of social comparison theory, in which a person's satisfaction and happiness are partially determined by how his or her situation compares with that of others. The factory worker seeing his coworkers receive a larger reward for an equal amount of work can become less satisfied with a formerly acceptable reward. Furthermore, it is reasonable to presume that, like the capuchins, the factory worker merely seeing the bigger reward (e.g., seeing a pile of money sitting on the factory owner's desk) would not be expected to have the same negative effect on satisfaction as would seeing coworkers being handed that reward.

TRUE HAPPINESS

If, as is often proposed, animals think and experience emotions only of the moment, happiness as a life-as-a-whole concept would not be expected to exist in animals. The key determinant would appear to be whether animals have the ability to assess life satisfaction in a broad view as humans do. What is the evidence that true happiness exists in animals as a long-term mood state—different from the ups and downs of emotional experiences felt on a moment-to-moment basis?

An anecdotal case may provide some preliminary answers to this question. Billy is a four-year-old male Beagle dog patient of mine. Billy behaves in a way that would lead the casual observer to say he is a happy dog. When he greets people, he doesn't just wag his tail but wags the whole back end of his body. But he doesn't act happy when he greets just people—he greets other animals such as dogs, cats, birds, and horses in the same way. He acts happy when he's playing, when he's on a walk, when he goes to the dog park, and when he's going to see the veterinarian. He acts happy when he gets a treat as well as when he gets an injection. He acts happy when he gets dirty and when he gets a bath. He acts just plain happy. He has what we would call in humans a happy disposition.

The numerous theories of happiness in humans have not resolved the question as to whether people with Billy's disposition experience happiness because good things happen to them, or do they judge things around them as good *because* they have happiness? In other words, because we regard an evaluation of one's own life to be strongly correlated with happiness, is the evaluation the *cause* of one's happiness level or the *result*? Not surprisingly, research in people provides evidence for both. Billy offers an interesting insight into the potential for animal happiness. Assuming a canine cognitive ability to assess one's own life as a whole (an assumption to be discussed shortly), how would Billy evaluate his life? Favorably, we could safely presume. However, the direction of causation of this evaluative process would be as unclear in Billy as it can be in humans.

But Billy's case has a more instructive lesson to offer regarding animal happiness. Billy's personality appears to provide an example of the well-recognized general stability of human happiness levels—the happiness set point. As previously discussed, people seem to have a base level of happiness from which each moment's emotions and moods cause only temporary deviation; in time, the individual's level of happiness gravitates back to the base level. Billy has an emotional makeup that reveals what, if he were a person, would be a regarded as a high happiness set point. Billy's owner has described to me the deviations he shows from his normal emotional state. He has occasional ups (rare, seemingly because his mood appears already so positive) and has shown several depressed mood states, such as when he was ill. However, within a short time, Billy would always return to his happy-looking self. The earlier story of Ben, the blinded Jack Russell terrier, and the study of paralyzed dogs appears to demonstrate in animals an adaptation process with an eventual return to a happiness set point that is not appreciably different than that seen in people. The emotional states associated with the adversity appear to eventually dissipate, and the animal recovers to the prior baseline emotional level, which, as in humans, differs from one individual to another. This set point seems to be so reliable that once the basic temperament of the individual animal is known, we can predict with great precision the happiness level that the animal will return to when the current transitory emotional state fades. If animals experience only emotions of the moment and have no long-term happiness mood state, what is this highly predictable level that they are they returning to after the emotional change of adversity, or good fortune, subsides?

Forming an evaluation of one's life overall as satisfactory or unsatisfactory would appear to require the cognitive capacity to conceptualize the future and the past. If the common view of nonhuman animals as only living in the present is true, then it would seem that animals lack the mental faculty to form a concept of life as a whole. Do animals have the ability to evaluate their lives as an overall experience? One answer to this question may be found in a concept discussed earlier: control and helplessness. In the learned helplessness model, the animal that lacks the ability to control the intensity of unpleasantness of an aversive situation may lapse into a mental state of helplessness and hopelessness and give up, unable to cope with even the simple tasks of life. Notably, the states of helplessness and hopelessness that arise do not remain confined to any specific event; rather, these mood states generalize to and permeate all aspects of the animal's life. Learned helplessness and the accompanying hopelessness are not transient emotions of the moment; animals suffering from them act as though they are mired in a depressed mood state with some permanence that now exerts a broad detrimental influence on the animals' reactions to future events. Helplessness seems to be an evaluative view of one's life condition. It is a distorted cognitive appraisal of the world overall; it is the animal seeing the world as an impossibly difficult set of challenges. Behavioral responses suggest that the helpless animal assesses its life as so hopeless that it has no reason to make any attempt at improvement. The animal appears to be thinking, "I can't do anything to change my miserable situation, so I'm not even going to try." A reasonable interpretation of this mental process is that learned helplessness is a cognitive and affective mental state that, in contrast to other mental states, involves cognitive evaluations and emotional affect regarding one's life *overall*. That is, it involves a life judged *and felt* to be unsatisfactory as a whole.

Helplessness suggests that animals have the capacity to think and form feelings about aspects of their lives over time, not to be "locked" in the present. Most importantly, if *unpleasant* mood states like helplessness and hopelessness can incorporate a life-as-a-whole view, it would seem logical to conclude that such a life view would be found in *pleasurable* mood states such as happiness.

The study of capuchin monkeys discussed above offers good evidence for the use by nonhuman primates of comparisons between their situations and others', and the relativity of satisfaction based on the results of such a comparison. This study, however, was evaluating comparisons for single incidents and resulting in apparent emotions of the moment. Although this supports the existence in animals of the capacity to react with negative emotions when comparing unfavorably to others, an immediate emotional reaction may not be the same as long-term happiness states. We need to search for evidence of social comparisons in animals in which an unfavorable comparison reflects a judgment of and effect on life overall.

One approach to this quest is to look for evidence that animals seek not an immediate affective reward but a better *life*. Can an animal strive for a better life? By attempting to create, or acquire, a better life, the animal would appear to be making a comparative assessment of overall lives. How might such a change of life be recognizable? First, we would have to observe the animal taking some action that changes its life in a substantial way. Second, that action would have to have no immediate reward; that is, there would have to be no payoff other than the new life itself. If, for example, a dog that lives in a house where he is physically abused leaps the fence and runs away, the dog might have made a cognitive judgment that a life elsewhere would be more favorable than his current abused life, or the dog may just be fleeing the punishment and gaining immediate relief from the pain. That a possible immediate reward for the flight exists means that we cannot attribute the action to the more complex cognitive process of assessing one's life as a whole and choosing to improve it. The behavior that leads to a better overall life would need to have as its only objective a better overall life.

Many animal species (including, in diverse and often subtle ways, human beings) form a social structure in which social status is ranked by dominance relationships. Once called "pecking orders" because of the early studies with chickens, such rankings are now termed *dominance hierarchies*. Dominance hierarchies appear to exist in almost all but the most solitary species of birds and mammals, including species as diverse as elephant seals, lions, mice, gorillas, domestic fowl, marmosets, gibbons, muskrats, and red deer. These hierarchical systems establish structure in animal societies by enforcing social order and greatly minimizing confusion, turmoil, social instability, and violent confrontations. Dominant status in these hierarchies is associated with numerous advantages. As compared to subordinates, dominant individuals generally have more freedom to move about, control the attention of group members, have priority of access to food and high-quality resting spots, attract higher quality

mates and favorable grooming relationships, can suppress others' reproductive activities, and have greater resistance to stress and disease. With these extensive "perks," any subordinate animal that can achieve dominant status clearly acquires a new life—one of substantially higher quality. The way in which a subordinate animal acquires dominant status is what is relevant to the issue of happiness. In some cases, a subordinate seizes a dominant position left vacant by the death of a dominant individual; however, the most common method by which a subordinate moves up the ladder in the dominance hierarchy is for the subordinate to challenge the dominant individual to a contest. These contests typically involve aggression in the form of highly ritualized displays of strength rather than actual violence, the winner being determined more by show than fight. Animals sometimes compete as forcefully and aggressively for social rank as they do for other highly desired resources such as food or mates (Serpell & Jagoe 1995), suggesting a strong motivation underlying the pursuit and protection of dominant status.

The key issue is the reason for the challenge itself. The important questions include: What is the psychological motivation for the challenge? Considering the potentially extreme risks associated with challenging a dominant individual for his position, what does the challenger see as the *reward* for the challenge? What, if any, immediate reward is the challenger aware of when he initiates the challenge? From the dominant animal's point of view, why, when he is challenged, does he fight so hard to defend his dominant position?

These questions currently lack answers. No identifiable immediate reward to dominance challenges appears to exist. With no such payoff, no motivation is apparent for the challenge other than to obtain a better *life*. If no immediate reward truly exists, this phenomenon—challenges within the dominance hierarchy—suggests the presence of the cognitive capacity to judge one's own life as satisfactory or unsatisfactory as compared to another's life and to take action to improve it. The only recognizable reward is a better life, implying, at the minimum, a judgment of dissatisfaction with one's current life (or, in the case of defending a dominant position, a judgment of satisfaction). This phenomenon, consistent with the social comparison theories of human happiness, also appears strikingly similar to the situation for human beings who strive for a better life (Lykken 1999), whether through the furthering of one's education, seeking a professional promotion, getting a better job, pursuing fame or fortune, or seeking the power of elective office.

As previously mentioned, gap theories in humans may involve comparisons between one's current and past situations. To identify this process in animals, we must find a situation in which an animal's life has undergone substantial change. Marine biologist Carol Howard (1996) recounts the story of two dolphins that were captured, studied extensively in captivity, and then released back into the ocean. Being tame and socialized to humans, the now-free dolphins continued interacting with researchers when the researchers went out in their boats to study the dolphins. Howard and her group noticed that once the dolphins were again living in the wild, the things that in captivity had elicited the greatest signs of pleasure and joy—such as being rubbed by a person and playing with Frisbees and other toys—no longer elicited interest from the dolphins. It is reasonable to surmise that the life change caused a relative change in the emotional reactions of the animals to pleasure-inducing stimuli, possibly by raising the threshold of joy once life overall became much more satisfying. This would be comparable to the lonely person who gets enjoyment from watching television, but, when surrounded by new friends, activities, and a much more fulfilling life, finds television programs to be much less rewarding. In these situations, the relative nature of the enjoyment derived from an activity appears to reflect a change in the satisfaction and happiness level in one's life overall.

Collectively, the above studies and anecdotal observations offer substantial evidence that animals form life-as-a-whole evaluations. These evaluations are likely not as cognitively complex as those in humans, but they do appear to represent an assessment of life satisfaction. Evidence supporting a happiness set point that functions similarly in animals and humans, control and helplessness contributing to a cognitive appraisal of the degree of hope in one's life, and satisfaction levels relative to how one's own situation compares to others' (the social comparison or gap theories of happiness) collectively support the existence of true happiness in animals that bears a strong resemblance to that in humans.

THE CHALLENGES OF ANIMAL HAPPINESS

Animal happiness, as the term is being used here, has not been a subject of serious study. Certainly, confirming the existence of happiness in nonhuman animals is a formidable challenge. A first step would be the development by cognitive scientists and animal behaviorists of testable hypotheses regarding animal happiness.

No consensus yet exists for an accurate way to measure emotional health, psychological well-being, quality of life, or happiness in any animal. Whether assessments of these differently named concepts are actually measuring the same thing is yet to be determined, but until terminology of the various mental states are standardized, it is at least likely that research in one area will lead to progress in the others.

Considering the vast interspecies differences, it is unreasonable to expect that prescriptions for promoting happiness (or any related psychological states) will have broad applicability across the diversity of species in the animal kingdom. Different animals have vastly different needs, live in different habitats, have social or solitary lifestyles, and use different modes of locomotion. Vast individual differences exist in humans as to what contributes to happiness. Given the enormous differences of needs and desires in animals—not just interspecies variation, but individual variation—it is likely that a specific factor that might promote happiness in one animal may fail to benefit another and may even work oppositely and adversely affect happiness (Novak & Suomi 1988).

Every animal—dog, cat, horse, sheep, rat, whale, beaver, hippopotamus, and human—is an individual with a unique set of needs and desires. Every animal, by virtue of genetic endowment and unique learning experiences, has an emotional makeup that responds differently to life's events. Therefore, in the final analysis, happiness is a highly individual matter and should be addressed at the level of the individual animal.

NOTES

1. It is worth noting that, at present, no consensus exists as to how, or even if, happiness differs from *quality of life* in humans. The issue has not yet been addressed in animals (see McMillan, this volume, Chapter 13).

REFERENCES

Anderson J, Chamove A. 1984. Allowing captive primates to forage. In: Universities Federation for Animal Welfare (ed), *Standards in laboratory animal science*, Vol. 2. Potters Bar, UK, Universities Federation for Animal Welfare:253–256.

Andreoni J, Brown PM, Vesterlund L. 2002. What makes allocation fair? Some experimental evidence. *Game Econ Behav* 40:1–24.

Anonymous. 1998. Dog's best friend. *People* 8/24/98:80.

Argyle M. 2001. *The psychology of happiness*, 2nd ed. New York: Taylor & Francis.

Averill JR, More TA. 1993. Happiness. In: Lewis M, Haviland JM (eds), *Handbook of emotions*. New York, The Guilford Press:617-629.

Averill JR, More TA. 2000. Happiness. In: Lewis M, Haviland-Jones JM (eds), *Handbook of emotions*, 2nd ed. New York, The Guilford Press:663–676.

Balasko M, Cabanac M. 1998. Motivational conflict among water need, palatability, and cold discomfort in rats. *Physiol Behav* 65:35–41.

Bauer M, Glickman N, Glickman L, et al. 1992. Follow-up study of owner attitudes toward home care of paraplegic dogs. *J Am Vet Med Assoc* 200:1809–1816.

Becher L. 1999. Personal communication. Brighton, Sussex, England.

Berridge KC. 1996. Food reward: Brain substrates of wanting and liking. *Neurosci Biobehav R* 20:1–25.

Bremner JD, Randall P, Scott TM, et al. 1995. Deficits in short-term memory in adult survivors of childhood abuse. *Psychiat Res* 59:97–107.

Brosnan SF, de Waal FBM. 2003. Monkeys reject unequal pay. *Nature* 425:297–299.

Brown HH. 1993. Ever indomitable, Secretariat thunders across the ages. *New York Times*, May 30:23.

Butler RA. 1953. Discrimination learning by rhesus monkeys to visual-exploration motivation. *J Comp Physiol Psych* 46:95–98.

Cabanac M. 1979. Sensory pleasure. *Q Rev Biol* 52:1-29.

Cabanac M. 1992. Pleasure: The common currency. *J Theor Biol* 155:173–200.

Cabanac M, Johnson KG. 1983. Analysis of a conflict between palatability and cold exposure in rats. *Physiol Behav* 31:249–253.

Clark JD, Rager DR, Calpin JP. 1997a. Animal well-being I. General considerations. *Lab Anim Sci* 47:564–570.

Clark JD, Rager DR, Calpin JP. 1997b. Animal well-being II. Stress and distress. *Lab Anim Sci* 47:571–579.

Colpaert FC, de Witte P, Maroli AN. 1980. Self-administration of the analgesic suprofen in arthritic rats: Evidence of *Mycobacterium butyricum*-induced arthritis as an experimental model of chronic pain. *Life Sci* 27:921–928.

Colpaert FC, Tarayre JP, Alliaga M, et al. 2001. Opiate self-administration as a measure of chronic nociceptive pain in arthritic rats. *Pain* 91:33–34.

Coren S. 1994. *The intelligence of dogs*. New York: Free Press.

Davis W. 1981. Pleasure and happiness. *Philos Stud* 39:305–317.

DeGrazia D. 1996. *Taking animals seriously*. Cambridge, UK: Cambridge University Press.

DeGrazia D, Rowan A. 1991. Pain, suffering, and anxiety in animals and humans. *Theor Med* 12:193–211.

Diener E, Larson RJ. 1984. Temporal stability and cross-situational consistency of affective, behavioral, and cognitive responses. *J Pers Soc Psychol* 47:871–883.

Diener E, Larsen RJ. 1993. The experience of emotional well-being. In: Lewis M, Haviland JM (eds), *Handbook of emotions*. New York, The Guilford Press:405–415.

Dodman N. 1997. *The cat who cried for help: Attitudes, emotions, and the psychology of cats*. New York: Bantam Books.

Fox MW. 1986. *Laboratory animal husbandry: Ethology, welfare and experimental variables*. Albany: SUNY Press.

Grill HJ, Berridge KC. 1985. Taste reactivity as a measure of the neural control of palatability. In: Sprague JM, Epstein AN (eds), *Progress in psychobiology and psychological psychology*, Vol. 11. Orlando, FL, Academic Press:115–135.

Hardy JD, Wolff HG, Goodell H. 1952. *Pain sensation and reactions*. Baltimore, MD: Williams & Wilkins.

Herzing DL. 2000. The pleasure of their company. In: Bekoff M (ed), *The smile of a dolphin: Remarkable accounts of animal emotions*. New York, Discovery Books:116–117.

Hobbs CJ, Hanks HGI, Wynne JM. 1993. *Child abuse and neglect: A clinician's handbook*. Edinburgh, Scotland: Churchill Livingstone.

Houpt KA. 1998. *Domestic animal behavior for veterinarians and animals scientists*, 3rd ed. Ames: Iowa State University Press.

Howard CJ. 1996. *Dolphin chronicles*. New York: Bantam Books.

Izard CE. 1977. *Human emotions*. New York: Plenum Press.

Kahneman D, Diener E, Schwarz N (eds). 1999. *Well-being: The foundations of hedonic psychology*. New York: Russell Sage Foundation.

Kavanau JL. 1967. Behavior of captive white-footed mice. *Science* 155:1623–1639.

Lascelles BDX. 1996. Advances in the control of pain in animals. *Vet Annu* 36:1–15.

Laudenslager ML, Ryan SM, Drugan RC, et al.1983. Coping and immunosuppression: Inescapable but not escapable shock suppresses lymphocyte proliferation. *Science* 221:568–570.

Lykken D. 1999. *Happiness*. New York: Golden Books.

McBain JF. 1999. Cetaceans in captivity: A discussion of welfare. *J Am Vet Med Assoc* 214:1170–1174.

McCobb EC, Brown EA, Damiani K, et al. 2001. Thunderstorm phobia in dogs: An internet survey of 69 cases. *J Am Anim Hosp Assoc* 37:319–324.

Mench JA. 1998. Thirty years after Brambell: Whither animal welfare science? *J Appl Anim Welf Sci* 1:91–102.

Michalos AC. 1985. Multiple discrepancies theory (MDT). *Soc Indic Res* 16:347–413.

Michalos AC. 1986. Job satisfaction, marital satisfaction, and the quality of life. In: Andrews FM (ed), *Research of the quality of life*. Ann Arbor, University of Michigan Institute for Social Research:57–84

Montgomery KC. 1954. The role of exploratory drive in learning. *J Comp Physiol Psych* 47:60–64.

Myers DG. 1992. *The pursuit of happiness*. New York: Avon Books.

Novak MA, Suomi SJ. 1988. Psychological well-being of primates in captivity. *Am Psychol* 43:765–773.

Overall KL. 2002. Treating depression in a cat after it loses a companion. *Vet Med* 9:508–510.

Panksepp J. 1998. *Affective neuroscience: The foundations of human and animal emotions*. New York: Oxford University Press.

Peterson C. 1999. Personal control and well-being. In: Kahneman D, Diener E, Schwarz N (eds), *Well-being: The foundations of hedonic psychology*. New York, Russell Sage Foundation:288–301.

Poole J. 2000. Family reunions. In: Bekoff M (ed), *The smile of a dolphin: Remarkable accounts of animal emotions*. New York, Discovery Books:122–123.

Poole T. 1997. Happy animals make good science. *Lab Anim* 31:116–124.

Pryor KW, Haag R, O'Reilly J. 1969. The creative porpoise: Training for novel behavior. *J Exp Anal Behav* 12:653–661.

Sapolsky RM. 1994. *Why zebras don't get ulcers: A guide to stress, stress-related diseases, and coping*. New York: W.H. Freeman.

Schuster CR, Thompson T. 1969. Self administration of and behavioral dependence on drugs. *Annu Rev Pharmacolog* 9:483–502.

Seligman ME. 1975. *Helplessness: On depression, development, and death*. San Francisco: W. H. Freeman.

Serpell J, Jagoe JA. 1995. Early experience and the development of behaviour. In: Serpell J (ed), *The domestic dog: Its evolution, behaviour and interactions with people*. Cambridge, UK, Cambridge University Press:79–102.

Shavit Y, Ryan SM, Lewis JW, et al. 1983. Inescapable but not escapable stress alters immune function. *Physiologist* 26:A64.

Siviy SM. 1998. Neurobiological substrates of play behavior: Glimpses into the structure and function of mammalian playfulness. In: Bekoff M, Byers JA (eds), *Animal play: Evolutionary, comparative, and ecological perspectives*. Cambridge, UK, Cambridge University Press:221–242.

Smith RH, Diener E, Wedell DH. 1989. Intrapersonal and social comparison determinants of happiness: A range-frequency analysis. *J Pers Soc Psychol* 56:317–325.

Suh EM, Diener E, Fujita F. 1996. Events and subjective well-being: Only recent events matter. *J Pers Soc Psychol* 70:1091–1102.

Vierck CJ. 1976. Extrapolations from the pain research literature to problems of adequate veterinary care. *J Am Vet Med Assoc* 168:510–513.

Visintainer MA, Volpicelli JR, Seligman MEP. 1982. Tumor rejection in rats after inescapable or escapable shock. *Science* 216:437–439.

Wemelsfelder F. 1990. Boredom and laboratory animal welfare. In: Rollin BE, Kesel ML (eds), *The experimental animal in biomedical research*. Boca Raton, FL, CRC Press:243–272.

Wemelsfelder F. 1993. The concept of animal boredom and its relationship to stereotyped behaviour. In: Lawrence AB, Rushen J (eds), *Stereotypic animal behaviour*. Wallingford, England, CAB International:65–95.

Wills TA. 1981. Downward comparison principles in social psychology. *Psychol Bull* 90:245–271.

17
Animal Happiness:
A Philosophical View

Bernard E. Rollin

Reading the preceding chapter on animal happiness (McMillan, this volume, Chapter 16) did a good deal for my own happiness, not only in the momentary experiential sense that McMillan describes of feeling something like joy, but in the long-term, evaluative sense that comes in humans from reflection on one's life as a whole. The joy came from realizing that I was reading a superb piece of philosophical argumentation and analysis that eloquently codified many of my own ideas. Not only that, but the piece moved effortlessly from science to common sense and back again, with the author easily shifting from data to anecdote, something no scientist concerned with his or her reputation would have attempted 20 years ago (Rollin 1989). The more reflective happiness evoked in me was occasioned precisely by the degree to which McMillan's sort of discussion is credible today and the degree to which what I have called scientific ideology, a major impediment to understanding both animal ethics and animal consciousness, has been overcome.

Beginning almost 25 years ago, I sought to develop a theory of our moral obligations to animals, one that went well beyond the traditional ethic enjoining the avoidance of cruelty. In the course of my analysis, I was clearly required to develop some notion of animal welfare, how it is determined, and, correlatively, some notion of animal happiness. At that time, most people in animal-using industries, particularly agriculture, saw the concept of "welfare" in strictly physicalistic terms, as objectively determinate and determinable, and thus as unrelated to either value judgments or animal subjectivity. Consider, for example, the statement of the first CAST Report, tellingly entitled "Scientific Aspects of the Welfare of Food Animals," published in 1981:

The principle criteria used thus far as indexes of the welfare of animals in production systems have been rate of growth or production, efficiency of feed use, efficiency of reproduction, mortality and morbidity. (CAST 1981)

In other words, according to the animal science community, animal welfare can be objectively determined from animal performance in the above categories. If an animal performs successfully, it is assumed to be in a state of good welfare. Disease or "stress," which impede fulfilling these criteria, are sources of negative welfare. Donald Broom's definition of welfare as being assessable in terms of an animal's coping with the challenges of its environment represents a more modern (and more sophisticated) iteration of this physicalistic account of welfare (Broom 1986).

The attempt to articulate the concept of welfare in such terms represented a special case of what I have elsewhere termed "Scientific Ideology" or the "Common Sense of Science," a set of philosophical assumptions that underfunded scientific thinking in the twentieth century (Rollin 1989). Though the thinking underlying this ideology can be traced back to Newton's "I do not feign hypotheses," the establishment of empirical verifiability and elimination of untestable concepts as a way of demarcating science from other areas such as metaphysics and theology peaked in the late nineteenth and early twentieth centuries. Though this dictum functioned salubriously to eliminate a good deal of fluff from science—aether, absolute space and time, entelechies, life force—it unfortunately led to a great deal of mischief that has been extremely harmful to society's view of science. Two key components of this ideology were, first, the notion that science was "value-free" and thus made no value judgments in general nor ethical judgments in particular, and, second, that one could not talk sensibly in science of subjective states in animals. This in turn militated in favor of the traditional view of animal welfare as measured by objective criteria and forestalled thought that went beyond such measures.

It is now clear that to effect a proper analysis of animal welfare, and *a fortiori* of animal happiness, one needs both of the areas proscribed by Scientific Ideology. In my work (Rollin 1981) and the work of other scholars such as Ian Duncan (1981) and Marian Dawkins (1980) in the early 1980s, we demonstrated that welfare had everything to do with the animal's subjective experience. An animal could be highly productive in objective ways yet still be experiencing negative welfare because of the nature of its experience—boredom, fear, frustration of basic needs, etc. Unlike nonconscious beings, animals have interests, not just needs (cars have needs, but not interests). As I put it in 1981:

> What is the difference marked by these terms? Very simply, "interest" indicates that the need in question *matters* to the animal. In some sense, the animal must be capable of being aware that the thwarting of the need is a state to be avoided, something undesirable. Any animal, even man, is not explicitly conscious of all or probably even most of its needs. But what makes these needs interests is our ability to impute some conscious or mental life, however rudimentary, to the animal, wherein, to put it crudely, it seems to care when certain needs are not fulfilled. Few of us humans can consciously articulate all of our needs, but we can certainly know these needs are thwarted and met. Pain and pleasure are, of course, the obvious ways these facts come to consciousness, but they are not the only ones. Frustration, anxiety, malaise, listlessness, boredom, anger are among the multitude of indicators of unmet needs, needs that become interests in virtue of these states of consciousness. Thus, to say that a living thing has interests is to suggest that it has some sort of conscious awareness, however rudimentary. (Rollin 1981)

Thus, to put it simply, welfare cannot be separated from the way the animal experiences or feels the satisfaction or thwarting of its interests.

Though thinkers such as Duncan and Dawkins did yeoman service in forcing the animal science community to focus on what the animal experiences, further potentiated by 1985 federal law for animals in experimentation mandating the control

of pain and distress, scientific ideology continued to forestall a full analysis of animal welfare and happiness by shunning talk of the relevance of value judgments to these concepts. A moment's reflection on the concepts of welfare and happiness, however, reveals that they are conceptually bound up with value judgments in general and ethical judgments in particular. The concepts of welfare, like the concepts of health and happiness, admit of gradations.

The ethical question that thus arises is this—given a spectrum of animal feeling running from abject misery to total euphoria, at what point have we fulfilled our moral obligation to the animal? Suppose we are talking about a horse, whose interests include running, or a pig, whose interests include foraging. (Stolba and Wood-Gush demonstrated that under extensive conditions, sows would cover about a mile a day foraging [Wood-Gush & Stolba 1981].) Clearly, a horse would be better off (subjectively) given a vast pasture to gallop in, as opposed to a relatively small corral, in which he can nonetheless run in circles. Are we fulfilling our obligations with the corral? If pigs prefer woodland loam, do we fulfill our obligations by letting them forage in desert terrain? We can certainly identify the ideal and the unacceptable extremes, but deciding where an acceptable mean is requires a moral judgment based on balancing expense, terrain availability, management considerations, and the like.

A similar point holds of health, which is clearly part of welfare. If we take seriously the World Health Organization definition of health (for humans) as "a complete state of mental, physical, and social well-being," very few, if any, of us are fully healthy. Furthermore, social policy must decide what degree of health society *ought* to guarantee to its members. This is *a fortiori* true of animal health, in which the social use of the animals and society's view of their values determine what counts as health and acceptable degrees of pain and suffering allowed to go untreated in animals.

As I have shown elsewhere (Rollin 1983), what counts as worthy of being treated in animals is not only what science deems it to be, but what society considers significant. When the role and value of animals in society is overwhelmingly economic, symptoms, syndromes, discomfort or abnormality that have no apparent relevance to animal productivity, marketability, or other human uses do not become of concern medically. Conditions that are not cost-effective to treat lead to euthanasia, hence the ignoring of animal pain by science and veterinary medicine during most of the twentieth century

(Rollin 1989, 1997). The only time animal pain was implicitly recognized in science was when it served human ends, as when pain was induced in animals to test analgesics in humans. No one ever thought to worry about animal pain *per se* and its control, and it was common to deny animal pain's existence. Anesthesia was called "chemical restraint." Food animal veterinarians typically didn't (and still don't) worry about the pain associated with cattle castration, dehorning, branding or other procedures; such worry was not perceived as economically viable. Similarly, laboratory animal veterinarians did not worry about post-surgical pain in animals until society declared in two laws in 1985 that control of pain in laboratory animals was part of their job. As a result, the field saw more papers on analgesia in animals in the ensuing five years than in the previous one hundred.

In an agricultural context, and in the society in general to whom agriculturists are accountable, the role and value of animals are defined in terms of the animals' productivity and the prices for their products. In this valuational context, animal welfare (and its study) is restricted to what has an effect on production and price. This is graphically illustrated in a letter I once saw from a government agricultural official supporting the principle of establishing a chair in animal welfare at a university. The official wrote that he viewed the job of the chairholder to be "the development of definitive criteria in assessing the amount of stress that animals are undergoing and the compatibility of the stress with the animal's productive life."

To recapitulate: the traditional view of animal welfare was purely physicalistic, and animal happiness was not discussed. If pressed, proponents of that view would probably say that an animal that is productive is happy, equating happiness with welfare. A more sophisticated view places the focus of welfare in animal consciousness and would presumably equate happiness with the presence of positive mental states and the absence of negative ones in animals. A yet more sophisticated view acknowledges the presence of value judgments, particularly ethical judgments in animal welfare, and admits that such judgments are necessary even if one is talking about welfare in terms of animal experience.

I wish to defend this third view of welfare, and I hope to deduce an explication of animal happiness from it. Clearly, the meaning of welfare changes with development of social ethics for animals. In today's world, where the companion animal is the paradigm for all animals, the old production view of welfare is socially unacceptable, as is the rejection of animal feelings. Thus, welfare today must be cast in terms of consciousness, and animals experiencing pain, suffering, distress, loneliness, and boredom grows increasingly morally unacceptable.

In other writings, I have stressed the nature of the emerging social ethic for animals. In my view, as buttressed by our Western cultural history over the past three decades, society has moved well beyond the traditional concern for deliberate, sadistic, intentional, willful cruelty to animals to concern about all animal suffering whether it is the result of cruelty or decent, legitimate motives such as providing cheap and plentiful food or curing disease (which most people see as accounting for 99 percent of animal suffering). The vehicle that society is using for conceptualizing the controlling of such suffering is drawn from our ethic for humans and is applied *mutatis mutandis* to animals. In human ethics, we must balance the good of the group against the good of individuals. Taxing the wealthy, for example, or sending someone to war, is good for society as a whole but not for the individual. Although we make most of our social decisions by reference to the general welfare, we protect the human individual from the general welfare and the "tyranny of the majority." These protective fences, called *moral/legal rights*, are fences we build around fundamental aspects of human nature—speaking one's mind, believing what one wishes, not being tortured—encoded in the Bill of Rights and in additional protections deduced therefrom. The basic interests protected by rights are thus derived from a reasonable view of human nature or, to use Aristotle's phrase, *telos*. But animals, too, have *telos*, the "pigness of the pig," the "dogness of the dog," which generates interests for the animal as important to it as speech, religion, and holding on to one's property are to us. Because modern uses of animals, such as factory farming or research, often fail to respect such basic animal interests, society is increasingly demanding that the legal system protects animal *telos*. The Swedish law of 1988, demanding for food animals environments that suit their natures, is a paradigm case of the legalization of animal rights based on *telos*.

The concept of animal welfare, therefore, in today's moral world, rests on legally protecting animal *telos* from the negative experiences occasioned by its violation. Correlatively, animal happiness, at least as an ideal, is presumed to be allowing the animal to actualize the interests dictated by its *telos*, where thwarting of those interests causes some form of suffering. The *degree* to which those who use animals in various ways must respect *telos* is still evolving, hence the move from zoos as prisons 50 years ago to animal quarters that at least attempt to respect animal interests (cf. the 1985 Animal Welfare Act amendment mandating that quarters for nonhuman primates used in research must "promote [their] psychological well-being").

One more important point must be noted. Virtually no one denies that animal mentation is far less sophisticated than human—indeed, various versions of the Cartesian claim that animals are machines are still flourishing today. But the consensus seems to have emerged that animals experience morally relevant states of awareness such as pain, pleasure, fear, boredom, loneliness, anxiety, and so on. (Ordinary common sense never denied this, and science seems to be "reappropriating common sense," as I have elsewhere characterized the situation.) In the area we are discussing—animal happiness—the relative simplicity of animal awareness seems to lead to the conclusion that we can be more certain of animal happiness than we can of human happiness, despite the presence of language in humans. If we observe animals in ideal conditions, allowing them to fully actualize their *telos*, we would have a hard time denying that these animals are happy—well-fed dogs frolicking in the park; groups of horses let out into lush green pastures kicking up their heels. Human consciousness allows for an infinite series of reflexivity, creating unhappiness. I may have everything I need or desire and yet be unhappy because I don't think I deserve it or because I worry about what might change or because I have some sort of survivor's guilt. Woody Allen and *Seinfeld* have made fortunes capitalizing on this sort of neurosis. It seems clear that animals do not fret at the meta-levels that we do. We may be morally certain that the horse gamboling on lush pastures is not feeling guilty that he is doing well while other horses are starving somewhere across the world.

Everything we have said thus far is quite compatible with the analysis provided by McMillan in his earlier chapter and should be viewed as an augmentation thereof. The proliferation of veterinary specialties—as well as the money spent on veterinary services and making pets happy—eloquently attests to the emerging, ever-increasingly sophisticated social notion of animal health, welfare, and happiness.

One problem exists with my and McMillan's discussion that needs to be addressed, however, which interestingly enough has been cast into prominence by the emergence of genetic engineering. Let us raise the issue by examining a hypothetical scenario.

My premise is that given an animal's *telos*, and the interests that are constitutive thereof, one should not violate those interests. But this is not to say that it would be wrong to change the *telos* itself. If, by changing their natures, animals could be made happier, I can see no moral problem in changing their natures. The *telos* is not sacred; the interests that follow from the *telos* are sacred.

Suppose, through advances in genetic technology, we had the ability to change an animal's *telos*. Consider a case in which it might seem desirable to engineer such a change—laying hens kept in battery cages. It is well-established that hens housed this way are often unable to carry out certain motivated behaviors that are readily performed by chickens in natural (non-caged) settings. Foremost among these is nesting behavior, for which chickens have a strong need and drive. From studies done on this behavior, we know that blocking or otherwise frustrating this drive results in a mode of suffering. Now suppose we acquired the technology to identify the gene or genes that code for the drive to nest and ablate that gene or substitute a different, non-nesting gene in its place. This would create a new kind of chicken—one not motivated to nest and hence content with housing that prevents nesting. As I then ask in my book on the implications of the genetic engineering of animals:

> If we identify an animal's *telos* as being genetically based and environmentally expressed, we have now changed the chicken's *telos* so that the animal that is forced by us to live in a battery cage is satisfying more of its nature than is the animal that still has the gene coding for nesting. Have we done something morally wrong?
>
> I would argue that we have not. Recall that a key feature, perhaps *the* key feature, of the new ethic for animals I have described, is concern for preventing animal suffering and augmenting animal happiness, which I have argued involved satisfaction of *telos*. I have also argued that the primary, pressing concern is the former, the mitigating of suffering at human hands given the proliferation of suffering that has occurred in the twentieth century. I have also argued that suffering can be occasioned in many ways, from infliction of physical pain to prevention of satisfying basic drives. So when we engineer the new kind of chicken that prefers laying in a cage and we eliminate the nesting urge, we have removed

a source of suffering. Given the animal's changed *telos*, the new chicken is now suffering less than its predecessor and is thus closer to being happy, that is, satisfying the dictates of its nature. (Rollin 1995)

In fact, the logic of reflecting on the possibility of changing the *telos* led me to consider a more practicable possibility—a sort of *Brave New World* scenario for animals—wherein animals were kept happy by the use of drugs, despite cavalier disregard for satisfying their *telos*. The question that arises is this: Is anything morally wrong with changing or drugging chickens so that fulfillment of their *telos* ceased to matter to them, either because they had a new *telos* or because of their altered state of consciousness? If the key feature of happiness is subjective experience, and the animals' subjective experiences are highly—even maximally—positive, what have we done wrong? (Let us for the sake of argument assume that biotechnologically changing the chickens or drugging them does not produce any unanticipated harms [e.g., disease] for the animals.)

To be sure, as I have pointed out elsewhere (Rollin 1995), we would consider such a move monstrous with regard to humans because our moral tradition has as "ur-values" preservation of freedom and reason. But we seem to have nothing similar regarding animals; the history of domestication is essentially a history of modifying animals to be compatible with the uses and habitats to which we put them.

Since I published my notion that modifying the animals to ensure their happiness is acceptable, be it by pharmacological or biological means, I have received a variety of criticisms. One criticism that is fairly widespread is the following: To genetically engineer diminished chickens, or to dope them, is to degrade the species, or to fail to respect the species, or something of that sort. My response to that is simple: Species are not the sorts of things one has moral obligations to. One does not have moral duties to entities where what we do to them doesn't matter to them. Second, if one accepts the modern scientific view of species, one realizes that what we call species are stop-time snapshots of a dynamic process of evolution, not the fixed natural kinds stipulated by the Bible or Aristotle.

It makes no sense to speak of harming a species, except perhaps metaphorically. However, we do deplore the extinction of species. But such a locution bespeaks our concern that humans will never, for example, enjoy the beauty of a snow leopard or

extract medicine from a fern if the organisms go extinct. Or perhaps our concern deplores the state of affairs perpetrated on other extant animals or plants or the ecosystem when a keystone species goes extinct; for example, if key predators vanish, deer proliferate beyond the land's carrying capacity, and many animals starve to death. But I do not believe that we can use the same moral notions about species that we do about sentient individuals.

To put it another way, if we genetically engineer new chickens (chickens$_1$) that have a less varied *telos* than current chickens so that chickens will no longer suffer in the impoverished environments in which we insist on raising them, and will indeed be happy, we have not harmed the species of chicken, because the chickens do not know that they belong to a "degraded" species. The essential point is that the individual chickens are happy and are not suffering.

But the fact remains that we are undoubtedly made uncomfortable by the process of genetically engineering chickens$_1$ to replace chickens just because we choose to continue to apply industrial methods to agriculture and put productivity and efficiency above all else. If we are not harming the species, why do we feel queasy about such behavior?

A number of possible explanations exist as to why we find such cavalier tinkering problematic, besides confusing individuals and species as objects of moral concern. One such explanation comes from discomfort at lowering the river, as it were, rather than raising the bridge. After all, we raised chickens for thousands of years without depriving them of the opportunity to actualize their *telos*—only in the past 50 or so years have we deliberately chosen to supplant the values of stewardship and husbandry in agriculture with the industrial model stressing efficiency and productivity. Americans spend only 11 percent of their income on food—the lowest in the world. Surely we can afford to spend a bit more to raise animals properly. Traditional husbandry agriculture worked well for most of human history—confinement, industrialized agriculture has not worked well for most of its 50 year history, exacting tremendous costs in animal welfare, environmental despoliation, food safety, and survival of small farmers and rural communities. For all of these reasons, our instincts condemn changing the chickens when we are perfectly capable of changing the system. It is *stupid* to lower the river when you can raise the bridge.

However persuasive this argument is (and I myself am in fact persuaded by it!) it does not prove that it is wrong to change the chickens or drug them *if* we insist on producing chickens primarily for efficiency and productivity. Chickens who don't suffer under those kinds of conditions are surely morally preferable to ones that do.

A subtle twist on the previous argument can also shed some light on this issue. If we approach this question from the point of view of virtue ethics, it generates the following sort of musings: Do we really want to be the kind of people who lower rivers rather than raise bridges simply for an extra ounce of profit? More accurately, is it seemly that we use our intellect—or at least our technical capability—to cavalierly subvert what has been worked out in hundreds of years of natural and careful artificial selection? Does it fit our views of human nobility and dignity to so cavalierly savage nature? What of the sentiment expressed so magnificently by David Hartley when he affirmed of animals that

> We seem to be in the place of God to them, to be his Vice-regents, and empowered to receive homage from them in His name. And we are obliged by the same tenure to be their guardians and benefactors. (Hartley 1749)

This is not a stupid argument, nor is it a trivial one. It should give us pause when considering doing things like genetically engineering chickens$_1$ or drugging animals. But in the end, it does not suggest that we are wronging or harming the animals if we choose to take this route. Indeed, the issue it raises is that we degrade *ourselves*; the issue is that *we* fail to behave with nobility, not that we are causing harm or even behaving immorally toward the animals. (Compare the reaction of witnessing someone wantonly trampling wildflowers in some remote area never visited by humans.)

All of these points go some way toward explaining why we feel morally uncomfortable about drugging or biotechnologically changing chickens. They can be supplemented with some additional arguments. For example, perhaps the intuitive distaste that we feel for the prospect of altering the animals is not ethical revulsion but rather aesthetic horror. Many of us grew up to images of farm animals, including chickens running happily in a barnyard. (Most Americans still do not realize that farms have radically changed and become factories.) The notion that we have moved so far from the pastoral ideal that we seriously contemplate using drugs and biotechnology to make life tolerable for farm animals is aesthetically jarring.

A friend of mine told me of a Canadian swine producer who had a very profitable, highly intensive, industrialized operation. When his daughter was eight years old, he showed her the system for the first time. She burst into tears, as did my small son when he first saw cattle being transported in double-decker trucks, urinating and defecating on top of other animals. A similar reaction occurs even among adults when they experience confinement systems for the first time. What is going on is not the *squeamishness* one sees when people first visit a slaughterhouse; rather it is a jarring sense that this is not what a farm should look like.

Perhaps this explains our sense of wrongness in using technology to make the animals happy in confinement—it does not sit well aesthetically. The solution, in its own way, is as ugly as the problem.

Finally, I can see an Aristotelian/functional/teleological explanation to our resisting drugging the chickens or replacing them with chickens$_1$. Insofar as we do either of these manipulations, we are certainly respecting the chickens as sentient beings, in that we are alleviating suffering and producing happiness for them in the subjective sense. At the same time, however, we are not treating them ethically *qua* chickens, the unique life form with the unique *telos* we are confronting. To create chickens$_1$ is to fail to address the issue of how we treat chickens; it is rather to avoid the issue. We are, after all, not addressing the question of our responsibilities to chickens; we are rather deftly side-stepping that question by creating chickens$_1$, where there is no issue in raising them in confinement. Rather than respecting *telos*, we are disregarding it. Rather than engaging a moral issue created by our practice, we deftly divide it.

To summarize: None of the arguments we have adduced give us solid grounds for the belief that we are morally wronging the animals by genetically manipulating them or drugging them to fit the questionable environments we insist on keeping them in for the sake of profit and productivity. To be sure, we appear to be infringing on our own nobility and sense of the sort of people we feel we should be at our best by undertaking such manipulations, but that does not mean that we are wronging the creatures we manipulate. As artificial and unnecessary and crazy and disrespectful of history and husbandry our drugging chickens or recreating them biotechnologically may be, we are still creating animals that are happy in the fundamental sense of having positive experiences subjectively. Though we are callously simplifying the animals for our own selfish needs, this does not cause unhappiness to these animals. (It might do so if chickens, or rather chickens$_1$, were of sufficient intellect to realize that we have stopped them from being all that they can be, but of course they are not of sufficient intellect to grasp this truth.) In the end, all we have done is create creatures that are happy, rather than animals that are miserable, and it is surely better to raise happy animals than miserable ones.

In conclusion then, though we are intuitively repelled at creating diminished or drugged chickens to satisfy our insatiable craving for profit, it is difficult to criticize such a practice morally from the point of view of the animal's well-being, if by hypothesis we are creating in them an experience of happiness and satisfaction, however artificial and contrived this feeling may be. Such a practice may be ugly, ignoble, selfish, and so on, but we seem nonetheless forced to conclude that from the perspective of what the animal phenomenologically experiences and lives, we have done nothing wrong and have promoted animal happiness.

REFERENCES

Broom DM. 1986. Indicators of poor welfare. *Brit Vet J* 142:524–526.

CAST (Council for Agricultural Science and Technology). 1981. *Scientific aspects of the welfare of food animals.* Ames, IA: CAST.

Dawkins MS. 1980. *Animal suffering: The science of animal welfare.* London: Chapman and Hall.

Duncan IJH. 1981. Animal rights—animal welfare: A scientist's assessment. *Poultry Sci* 60:489–499.

Hartley D. 1749. *Observations on man, his frame, his duty and his expectations*, 2 Vols. Reprinted 1976. Delmar, NY: Scholars Facsimiles and Reprints.

Rollin BE. 1981. *Animal rights and human morality.* Buffalo, NY: Prometheus Books.

Rollin BE. 1983. The concept of illness in veterinary medicine. *J Am Vet Med Assoc* 182:122–125.

Rollin BE. 1989. *The unheeded cry: Animal consciousness, animal pain, and science*, 2nd ed. Ames: Iowa State University Press.

Rollin BE. 1995. *The frankenstein syndrome: Ethical and social issues in the genetic engineering of animals.* New York: Cambridge University Press.

Rollin BE. 1997. Pain and ideology in human and veterinary medicine. *Semin Vet Med Surg* 12:56–60.

Wood-Gush DGM, Stolba A. 1981. Behavior of pigs and the design of a new housing system. *Appl Anim Ethol* 8:583–585.

Part IV
Special Populations

18

Mental Well-Being in Farm Animals: How They Think and Feel

Temple Grandin

As a person with autism, I can provide a unique perspective on how an animal may perceive the world. Autism is a developmental disorder in which there is immature development in some parts of the brain with the visual parts developing normally (Bauman & Kemper 1994, Courschesne et al. 2001). Most people think in language, but I think in pictures instead of words. Some people have difficulty imagining how an animal would think or feel because they cannot escape from the way words shape their thoughts. The animal's world is a world without words. It is a world where thoughts would be images, smells, sounds, or touch sensations. Feelings would be associated with sensations instead of words.

In this chapter I am going to interweave the scientific literature and my own experiences with autism in a discussion of mental well-being in farm animals.

VISION AND HANDLING

Cattle, horses, pigs, sheep, and chickens are all species whose wild ancestors survived by being vigilant and avoiding predators. Vision is the dominant sense for spotting predators, and animals notice visual details that people will ignore. The attention of an animal is instantly attracted to things that move quickly and objects with high contrast. All animals are sensitive to rapid movement (Rogan & LeDoux 1996). Such motion makes prey species such as grazing animals run away and it induces predatory animals to chase. Controlling what a grazing animal sees when it is handled for procedures such as vaccinations can keep it calmer.

When cattle, sheep, or pigs are moved through a chute for veterinary procedures, they often balk and back up when they are driven toward an object that looks "out of place." A white paper cup on the floor of a chute or a shadow will make them stop. They may refuse to enter a chute if a small piece of chain is dangling down and moving at the entrance. Little visual details and distractions that people do not notice will attract an animal's attention. The lead animal will orient and point its eyes and ears at the swinging chain and look at the chain to determine if it is dangerous before moving forward. People handling animals often make the mistake of rushing the leader and not allowing him enough time to look at the chain or other distracting objects. The leader needs time to look to determine whether it is safe to move forward. After the leader walks past the moving chain, the other animals will usually follow. In large feedlots and slaughter plants, not enough time exists to allow cattle or pigs to inspect every puddle, sparkling reflection, or dangling chain. These distractions need to be identified and eliminated. Removing distractions such as dangling chains will improve animal movement through handling facilities. Simple changes in lighting can eliminate reflections that make animals balk (Grandin 1996). When the distractions that animals are afraid of are removed from a facility, the animals will move quickly and easily. It has been shown that high speed cattle slaughter plants that have removed distractions and have well-designed chutes can move 95 percent of the cattle without an electric prod. Until the distractions were removed, doing this would have been impossible. I was amazed that such simple changes in facilities could have such a great positive effect. This is the power of reducing fear by preventing the animals from seeing things that scare them.

In the 1970s, many cattlemen in Arizona thought I was crazy when I got inside the cattle chute to see why the cattle sometimes refused to move through a facility. Because I am a visual thinker it seemed a logical way for to me to see what the animals were seeing. This is when I discovered that they were afraid of shadows, dark places, shiny reflections, and seeing people moving around ahead.

In my work on improving how pigs and cattle were handled, both research and practical experience have shown that blocking an animal's vision with either solid fences on a chute or with a blindfold will calm animals (Grandin 1980, 2000; Andrade et al. 2001). In many slaughter plants, installation of a sheet of plywood to prevent animals from seeing moving people ahead reduced backing up and balking in the chute. A combination of high visual contrast and rapid movement will stop animals in the chute. At one plant, approaching animals could see people in white coats that contrasted greatly with the gray walls. Replacing white coats with dark blue coats, which reduced contrast with the gray concrete wall, improved animal movement. If a plant had white walls, however, white coats would be better. Animals may also refuse to walk over a drain or the point where a concrete floor changes to a metal floor.

All grazing animals have eyes on the sides of their heads, which gives them 360°-wide panoramic vision (Prince 1970). Contrary to popular belief, horses and cattle can see color (Gilbert & Arave 1986, Arave 1996). Cattle and sheep are dichromats and are partially color blind. They are most sensitive to yellowish green (553–555 nm) and blue-purple light (444–455 nm) (Jacobs et al. 1998). Having dichromatic vision is probably one reason that grazing animals are so sensitive to contrasts of light and dark colors.

Animals are very sensitive to small changes in illumination in a handling facility. They often refuse to enter a dark chute or a dark building. Adding lamps to light up the entrance will improve movement. Moving a lamp a few feet to eliminate a sparkling reflection on a wet floor will sometimes make it possible to almost eliminate the use of electric prods. The use of white translucent skylights to admit bright, shadow-free daylight will often improve cattle movement into buildings. The ideal illumination should look like a bright, cloudy day with no shadows.

In my work designing cattle handling facilities, I am frustrated because it is difficult to teach some people the importance of design features on equipment that has a strictly behavioral purpose (Grandin 2003). People in the metal shops that built a restrainer system I designed for slaughter plants thought they could improve the design by removing some metal panels. They could not see the need for the panels; to them, the panels were just extra metal. The purpose of the panels was to prevent the cattle from seeing things that scared them.

ANIMAL HEARING

Animals have much more sensitive ears than do people. Two studies have shown that being yelled at increases animals' heart rates and is highly aversive (Rushen et al. 1999, Waynert et al. 1999). I can closely relate to this sensitivity. When I was a child, the ringing school bell hurt my ears like a dentist drill hitting a nerve; sound sensitivity is a common symptom for people with autism. It is likely that loud noises hurt an animal's ears. Animals will remain calmer when people are quiet. Grazing animals can hear much higher frequencies than people. People are most sensitive at 1000–3000 hz, and cattle are most sensitive at 8000 hz (Ames 1974, Heffner & Heffner 1983). A high-pitched intermittent sound will cause an animal to react more than will a steady sound (Talling et al. 1998). The cattle most likely to become agitated and run into fences in an auction ring were the sound-sensitive individuals that flinched when people yelled or waved their arms (Lanier et al. 2000). High-pitched sounds will increase a pig's heart rate more than will low-pitched sounds (Talling et al. 1998). In my work with handling equipment, I have observed that systems designed to reduce noise, especially high-pitched whining noises, will keep animals calmer. I believe that ventilation fans in animal houses should be designed to reduce high-pitched sounds.

An agitated cow in an auction ring probably feels like an autistic child in a large supermarket. The noise and the stimuli may be overwhelming. It would be like being inside the speaker at a rock concert. To the animals, the sound volume of the auctioneer and the frantic activity of the ring men taking bids would be as loud as a jackhammer would be to humans.

I can also relate to why intermittent high-pitched sounds are disturbing. It is very difficult for me to sleep if I hear high-pitched intermittent noise such as a backup alarm on a dump truck. Every time it beeps, my heart rate increases. I know that the truck will not harm me, but the old anti-predator circuits in my brain are setting off alarms (Grandin 1995). I speculate that my brain reacts to certain sounds more like that of a nonhuman than a human brain.

SENSE OF TOUCH

In my work with cattle I have designed systems for holding animals during regular and kosher slaughter. The big mistake that many people make when they restrain an animal is to squeeze it tighter and tighter when it struggles, simply applying more and more force. My personal experiences with autism helped give me insight into how to restrain animals and keep them calm. Children with autism often seek deep pressure by wrapping themselves in blankets or getting under a pile of cushions. I used to do this to calm my nervous system. Light touches from people set off a panic response, and I would pull away when people hugged me because the stimulation was too overwhelming. I was like a wild horse jerking away when I was touched.

While visiting my aunt's ranch, I observed that some cattle would appear to relax when they were put in a squeeze chute for vaccinating. A squeeze chute applies pressure to both sides of the animal's body by two large, flat metal panels. Due to defects in my nervous system, I had the hyped up flightiness of a wild deer and was desperate for relief from constant panic attacks. I got in the squeeze chute and found that the pressure calmed me. At first I tried to pull away from it in a panic, and then a wave of relaxation set in. To calm myself, I built a padded squeeze chute for human use in which I could control the pressure to relax myself (Grandin 1995).

From my own experiences and observations of cattle and other animals, I have developed four behavioral principles of restraint that are most supportive of mental well-being. They are (1) blocking vision, (2) applying optimal pressure, (3) making slow, steady movement, no jerky sudden movement, and (4) do not trigger the righting reflex "fear of falling." Blocking vision has been discussed. Optimal pressure is very important. An animal must be held tightly enough so that it gets a feeling of restraint but not so tightly that it hurts. Restraint devices that apply even pressure to a large area of the body are best. Deep pressure is calming, but tickle touches may cause an alerting alarm reaction. Therapists who work with autistic children have observed the same response to pressure and touching (Ayres 1975). Pinch points or sharp edges will cause vocalization or struggling. When an animal is being held by either a device or a person, no sudden jerky motion should occur. I have observed that sudden jerky motion scares the animals and will cause them to resist. Principle 4 is very important. If an animal gets off balance and gets the sensation that it will fall, it will often struggle. Nonslip flooring is essential to prevent slipping that can cause panic. Restraint devices that hold an animal with its feet off the floor must fully support the body in a balanced upright position. More information on restraint devices has been described by Grandin (1992, 1994, 2000, 2003), Hutching (1993), Matthews (2000), and Panepinto (1983). When small animals are held in a person's hands, the animal's body should be supported. Veterinarians who work with puppies have learned to hold them so that they do not struggle. The principle is to release pressure when the animal relaxes and to gently increase pressure when it resists. This method has been explained by Gates (2003).

SENSE OF SMELL

I am often asked if animals are afraid of the slaughter and smells at a slaughter plant. This might intuitively seem to be the case; however, I have observed that cattle and pigs moving up a chute at slaughter plants behave exactly the same when they are moved through a chute on the farm for truck loading or vaccinations (Grandin 2001). With specific regard to the smells, it is known that any strange new smell will make animals stop. Paint sprayed on a chute will stop cattle movement. In kosher plants, I have observed hundreds of cattle calmly walking into a restrainer that is covered with blood. Visual contrast appears to have a greater effect on their behaviors than does the mere sight or smell of blood. In fact, animals may refuse to walk over a portion of the floor where blood has been wiped off and the silver floor has been exposed. Because of the effect of visual contrast, a silver spot against a red background attracts their attention.

Blood or other secretions from a stressed animal *does* have an effect, however. During startups of new equipment, I have observed that if an animal got stuck in the equipment for 10–15 minutes, the next animals in line would refuse to enter. Research indicated that cattle and pigs would often refuse to enter an area where an animal had been highly stressed for 15–20 minutes (Vicville-Thomas & Signoret 1992, Boissy et al. 1998). The stress substance apparently takes several minutes to be secreted. An experiment with rats indicated that blood from stressed animals was avoided (Stevens & Gerzog-Thomas 1977). The appearance of avoidance behavior follows the same time interval as release of cortisol. A review of the literature by Grandin (1997a) indicated that cortisol secretion during handling on the farm was similar to handling at the slaughter plant.

Could calm behavior be due to learned helplessness? This is a condition in which an animal under uncontrollable aversive conditions gives up (Seligman 1975). It is not learned helplessness because at both places the animal sometimes makes active attempts to jump fences. Active attempts to escape occur more often when cattle are shocked with electric prods. The way people handle the cattle has a much greater effect on their behavior than does the location where handling occurs.

THE FEAR FACTOR

Veterinarians, animal scientists, and industry people often like to use the vague word "stress." The word "fear" is often avoided. When a steer in a slaughter plant refuses to move on seeing a shiny reflection, the emotion would be fear. Numerous studies by Paul Hemsworth and his colleagues have shown that pigs and dairy cattle that fear people are less productive (Hemsworth & Coleman 1998). Pigs and cattle treated in an aversive manner such as being slapped or shocked will have lower productivity. Dairy cows that had been treated in an aversive manner had larger flight zones and lower milk production (Hemsworth et al. 2002). Voisinet et al. (1997) found that cattle that became highly agitated in squeeze chutes had lower weight gains, and Fell et al. (1999) reported that cattle that run fast out of squeeze chutes gain less weight.

Reducing an animal's fearfulness during handling and transport is an easy thing to do and requires no expensive equipment. During a 30-year career as a designer of livestock handling equipment, I have observed that people are often much more willing to make an expensive investment in equipment rather than learn behaviorally based, low stress animal handling methods. Animal handling has improved greatly during the past 10 years, but there are still some people who continue to yell at animals and frequently use electric prods. Why do they continue to do this when both research and practical experience show that it costs money? I speculate that this may be partly because of verbal, language-based thinking. In addition, it is difficult for many people to comprehend that what the animal experiences is important. I have observed that highly verbal people who have poor visual skills are often the ones who have the most difficulty understanding how an animal may think or feel. It is hard for them to imagine that the animal feels fear in a manner similar to people. Research shows very clearly that the brain circuits that control fear are very similar in people and animals (LeDoux 1996, Rogan & LeDoux 1996).

FEAR CIRCUITS IN THE BRAIN

Fear is a universal emotion in the animal kingdom (Boissy 1995, LeDoux 1996). Fear motivates animals to avoid predators and survive in the wild. All mammals and birds can be conditioned to fear things that are perceived as dangerous. The amygdala is the location of the central fear system involved in both fear behavior and learning to fear certain things or people (Davis 1992). In humans, electrical stimulation of the amygdala elicits feelings of fear (Gloor et al. 1981). Stimulating the amygdala in the animal brain elicits nervous system responses similar to fear responses in humans (Redgate & Faringer 1973). Destroying the amygdala will block both unconditioned (unlearned) and conditioned (learned) fear responses (LeDoux 1996, Rogan & LeDoux 1996). An example of an unlearned fear response would be a horse being spooked at the sound of a firecracker. A learned fear response has occurred if the horse refuses to enter the place where the firecracker went off. Lesioning of the amygdala also had a taming effect on wild rats (Kemble et al. 1984). Fear learning takes place in a subcortical pathway; extinguishing a learned fear response is difficult because it requires the animal to suppress the fear memory via an active learning process. A single, very frightening or painful event can produce a strong learned fear response, but eliminating this fear response is much more difficult (LeDoux 1996). Animals may develop fear memories that are difficult to eliminate.

GOOD FIRST EXPERIENCES ARE IMPORTANT

My observations on cattle ranches have shown that to prevent cattle and sheep from becoming averse to and fearful of a new squeeze chute or corral system, painful or frightening procedures that cause visible signs of agitation should be avoided the first time the animals enter the facility (Grandin 1997a). It is important that an animal's first experience with a new corral, trailer, or restraining chute be pleasant in nature. Practical experience has shown that if a horse has a frightening or painful experience the first time he goes into a trailer, it may make teaching him to get in a trailer difficult. This happens because he has developed a fear memory. First experiences with new things make a big impression on animals. When an animal is first brought in to a new farm or laboratory, its first experiences should be made pleasant by feeding it and giving it time to settle down. Nonslip flooring is essential because slipping and falling in the new facility may create a fear memory.

SENSORY-BASED ANIMAL FEAR MEMORIES

Because I think in pictures rather than language, my autism allows me to closely relate to how an animal may think or feel (Grandin 1995, 1997b). Many practical experiences with animals indicate that fear memories are stored as pictures or sounds. Fear memories are often very specific. I observed a horse that was afraid of black cowboy hats because he had been abused by a person wearing a black cowboy hat. White cowboy hats and baseball caps had no effect on this horse. The black hat was most threatening when it was on a person's head and somewhat less threatening when it was on the ground.

Animals that had been darted by the zoo veterinarian were able to recognize his voice, and they would run and hide. Ranchers have learned, however, that fearful cattle will often quiet down when they hear the voice of a familiar person who is associated with previous positive experiences. Animals have the ability to recognize the voices of individual people. Their auditory memories are hyperspecific.

Research on animal perception indicates that cattle are able to differentiate between "good" and "bad" people. At a zoo an elephant with a fear of bearded men became aggressive toward a new keeper who had a beard. The new keeper was accepted after he shaved off the beard. Animals have a tendency to associate bad experiences with prominent visual features on people such as beards or lab coats, or they may associate a scary or painful experience with a specific place. Pigs and cattle can recognize a person by the color of their clothing (Koba & Tanida 1999, Rybarczyk et al. 2003) and can also learn that some places are safe and others are scary and bad. Cattle can learn that a certain person is scary or dangerous when he is in a certain place (Rushen et al. 1999). For example, the animal may see the person as bad only when that person is in the milking parlor because he gave injections there.

It is also possible for an animal to associate a painful or scary experience with a prominent feature in the environment. In one case, a young stallion fell down and was whipped during his first attempt to mount a dummy for semen collection. He developed a fear of overhead garage doors because he had been looking at one when he fell. A future collection was done easily when it was done outdoors away from buildings and garage doors. Unfortunately, a fear of something as common and unavoidable as garage doors creates problems when a horse is ridden.

Sometimes, problems with bucking or rearing in horses can be stopped by changing the type of bridle or saddle because the horse has a fear memory associated with the feeling of certain equipment. A different bridle or saddle feels different. In this case, the fear memory may be a "touch" picture. For example, if a horse was abused with a jointed snaffle bit, he may tolerate hackamore or a standard one-piece western bit. One horse had a sound fear memory because he had a bad experience with a canvas tarp; horse blankets that sounded like a tarp were scary, but a wool blanket that made little sound was well tolerated.

Animal fears can generalize. A common generalization is that men are a threat to be avoided and women are safe. Fear of a man in blue coveralls will generalize to other people wearing blue coveralls. I was once asked how a fear memory can be a specific visual image if it can spread and generalize. I observed an example of both generalization and specificity in a dog. Red Dog was afraid of hot air balloons because one flew over the house and its burner roared. Red Dog's fear then spread to round plastic balls on electric lines. A few months later when she was riding in a car, she became afraid of the round rear end of a tanker truck and a round street light. I was puzzled why other round objects such as traffic lights and round globe lights on a building were tolerated. I finally figured out that the dog had made a very specific generalization. Round objects with the sky as a background had become feared because the original hot air balloon was a round object against the sky. The globe lights on the building had a brown brick background, and the traffic lights were mounted on a black metal rectangle; therefore, they were not round objects with a sky background.

HANDLING TRAINING

Training animals to handling procedures can greatly reduce agitation and make animal handling easier (Hutson 1985). When an animal becomes accustomed to a procedure, fear will be reduced. Pigs will become easier to handle and transport if they become accustomed to people walking through their pens (Grandin 1993). In my work, I have found that getting pigs accustomed to people walking among them makes it possible to greatly reduce electric prod use. Electric prods are highly detrimental to pig welfare (Benjamin et al. 2001). Pigs that have been walked in the aisles during finishing are easier to handle (Geverink et al. 1998). Moving pigs a month prior to slaughter improved their willingness to move (Abbott et al. 1997).

Australian researchers have found that walking quietly among calves produced calmer adult cows (Binstead 1977, Fordyce 1987, Fordyce et al. 1988). During the training, the animals were walked through the corrals and chutes and taught to follow a lead horseman. Becker and Lobato (1997) also found that handling zebu cross calves produced calmer adults.

Even adult animals can be trained to move through chutes and to voluntarily enter a restrainer device (Grandin 1989b) for blood tests or injections. Bongo antelope that had been trained to voluntarily enter a box for blood testing had almost baseline cortisol levels (Phillips et al. 1998). The antelope that had been immobilized with a dart had significantly higher glucose levels than trained animals (Phillips et al. 1998). Training the animal to cooperate reduces both physiological and behavioral indicators of stress.

THE PARADOX OF NOVELTY

Animals become highly fearful when something new is suddenly introduced, but that same object may be attractive if the animal is allowed to voluntarily approach it. For example, cattle will run away from a flag that is suddenly waved at them but will approach it and investigate the same flag if it is put out in a pasture. New things are both scary and attractive (Grandin & Deesing 1998). To prevent a fear of new things, handlers should gradually expose animals to many different people and vehicles. This will help prevent panic when the animals are taken to new places. Working with sheep, Reid and Mills (1962) were the first researchers to suggest that animals could become accustomed to variations in their routine. I have observed that cattle differentiate between a person on a horse and a person walking on the ground. Cattle that have been handled exclusively by people on horseback may panic if they are suddenly confronted with a person on the ground. It is important to train cattle that both people walking on the ground and people on horses are safe. Because cattle are visual thinkers, people on horses and people on the ground are perceived as different things. New things should be introduced gradually in a nonthreatening manner. If animals are gradually exposed to a wide variety of new things, new experiences are less likely to elicit fear. An animal's thinking can be remarkably specific.

Producers have observed that playing a radio in the barn will help produce pigs that are less likely to startle at every small sound. Providing pigs in a bar-ren environment with objects to chew and manipulate produced calmer animals that were less easily startled (Grandin et al. 1987). It is best to have a variety of music and talk. However, it is important to not subject the animal to noise overload.

THE NEED FOR NOVELTY

Many farm animals are reared in environments where little stimulation and novelty exist. As mentioned, novelty is feared when it is suddenly introduced, but animals will actively seek new things to investigate and manipulate. Varied environmental stimulation is beneficial to nervous system development. Walsh and Cummins (1975), Melzack and Burns (1965), and Schultz (1965) all concluded that when the variety of stimuli is reduced, the nervous system becomes sensitized and sensory thresholds become lower. This would explain why pigs reared on a concrete floor will startle more easily than pigs reared on straw. Melzack and Burns (1965) learned years ago that rearing puppies in barren kennels produced dogs that still showed signs of hyperexcitability in their adulthoods. The changes in the nervous system remained permanent even after the dogs had been returned to a farm family environment. In my doctoral research, I found that pigs reared in barren pens were more excitable and had abnormal dendritic growth of neurons in the brain as compared to pigs reared on straw with a variety of objects to manipulate (Grandin 1989a). Pigs in the barren pens spent significantly more time rubbing their noses on the floor and on each other as compared to pigs in the straw pens. This excessive rubbing resulted in an abnormal growth of extra dendrites on the neurons of the somotosensory cortex. I had to use video cameras to observe the abnormal nosing activity, as most of the behavior occurred at night when nobody was around to observe. When people entered the room, the pigs housed in the barren pens became hyperexcited.

The pigs in the barren pens were both highly fearful and high in novelty-seeking as compared to my straw-bedded pigs. During the first few days of pen washing, the pigs in the barren pens were afraid of the hose. After a few days they changed from being fearful to hyperactively seeking novelty. They would continuously bite at the water and the hose. When I cleaned feeders, the barren-environment pigs repeatedly bit my hands, whereas the straw-bedded pigs could be easily moved away. They were not attracted to chewing on hands because they had straw to chew on.

Regrettably, I saw that my attitude toward the two groups of pigs differed even though they were litter-mate pairs. While I enjoyed working with the calm, straw-bedded pigs, I disliked working with the bar-ren environment pigs that constantly bit at the hose and at my hands. The latter pigs were starving for stimulation and were also the first pigs to start jumping in fear when they heard a plane fly over the building.

WHAT DO ANIMALS PERFORMING STEREOTYPIES EXPERIENCE?

Drawing on my autistic experience, I would like to speculate on what the pigs are experiencing when they engage in repeated belly nosing. Interestingly, the repetitive and stereotypical behavior of an autis-tic child is similar to the behavior of an animal per-forming repetitive pacing or bar biting. I used to engage in several repetitive stereotypies, and I can remember how they felt. For hours, I would dribble sand through my hands or spin a brass plate that covered up a bolt on the bed frame. When I did this, I became hypnotized and mesmerized. It was like taking a psychoactive drug or feeling the high that runners experience. When I performed the repetitive behavior, I could tune out the noises that hurt my ears. Research with pigs and other animals indicates that the brains of animals performing repetitive stereotypies may have an elevation in endorphins (Cronin et al. 1985, Dodman et al. 1987, Rushen et al. 1990). The animal may be performing the stereo-typy to cope with the barren environment, and the autistic child does it to escape from an environment that causes a cacophony of sensory overload in an immature nervous system.

One could argue that if stereotypies enable a sow to cope with living in a sow stall, then she would not suffer if she becomes "zonked" on her own endor-phins. Some research has shown that pigs living in tether housing that perform high levels of stereotyp-ies show differences in the density of endogenous opioid receptors in the brain compared to pigs that perform low levels of stereotypies (Loijens et al. 2002). Ethically, stereotypies are not acceptable because animals that perform them have abnormal changes in the brain. Research at University of California, Davis (UCD) indicated that the basal ganglia may be damaged (Knight 2001), and my own dissertation research indicated that the pigs in the barren environment had abnormal dendritic growth in the region of the brain that processes sen-sory information from the snout (Grandin 1989a). Further research by Joseph Garner and his col-leagues at UCD indicates that rodents with greater amounts of stereotypies have a greater degree of brain dysfunction than those showing no or few stereotypies (Garner & Mason 2002). The brains of animals performing stereotypies have been forced into a completely abnormal mode of operation. Animals that have been performing stereotypies for long periods of time are difficult to rehabilitate. By placing the animals in a more enriched environ-ment, we will cause some of the abnormal behavior to disappear, but the changes in the brain are likely permanent. The proper approach to animal stereo-typies must emphasize the prevention of stereotyp-ies from starting rather than treating the behavior once it has become established. Cribbing in horses is a common stereotypy. Stopping a horse from crib-bing is difficult unless one gives the horse drugs to block the secretion of endorphins. The drug naltrex-one will stop stereotypic behaviors in horses; how-ever, a better approach is to prevent the stereotypy by providing appropriate environmental enrich-ment. Both farm animals and laboratory rodents may be performing stereotypies that people never see. Mice in standardized lab cages appeared nor-mal during the day, but at night when nobody was around, they performed bizarre stereotypies such as somersaults (Wurbel 2001, 2002). To discover their behavior, lab workers had to rely on videotape.

MOTIVATION OF ABNORMAL BEHAVIOR

Animals have motivations to perform specific behaviors. The strength of the motivation is deter-mined by a complex interaction of genetics and environment. Stereotypies are more likely to occur in genetically nervous animals. My observations on farms indicated that lean type pigs bred for rapid gain will engage in more belly rubbing than a fatter genetic line. Egg-laying hens genetically selected for high egg production engage in more feather pecking and cannibalism than less prolific strains (Craig & Muir 1993). Animals with more excitable temperaments are more prone to developing abnor-mal behavior than animals from calmer genetic lines.

Species type will determine the nature of stereo-typies performed. Pigs spend large amounts of time rooting, so they tend to develop oral stereotypies. Because big cats in their natural environments spend large amounts of time walking, they develop motor stereotypies such as pacing. Parrots that are isolated will engage in picking out their own feathers, which may be grooming behavior that is grossly exaggerated. Rodents may be motivated to perform motor activities because they cannot find a place to hide in a plastic cage.

Each species has species-specific behaviors. Hens have a high motivation for finding a nesting place that is behind a visual barrier. They are also motivated to perform dust bathing. How important are these behaviors to the hen, and does she suffer if she is prevented from performing them? Ian Duncan, at the University of Guelph, has developed a simple way to quantify motivation strength. A hen is taught to push open a "doggie door" to obtain things such as a dust bath or a secluded nest box. The strength of the motivation can be measured by adding weights to the door to determine how hard the hen is willing to work to obtain the dust bath (Widowski & Duncan 2000). Hunger motivation can be measured with operant conditioning methods (Lawrence et al. 1989).

This system measures the strength of motivation but not how the animal feels. Fear may be the motivator for the secluded nest box. In the wild, a hen laying her eggs in a secluded hidden place would be less likely to be eaten by predators. However, fear would not be the main motivator for dust bathing. Dust bathing helps to maintain good feather condition, and it is possible that pleasure may be the main motivator (Widowski & Duncan 2000). Studies of the neurotransmitters in the animal's brain may help answer these questions.

Hungry animals are also more likely to engage in stereotypies than are satiated animals. Modern sows and broiler chickens are bred for rapid growth. The young animals are allowed to eat all they want, but the breeding sows and hens are kept on a restricted diet to prevent them from becoming overweight. They have been genetically selected for a vast appetite that they cannot satisfy. Gestating sows on grain are fed about 60 percent of their *ad lib* intake (i.e., the amount of feed an animal will eat if it is provided with an unlimited supply of feed) (Lawrence et al. 1988). Lawrence and Terlouw (1993) reviewed numerous studies that showed that many abnormal behaviors and stereotypies occur in animals that are feed-restricted. Several studies have shown that stereotypies develop when not enough feed exists to satisfy the hunger drive (Appleby & Lawrence 1987, Bergeron & Gonyou 1997). Having straw to eat and root in may be more important to

the sows than is straw to sleep on. Providing sows in tether stalls with small amounts of straw to eat and root reduced stereotypic behavior (Fraser 1975). Sows on a restricted diet will eat significant quantities of straw, which presumably helps them feel full without gaining weight. Animal well-being in totally slotted floor buildings could likely be improved by providing straw, hay, or hay cube as roughage—a bulky feed supplement.

ENVIRONMENTAL ENRICHMENT

Environmental enrichment must be appropriate for the animal's species-specific behaviors. It is beyond the scope of this chapter to review the subject of environmental enrichment, but it is well established that different methods are important to different animals. An enrichment device that is appropriate for one animal may not be appropriate for another species or individual. Pigs need materials that they can chew up and destroy, such as straw or cornstalks. Feeding roughages such as straw to sows or long hay to horses helps to prevent stereotypies such as cribbing or bar biting (Fraser 1975, Gillham et al. 1994). In my dissertation research, I found that pigs housed in barren pens preferred cloth or rubber objects over chains (Grandin 1989a). Rodents need places where they can hide, such as toilet paper tubes and crumpled paper towels; primates need many interesting things to climb on.

GENETICS AND MENTAL WELL-BEING

Some of the worst animal welfare problems I have observed have been made worse by genetics. Breeders selecting animals for a narrow range of production traits have sometimes neglected to also select for structurally sound feet and legs in pigs, chickens, and dairy cattle. These leg problems are an important cause of pain. Other genetic problems I have observed in animals are an excitable, flighty temperament that makes them difficult to handle (Grandin 1993). Animals bred for both high productivity and good feed conversion are often hyperactive, as well as more nervous and fearful. In layer hens, large differences in temperament exist between genetic lines. I have observed that brown hybrids are calmer than white hybrids. Craig and Muir (1989) discussed genetic effects on fearful behavior in hens. Certain genetic lines of white hybrids will react to a strange person by flapping and attempting to escape from their cages for a full five minutes. Breeding an animal with this much fear is detrimental to the animal's mental health and well-being.

Breeding and genetics could conceivably be used to reduce discomfort by breeding chickens that have low motivation to dust bathe. Broodiness has been bred out of commercial layers for decades. By using genetic selection to reduce the motivation for certain behaviors, discomfort and suffering associated with frustrated attempts to perform the behavior are alleviated. When I went to Japan, I observed that their older, fatter genetic line of pigs was free of stereotypies and other abnormal destructive behaviors such as tail biting. The pigs seemed content to just lay around on a totally slotted floor and eat. Barren environments may be tolerated better by calmer, less active genetic lines. Minero et al. (1999) reported that crib-biting horses had a higher heart rate when they were suddenly exposed to a novel inflating balloon. Horses that are prone to cribbing may be more sensitive to stress (Bachmann et al. 2003).

STRESS—IS IT FEAR OR SOME OTHER MOTIVATOR?

In addressing how an animal perceives and feels in different situations, we need to get away from vague references to stress. Any person can tell you that feeling hungry is a different feeling than feeling fear. Anger is also a different feeling than fear. When animals struggle, kick, or bite during handling and restraint, many people assume that the animals are motivated by anger. In situations associated with handling and restraint, the kicking is most often because of fear. In other situations, the animal may be truly angry. A bull that chases a person in a pasture is motivated by anger, but a bull that struggles or bellows in a squeeze chute is likely motivated by fear or pain. Restraint alone is most likely to cause fear, but a procedure such as dehorning would cause pain. It is important to determine the motivation (see McMillan, this volume, Chapter 7). Pinker (1997) has said that there are four basic drives for animal behavior. Often referred to as the "Four F's," they are (1) food (hunger), (2) fear (and fleeing from predators), (3) fighting, and (4) reproduction (I will leave it to the reader to figure out the fourth "F").

Interestingly, many stereotypies start out as either feeding or antipredator activities. Fear and hunger are the two prime motivators. A hen's need for a secluded nesting area and a rodent's need for a place to hide are motivated by fear. Many farm animals engage in oral stereotypies that are motivated by either hunger or species-specific foraging and grazing behaviors. The stereotypies start after the animal has been frustrated by not being able to perform the species-typical behavior. My own experience with autism allows me to relate to the lab mice that have no place to hide. I have an extremely high-fear nervous system. In the wild, the mouse is going to both feel and be safe from a hawk if he is under a leaf where he cannot be seen. In the lab, being inside the toilet paper tube will make the mouse feel safe even when the lab technician can still reach in and grab him. Hiding behind a visual barrier is a hardwired species-typical behavior that will make the mouse feel safe.

DIFFERENTIATING PAIN FROM FEAR

Fear and pain are often mixed up in the scientific literature under the term "stress." Fear and pain are different things. Think about your own experiences. Here is a personal example of a highly stressful event that was all fear and no pain. When I was in high school, I was in a plane that had to make an emergency landing, and all the passengers had to go down the escape chute. I had no pain but lots of fear. When I sprained my ankle by stepping on a pipe, it was all pain and no fear. Other situations exist in which one can have both fear and pain. Major surgery would be a good example. When an animal is approaching a place where it had either a painful or scary experience, its emotion is likely to be fear. Fear can occur when an animal anticipates that something painful will occur. For example, dairy cows that had been shocked in a chute remember the painful experience and six months later when brought back to the same chute, the shocked cows had higher heart rates as compared to unshocked cows (Pascoe 1986).

Research has demonstrated clearly and convincingly that birds and nonhuman mammals perceive pain. All of these animals will pain-guard and avoid putting weight on an injured limb. Duncan et al. (1989) and Gentle et al. (1990) report that chicks will peck less after beak trimming. Research by Colpaert et al. (1980, 2001) illustrates very clearly that animals will actively seek relief from pain. Rats with arthritic legs will drink unpalatable water containing an opiate analgesic. As the legs heal, the rats will drink progressively less water containing the analgesic and more and more highly palatable sugar water from a second dispenser. When the rats' legs were inflamed, they switched from the preferred sugar water to the noxious-tasting analgesic water. This study clearly shows that rats could seek out and drink a substance that tasted bad to reduce pain. It is my opinion that this self-medication experiment is the gold standard for demonstrating that rats with painful legs have a disagreeable sensation that they are highly motivated to alleviate.

PAINFUL PROCEDURES

In the classroom, a veterinary student asked me why she had to give a dog an anesthetic when it was castrated but a calf undergoing the same procedure would receive no anesthesia. I explained that from a strictly biological standpoint, they both would benefit from pain relief. Many studies show that giving local anesthetics after the surgery reduces both behavioral and physiological indicators of pain and stress (McGlone & Hellman 1988, Molony & Kent 1997, Sutherland et al. 2002). I used the vague term stress because surgery causes both pain and damage to tissue. Both pain and tissue damage will have an effect on physiological measures such as cortisol. Providing pain relief with an anti-inflammatory analgesic may have an effect on physiological measures that may be at least partially independent of pain or fear. In other words, surgery would have both emotional and physical effects. Further studies have shown that farm animals should be given an analgesic in addition to local anesthetics to reduce pain after the operation. Calves that were dehorned with both a local anesthetic and given ketoprofen, a non-steroidal anti-inflammatory analgesic, had lower blood cortisol levels than the controls or calves given only the local anesthetic (McMeekan et al. 1998). Studies by Ting et al. (2003) and Faulkner and Weary (2000) support the use of analgesics after dehorning or castration.

When wild cattle that are not accustomed to being handled are restrained, fear-stress will be greater than in tame dairy animals. Lay et al. (1992a, 1992b) reported that cortisol levels and heart rates were higher after restraint in a squeeze chute as compared to dairy cows. Handling an animal that is not accustomed to restraint can cause high levels of fear-stress.

When evaluating common husbandry practices such as ear tagging or dehorning, one has to look at the relative contribution of pain and fear. Dehorning of adult cattle would be a highly painful procedure for which the use of a local anesthetic substantially

reduces distress. The additional handling-stress from administering the anesthetic would probably be minor compared to the pain of the dehorning procedure. On the other hand, ear tagging is a minor procedure—comparable to ear-piercing in people— and the extra handling associated with giving an anesthetic would cause more fear than the little prick from an ear tagging procedure.

Large individual differences appear to exist in how animals experience pain. I observed a group of bulls that were castrated with a high-tension rubber-band. After the band was applied, some bulls appeared behaviorally normal, a few stamped their feet, and one bull laid on the ground and moaned. I was able to observe their behavior because I hid in the scalehouse. Grazing animals will "act normal" when they are in pain to avoid attracting a predator's attention. To see pain-related behaviors, one needs to observe them from either a hidden location or via the recordings of a video camera.

CONCLUSION

The way farm animals feel is both similar and different when compared to human feelings. Animals fear little things that people do not notice. Rapid movement and objects with high visual contrast attract their attention because in the wild, these things may mean danger. Cattle and pigs will walk quietly into a slaughter plant but will stop instantly if they see a sparkling reflection or jiggling chain. Elimination of these distractions will lessen fear and facilitate animal movement. The fear circuits in an animal's brain are similar to those in people. To prevent fear memories, animal caregivers should make an animal's first exposure to a new thing be a positive experience. Animals have sensory-based memories. They may associate certain people or places with either painful or frightening experiences. They will often associate a prominent feature on a person, such as a beard or blue coveralls, with aversive experiences such as injections. Training and habituating animals to handling and restraint will reduce fear.

New experiences are both frightening and attractive. Novel objects are frightening when they are suddenly introduced but attractive when the animal can voluntarily approach them. The animal's nervous system needs a certain amount of environmental novelty to function normally. Animals in barren environments will often engage in repetitive stereotypies. Stereotypies can be largely prevented by providing environmental enrichment that allows an animal to perform species-typical behaviors. There is a need to differentiate fear- and pain-stress. The feelings of fear and pain are different.

REFERENCES

Abbott TA, Hunter EJ, Guise JH, et al. 1997. The effect of experience of handling on pig's willingness to move. *Appl Anim Behav Sci* 54:371–375.

Ames DR. 1974. Sound stress and meat animals. *Proc Internat Livestock Environment Symp Amer Soc Agri Eng* SP-01174:324.

Andrade O, Orihuela A, Solano J, et al. 2001. Some effects of repeated handling and use of a mask on stress responses in zebu cattle during restraint. *Appl Anim Behav Sci* 71:175–181.

Appleby MC, Lawrence AB. 1987. Food restriction as a course of stereotypic behavior in tethered gilts. *Anim Proc* 45:103–110.

Arave CW. 1996. Assessing sensory capability of animals using operant technology. *J Anim Sci* 74:1996–2000.

Ayres JA. 1975. *Sensory integration and the child.* Los Angeles: Western Physiological Services.

Bachmann T, Bernasconi P, Herrmann R, et al. 2003. Behavioral and physiological responses to an acute stressor in crib biting and control horses. *Appl Anim Behav Sci* 82:297–311.

Bauman ML, Kemper TL. 1994. Neuroanatomic observations of the brain in autism: In: Bauman ML, Kemper TL (eds), *The neurology of autism.* Baltimore, MD, Johns Hopkins University Press:119–145.

Becker BG, Lobato JFP. 1997. Effect of gentle handling on the reactivity of the zebu cross calves to humans. *Appl Anim Behav Sci* 53:219–224.

Benjamin ME, Gonyou HW, Ivers DL, et al. 2001. Effect of animal handling method on the incidence of stress response in market swine in a model system. *J Anim Sci* Suppl. 1 79:279 (Abstract).

Bergeron R, Gonyou HW. 1997. Effects of increasing energy intake and foraging behaviors on the development of stereotypies in pregnant sows. *Appl Anim Behav Sci* 53:259–270.

Binstead M. 1977. Handling cattle. *Queensland Agric J* 103:293–295.

Boissy A. 1995. Fear and fearfulness in animals. *Q Rev Biol* 70:165–171.

Boissy A, Terlouw C, LeNeindre P. 1998. Presence of cues from stressed conspecifics increases reactivity to aversive events in cattle: Evidence for the existence of alarm substances in urine. *Physiol Behav* 63:489–495.

Colpaert FC, deWitte PC, Maroli AN, et al. 1980. Self-administration of the analgesic suprofen in arthritic rats: Evidence of *Mycobacterium butyricum*-induced arthritis as an experimental model of chronic pain. *Life Sci* 27:921–928.

Colpaert FC, Tarayre JP, Alliaga M, et al. 2001. Opiate self-administration as a measure of chronic nociceptive pain in arthritic rats. *Pain* 91:33–34.

Courchesne E, Karns CM, Davis HR. 2001. Unusual brain growth patterns in early life in patients with autistic disorders. *Neurology* 57:245–254.

Craig JV, Muir WM. 1989. Fearful and associated responses of caged White Leghorn hens. Genetic parameter estimates. *Poultry Sci* 68:1040–1046.

Craig JV, Muir WM. 1993. Selection for reduction of beak-inflicted injuries among caged hens. *Poultry Sci* 72:411–420.

Cronin GM, Wiepkema RR, Van Ree JM. 1985. Endogeneous opioids are involved in abnormal stereotype behaviors in sows. *Neuropeptides* 6:527–530.

Davis M. 1992. The role of the amygdala in fear and anxiety. *Annu Rev Neurosci* 15:353–375.

Dodman NH, Shuster L, Court MH, et al. 1987. Investigation into the use of narcotic antagonists in the treatment of stereotypic behavior pattern (crib biting) in the horse. *Am J Vet Res* 48:311–319.

Duncan IJ, Slee GS, Seawright E, et al. 1989. Behavioral consequences of partial beak amputation (beak trimming) in poultry. *Brit Poultry Sci* 30:479–488.

Faulkner PM, Weary DM. 2000. Reducing pain after dehorning in dairy calves. *J Dairy Sci* 9:2037–2041.

Fell LR, Colditz KH, Watson DL. 1999. Associations between temperament, performance and immune function in cattle entering a commercial feedlot. *Aust J Exp Agr* 39:795–802.

Fordyce G. 1987. Weaner training. *Queensland Agr J* 6:323–324.

Fordyce G, Dodt RM, Wythes JR. 1988. Cattle temperaments in extensive herds in northern Queensland. *Aust J Exp Agr* 28:683–688.

Fraser D. 1975. The effect of straw on the behavior of sows in tether stalls. *Anim Prod* 21:59–68.

Garner JP, Mason GJ. 2002. Evidence for a relationship between cage stereotypies and behavioural disinhibition in laboratory rodents. *Behav Brain Res* 136:83–92.

Gates G. 2003. *A dog in hand, teaching a puppy to think.* Irving, TX: Tapestry Press.

Gentle MJ, Wadington D, Hunter LN, et al. 1990. Behavioral evidence for persistent pain following partial beak amputation in chickens. *Appl Anim Behav Sci* 27:149–157.

Geverink NA, Kappers A, Van deBurgwal E, et al. 1998. Effects of regular moving and handling on the behavioral and physiological responses of pigs to pre-slaughter treatment and consequences for meat quality. *J Anim Sci* 76:2080–2085.

Gilbert BJ, Arave CW. 1986. Ability of cattle to distinguish among different wavelengths of light. *J Dairy Sci* 69:825–832.

Gillham S, Dodman NH, Shuster L, et al. 1994. The effect of diet on cribbing behavior and plasma ß-endorphin in horses. *Appl Anim Behav Sci* 41:147–153.

Gloor P, Oliver A, Quesney LF. 1981. The role of the amygdala in the expression of psychic phenomenon in temporal lobe seizures. In: Ben Avi Y (ed), *The amygdaloid complex*. New York, Elsevier:489–507.

Grandin T. 1980. Observations of cattle behavior applied to the design of handling facilities. *Appl Anim Ethol* 6:19–33.

Grandin T. 1989a. Effect of rearing environment and environmental enrichment on behavior and neural development of young pigs. Doctoral dissertation. University of Illinois, Urbana-Champaign, IL.

Grandin T. 1989b. Voluntary acceptance of restraint in sheep. *Appl Anim Behav Sci* 23:257–261.

Grandin T. 1992. Observations of cattle restraint devices for stunning and slaughtering. *Anim Welfare* 1:85–91.

Grandin T. 1993. Environmental and genetic factors which contribute to handling problems at pork slaughter plants. In: Collins E, Boone C (eds), *Livestock environment IV*. St. Joseph, MI, American Society of Agricultural Engineers:116–145.

Grandin T. 1994. Euthanasia and slaughter of livestock. *J Am Vet Med Assoc* 204:1354–1360.

Grandin T. 1995. *Thinking in pictures*. New York: Doubleday. Currently published by Vintage Press, New York.

Grandin T. 1996. Factors that impede animal movement at slaughter plans. *J Am Vet Med Assoc* 209:757–759.

Grandin T. 1997a. Assessment of stress during handling and transport. *J Anim Sci* 74:249–257.

Grandin T. 1997b. Thinking the way animals do. *Western Horseman* November:140–145.

Grandin T. 2000. *Livestock handling and transport*. Wallingford, UK: CAB International.

Grandin T. 2001. Welfare of cattle during slaughter and the prevention of non-ambulatory (downer cattle). *J Am Vet Med Assoc* 219:1377–1382.

Grandin T. 2003. Transferring results of behavioral research to industry to improve animal welfare on the farm, ranch and the slaughter plant. *Appl Anim Behav Sci* 81:215–228.

Grandin T, Curtis SE, Taylor IA. 1987. Toys, mingling and driving reduce excitability in pigs. *J Anim Sci* 65 (Suppl. 1):230 (Abstract).

Grandin T, Deesing MJ. 1998. Behavioral genetics and animal sciences. In: Grandin T (ed), *Genetics and the behavior of domestic animals*. San Diego, Academic Press:1–32.

Heffner RS, Heffner HE. 1983. Hearing in large mammals: Horse (*Equus caballus*) and cattle (*Bos Taurus*). *Behav Neurosci* 97:299–309.

Hemsworth PH, Coleman GJ. 1998. *Human livestock interactions*. Wallingford, UK: CAB International.

Hemsworth PH, Coleman GJ, Barnett JL, et al. 2002. The effects of cognitive behavioral intervention on the attitude and behavior of stock persons and the behavior and productivity of commercial dairy cows. *J Anim Sci* 80:68–78.

Hutching B. 1993. Deerhandlers. *The Deer Farmer* 105:39–47.

Hutson GD. 1985. The influence of barley food rewards on sheep movement through a handling system. *Appl Anim Behav Sci* 14:263–275.

Jacobs GH, Deegan JF, Neitz J. 1998. Photopigment basis for dichromatic colour vision in cows, goats and sheep. *Visual Neurosci* 15:581–584.

Kemble ED, Blanchard DC, Blanchard RJ, et al. 1984. Taming in wild rats following medial amygdaloid lesions. *Physiol Behav* 32:131–134.

Knight J. 2001. Animal data jeopardized by life behind bars. *Nature* 412:669.

Koba Y, Tanida H. 1999. How do miniature pigs discriminate between people? The effect of exchanging cues between a non-handler and their familiar handler on discrimination. *Appl Anim Behav Sci* 61:239–252.

Lanier JL, Grandin T, Green RD, et al. 2000. The relationship between reaction to sudden intermittent movements and sounds to temperament. *J Anim Sci* 78:1467–1474.

Lawrence AB, Appleby MC, Illius AW, et al. 1989. Measuring hunger in the pig using operant conditioning. The effect of dietary bulk. *Anim Prod* 48:213–220.

Lawrence AB, Appleby MC, McLeod HA. 1988. Measuring hunger in the pig using operant conditioning: The effect of food restriction. *Anim Prod* 47:131–137.

Lawrence AB, Terlouw EMC. 1993. A review of behavioral factors involved in the development and continued performance of stereotypic behaviours in pigs. *J Anim Sci* 71:2815–2825.

Lay DC, Friend TH, Bowers CC, et al. 1992a. A comparative physiological and behavioral study of freeze and hot iron branding using dairy cows. *J Anim Sci* 70:1121-1125.

Lay DC, Friend TH, Randel RD, et al. 1992b. Behavioral and physiological effects of freeze and hot iron branding on crossbred cattle. *J Anim Sci* 70:330–336.

LeDoux JE. 1996. *The emotional brain*. New York: Simon and Schuster.

Loijens LWS, Schouten WGP, Wiepkema PR, et al. 2002. Brain opioid response reflects behavioral and heart rate response in pigs. *Physiol Behav* 76:579–598.

Matthews LH. 2000. Deer handling and transport. In: Grandin T (ed), *Livestock handling and transport*. Wallingford, UK, CAB International:331–362.

McGlone JJ, Hellman JM. 1988. Local and general anesthetic effects on the behavior and performance of 2 and 7 week old castrated and uncastrated piglets. *J Anim Sci* 66:3049–3058.

McMeekan CM, Stafford KJ, Mellor DJ, et al. 1998. Effects of regional analgesia and/or a nonsteroidal anti-inflammatory analgesic on acute cortisol response to dehorning in calves. *Res Vet Sci* 64:147–150.

Melzack R, Burns SK. 1965. Neurophysiological effects of early sensory restriction. *Exp Neurol* 13:163–175.

Minero M, Canali E, Ferrante V, et al. 1999. Heart rate and behavioral response of crib biting horses to two acute stressors. *Vet Rec* 145:430–433.

Molony V, Kent JE. 1997. Assessment of acute pain in farm animals using behavioral and physiological measurements. *J Anim Sci* 75:266–272.

Panepinto LM. 1983. A comfortable minimum stress method of restraint for Yucatan Miniature Swine for laboratory procedures. *Lab Anim Care* 18:584–587.

Pascoe PJ. 1986. Humaneness of an electroimmobilization unit for cattle. *Am J Vet Res* 10:2252–2256.

Phillips MT, Grandin T, Graffam W, et al. 1998. Crate conditioning of bongo (*Tragelaphus eurycerus*) for veterinary and husbandry procedures at Denver Zoological Garden. *Zoo Biol* 17:25–32.

Pinker S. 1997. *How the mind works*. New York: W.W. Norton.

Prince JH. 1970. The eye and vision. In: Swenson MJ (ed), *Duke's physiology of domestic animals*. New York, Cornell University Press:696–712.

Redgate ES, Fahringer EE. 1973. A comparison of pituitary adrenal activity elicited by electrical stimulation of preoptic amygdaloid and hypothalamic sites in the rat brain. *Neuroendocrinology* 12:334–343.

Reid RL, Mills SC. 1962. Studies of carbohydrate metabolism of sheep. XVI. The adrenal response to physiological stress. *Aust J Agr Res* 13:282–294.

Rogan MT, LeDoux JE. 1996. Emotion: Systems, cells and synaptic plasticity. *Cell* 85:469–475.

Rushen J, dePassille AM, Schouten W. 1990. Stereotypic behavior, endogenous opioids and post feeding hypoalgesia in pigs. *Physiol Behav* 48:91–96.

Rushen J, Taylor AA, dePassille AM. 1999. Domestic animals' fear of humans and its effect on welfare. *Appl Anim Behav Sci* 65:295–303.

Rybarczyk P, Rushen J, dePassille AM. 2003. Recognition of people by dairy calves using color of clothing. *Appl Anim Behav Sci* 81:307–319.

Schultz D. 1965. *Sensory restriction*. New York: Academic Press.

Seligman ME. 1975. *Helplessness: On depression, development, and death*. San Francisco: W.H. Freeman.

Stevens DA, Gerzog-Thomas DA. 1977. Fright reactions in rats to conspecific tissue. *Physiol Behav* 18:47–51.

Sutherland MA, Mellor DJ, Stafford KJ, et al. 2002. Effect of local anesthetic combined with wound cauterization on the cortisol responses to dehorning in calves. *Aust Vet J* 80:165–167.

Talling JC, Waran NK, Wathes CM, et al. 1998. Sound avoidance by domestic pigs depends on characteristics of the signal. *Appl Anim Behav Sci* 58:255–266.

Ting ST, Early B, Hughes JM, et al. 2003. Effect of ketoproten, lidocaine local anesthesia and combined xylazine and lidocaine caudal epidural anesthesia during castration of beef cattle on stress responses, immunity, growth and behavior. *J Anim Sci* 81:1281–1293.

Vicville-Thomas RK, Signoret JP. 1992. Pheromonal transmission of aversive experiences in domestic pigs. *J Chem Endocrinol* 18:1551–1557.

Voisinet BD, Grandin T, Tatum JD, et al. 1997. Feedlot cattle with calm temperaments have higher average daily gains than cattle with excitable temperaments. *J Anim Sci* 75:892–896.

Walsh RN, Cummins RA. 1975. Mechanisms mediating the production of environmentally induced brain changes. *Psychol Bull* 82:986–1000.

Waynert DE, Stookey JM, Schwartzkopf-Gerwein JM, et al. 1999. Response of beef cattle to noise during handling. *Appl Anim Behav Sci* 62:27–42.

Widowski TM, Duncan IJ. 2000. Working for a dust bath: Are hens increasing pleasure rather than reducing suffering? *Appl Anim Behav Sci* 68:39–53.

Wurbel H. 2001. Ideal homes? Housing effects on rodent brain and behavior. *Trends Neurosci* 24:207–211.

Wurbel H. 2002. Behavioral phenotyping enhanced beyond environmental standardization. *Genes Brain Behav* 1:3–8.

19

The Mental Health of Laboratory Animals

Lesley King and Andrew N. Rowan

INTRODUCTION

The mental health of laboratory animals is an important topic not only for those directly involved in animal-based scientific research but also for every member of society in whose name scientific research is conducted. The wide concern for laboratory animal welfare stems in part from the public funding of much basic, biomedical, and toxicological research; the impact of the results of such research on the development of medical treatments and procedures; and the widespread public concern that harms to animals used in research be minimized. The utility of animal-based research and the validity and accuracy of the scientific results generated are also a matter of concern both for the public and for those who perform or commission such research.

Debates about the ethical importance of animal welfare and what constitutes animal well-being are not new in the field of biomedical research. In the past 30 years, an increasing emphasis has been placed on the minimization of pain, suffering, and distress. This concern has led scientists and philosophers to try to define "animal welfare" and to develop practical, operational means for its assessment. What is relatively new, however, is the growing understanding that laboratory animal welfare is not just about the physical health of research animals. Indeed, the animal's mental health and psychological well-being is central to the modern concept of animal welfare. Some scientists even argue that the only aspect of welfare that is important is how the animal feels—whether the animal is suffering from pain or emotional distress such as fear—rather than any physical injury or damage that is associated with the state.

Recent evidence (summarized later) suggests that some animals used in research may develop psychological dysfunction when maintained in standard (and environmentally and socially impoverished) laboratory housing. Therefore, the experimental protocol is not the only aspect of animal research that needs to be addressed when considering animal welfare. Consideration should also be given to the effects of animal housing and husbandry. If there really is more to animal distress than "meets the eye" in terms of insults to physical health, then better assessment of animals' mental states and improved provisions for their psychological well-being in the laboratory may require substantial re-evaluation.

This chapter aims to provide an overview of the scientific and regulatory bases on which laboratory animal mental health is considered and to draw out some implications for the care and use of animals in research. It will examine what we do and can know about whether laboratory animals are capable of mental suffering. It will look at the consequences of current housing and care techniques for animal mental health; in so doing, it will highlight how an improved understanding of the mental well-being of animals can affect the quality and accuracy of data derived from animal models in scientific and biomedical investigation. Possible future developments in animal welfare knowledge are also proposed.

THE USE OF ANIMALS IN RESEARCH: A BRIEF OVERVIEW OF REGULATIONS AND PRACTICE

Animals are used in a diverse range of research procedures including the development of basic scientific knowledge, the development and assessment of drugs and biologicals, the development of biomedical and surgical procedures, the toxicological evaluation of chemical compounds, and the education and training of students entering the medical, veterinary, and other scientific professions. The direct negative consequences of potential research protocols for the animals involved are quite varied. For example, an animal may experience sickness and malaise as a result of exposure to toxic chemicals or infectious agents, pain or sickness from the induction of specific medical conditions such as diabetes or coronary failure, alteration of cognitive function leading to suffering through psychopharmacological treatments, and suffering as a result of exposure to adverse stimuli such as electric shocks or extremes of heat or cold.

The experimental protocol may also have indirect influences on the animal's well-being. For example, a protocol may require an animal to complete a benign cognitive or motor response task such as pressing a button or touching a computer screen for a reward such as a palatable drink. However, the animal may be trained to complete the task through the use of water deprivation. If the research protocol requires the animal to remain very still during the test session (e.g., as in the tracking of eye movements), the animal may be restrained for lengthy periods. During the restraint, the animal may suffer because it is unable to stretch, move about freely, or perform normal behaviors and postural adjustments. Table 19.1 lists only a few of the possible pain and non-pain sources of distress and suffering in laboratory protocols. Some of the sources will be relatively rare (e.g., muricide as a model of aggressive behavior), but others are common (e.g., toxicology studies may account for 10–15 percent of all laboratory animal use and high degrees of distress; Canada reports that more than 60 percent of animals used in such studies experience moderate to significant distress).

In many cases, the majority of the research animal's life is spent in its "home" cage. The animal

Table 19.1. Causes of distress and suffering in research protocols involving pain and non-pain experiences.

Source	Description and examples
Pain sources of distress and suffering	
Arthritis models	Can involve single or multiple joints. Pain on ambulation or other use of joint(s).
Burn research	Acute and chronic pain.
Cancer research	Cancer pain—may be severe.
Chronic pain studies	Acute pain should not be a problem if IASP[1] guidelines are followed.
Inflammation studies	Can involve all areas of the body. Some, such as meningitis and pancreatitis, can be associated with extreme pain.
Experimental surgery	Pain can be from immediate post-operative effects or longer-term consequences (e.g., ischemic pain from ligated coronary arteries or induced bowel obstruction).
Muricide	May result from models of aggression, neophobia, etc.
Orthopedic studies	Prosthetic joints, fracture repair, bone transplant studies, amputations, salvage procedures.
Trauma research	Wide range of studies, e.g., gunshot wounds, impact trauma, head and spinal trauma, etc.
Non-pain sources of distress and suffering	
Aggression models	Emotional suffering of being aggressor or being victim.
Anxiety models	E.g., the Vogel conflict-drinking model. Chronic anxiety presumed to be extremely distressful.
Cancer	Tumor burden, nausea, toxic effects, cachexia, chemotherapy trials, carcinogenicity testing.
Depression models	Models include learned helplessness, forced swimming, and mother-infant separation.
Diabetes models	Disease effects, tests, and treatments.
Drug addiction/ withdrawal models	Signs of withdrawal appear to involve distress and suffering comparable to humans.

Source	Description and examples
Environmental stress	Environmental heat and cold, pollution studies, population crowding studies.
Fear models	Fear is believed by many to have more potential for distress and suffering than does physical pain.
Immunological research	Vaccine efficacy testing, antigen exposure for immunoglobulin production.
Infectious disease	Nausea, toxic feelings, fever, dehydration. Includes studies of bioterrorism agents.
Isolation models	Social deprivation in social animals may cause extreme suffering.
Motion sickness models	Nausea, disorientation.
Nutrition research	Deprivation and excessive intake of nutritional factors.
Panic models	Includes post-traumatic stress disorder models.
Pharmacology (some)	E.g., research using tumor necrosis factor or capsaicin.
Psychological stress models	Emotional distress and suffering, overlapping some of the above models (e.g., social isolation, fear, and anxiety).
Psychopathology	Other than anxiety, fear, depression, stress, etc., otherwise mentioned. Includes models of bipolar disease, schizophrenia, sociopathic personality.
Radiation research	Nausea from loss of GI epithelium, burned tissues, sloughed skin and flesh.
Renal failure models	Suffering from uremic poisoning, GI ulceration, uremic encephalopathy.
Models of respiratory disorders	Models of airway obstruction, emphysema, asthma, pulmonary edema, pulmonary thromboembolism, pleural effusion, pneumothorax, lung lobe torsion, and bronchitis. Distress and suffering associated with hypoxia and dyspnea considered among the most severe of all disorders.
Toxicology	Extreme distress and suffering potential in wide variety of body systems, e.g., anticoagulation, neurotoxicity, GI destruction, dehydration.
Transgenic studies	Many new transgenics are significantly compromised and unable to properly respond to physical and emotional challenges.

[1] IASP: Report of International Association for the Study of Pain; Subcommittee on taxonomy.

may be housed singly or with conspecifics. The cage environment would include food (usually only in standardized pellet form), water, and, in many cases, some form of bedding. Additional enrichments may be provided such as nesting material or shelters, activity resources such as ropes for climbing in primate enclosures, or hide-away containers and running wheels for rodents. Typically, primates, dogs, and cats are provided more enrichment in their cage environments than are rodents, although providing special housing (a very important source of enrichment) for rodents is much less costly than for these other animals. The cage environments and social groupings of the animals are usually much more limited than and quite different from the "natural" environments in which the species evolved.

Other aspects of the laboratory environment are also very different from the "natural" environment. These include the light intensity, light spectra, and daylength; the ambient temperature; the presence or absence of certain aural stimuli (e.g., ultrasound from running water, transistor radios, or fluorescent

tubes); and the presence, location, and stability (disrupted by frequent cleaning) of olfactory stimuli such as food or more-dominant conspecifics. Some of these factors may be important for mental welfare, as will be discussed later in the chapter.

The welfare of animals used in research is regulated in the United States under two main provisions: the Animal Welfare Act, a federal law enforced by the United States Department of Agriculture, and Public Health Service policy guidelines on the use of animals in scientific research, overseen by the National Institutes of Health's (NIH) Office for Laboratory Animal Welfare (Institute for Laboratory Animal Research 2003). These laws and guidelines require oversight of animal welfare issues mainly via institutional animal care and use committees at each research facility. The Animal Welfare Act excludes oversight of birds, mice, and rats; the Public Health Service policy does cover these species, but only for those institutions receiving public sources of funding for research.

Both the federal law and the Public Health Service policy specifically address pain and distress (animal "suffering" is not addressed in US regulatory oversight), although the focus of both oversight mechanisms has been mainly on pain. Distress is not defined in either oversight system. Both oversight systems acknowledge indirectly or directly the public concern to minimize animal pain and distress. In terms of mental well-being, the Animal Welfare Act also requires that institutions provide for certain psychological and behavioral needs in two species—specifically, environmental and social enrichment to allow for the psychological well-being of nonhuman primates and exercise requirements for dogs (Institute for Laboratory Animal Research 1998; for more information on US regulation, see Humane Society of the United States 2002). Finally, the Animal Welfare Act, US Government policies, and various guidance documents on the use of animals in research all emphasize the responsibility of the researcher, institution, or both to minimize pain and distress.

DEFINING TERMS: WHAT IS ENCOMPASSED IN THE "MENTAL HEALTH" OF LABORATORY ANIMALS?

Before trying to identify how to measure or accommodate the "mental health" of laboratory animals, we must determine what elements might be incorporated in such a term. For humans, the World Health Organization (WHO) defines mental health as "a state of well-being, in which the individual realizes his or her own abilities, can cope with the normal stresses of life, can work productively and fruitfully and is able to make a contribution to his or her community" (World Health Organization 2001).

The WHO's concept of mental well-being lies within a wider definition of health, which is defined as "a state of complete physical, mental and social well-being and not merely the absence of disease or deformity" (World Health Organization 2003).

These definitions of what mental health comprises have four key components to them. They are broad in scope and reflect global concepts that make intuitive sense to us as humans; if we ourselves were in a state of poor mental well-being we might be able to report at a particular time, on a scale of 1–10 perhaps, how our mental state was faring. We thus have access to and an understanding of our own mental experiences, so the idea of assessing and measuring mental well-being among ourselves and

others is neither an alien nor a ludicrous concept.

Nevertheless, these definitions of mental health contain a number of abstract concepts. If we are to measure mental health more carefully and definitively, we must divide "mental health" into separate, measurable items that may be "operationalized." For example, in assessing whether a person is depressed, we might ask him or her to respond to a battery of attitude or emotional statements, assess his or her activity levels at different times of day or when dealing with stress, and assess the extent of his or her sleep disruption or cognitive impairment. Such measures, when put together and validated, provide a picture of the person's mental state.

A description of somebody's mental health refers to a subjective state in another person. Because we cannot directly access the mental or emotional states of others, we can never obtain a fully objective measurement of such states in the way that we might measure a physical attribute such as height or weight. We do not deny that other humans have these mental states just because we cannot fit a tape measure around them. We reason by analogy that, based on the similarity of the biology and neurophysiology of other humans to ourselves, they will likely have feelings similar to ours.

Wittgenstein demonstrated this idea very clearly. His view is summarized succinctly by Kemerling (2001):

> If any of my experiences were entirely private, then the pain that I feel would surely be among them. Yet other people commonly are said to know when I am in pain. Indeed, Wittgenstein pointed out that I would never have learned the meaning of the word "pain" without the aid of other people, none of whom have access to the supposed private sensations of pain that I feel. For the word "pain" to have any meaning at all presupposes some sort of external verification, a set of criteria for its correct application, and they must be accessible to others as well as to myself.

Wittgenstein illustrated this idea with an elegant thought experiment. If we all had a small box in which we carried an item, say a small beetle that only we and nobody else had seen, then we could only develop a dialogue on what a beetle is and talk sensibly among ourselves about the qualities of "beetleness" if all our beetles were very similar to make the resulting conversation comprehensible.

Finally, and most importantly, the concept of mental well-being is seen as a key component in a broader idea of health. As such, mental and physical health are not viewed as separate parts of a dualism but are integrated components within the individual. Thus, evaluation of mental well-being is essential to understanding overall health.

Can we conceive of or assess an animal's mental state in the same way? Initially, this might seem a silly idea. How can an animal housed in a laboratory "make a contribution to his or her community" or "realize his or her own abilities"? Yet, with appropriate flexibility, the WHO definition could certainly apply to animals. For example, in evolutionary terms, animals could "realize [their] own abilities" in terms of the extent to which they are able to fulfill their evolutionarily based, genetically determined phenotypes. Bernard Rollin (1990; this volume, Chapter 1) encapsulated this idea when he described animals as having a nature or "telos," which is an inherent part of their design and is recognizable as a set of propensities to behave in certain ways or develop certain physical traits.

The WHO definition of mental health also emphasizes the individual's ability to cope with the normal challenges and stresses of life. It emphasizes that the ability to respond appropriately to these challenges is part of well-being and suggests that health is compromised when the stressor (the cause of the stress), or the stress response itself, leads to the experience of more than short-term, low-intensity emotional distress or, worse, mental or physical impairment or even damage. This idea of coping is directly mirrored in concepts and definitions of animal welfare that refer to evolutionary theories of adaptive behavior and that call on research in stress physiology involving activation of the hypothalamic-pituitary-adrenal (HPA) axis, which readies the animal for action (see Moberg & Mench 2000). Certain definitions of animal distress are based on the idea that distress occurs when the animal is no longer able to respond adaptively or cope with (in physiological and behavioral terms) the environmental challenge (Broom & Johnson 1993; McMillan, this volume, Chapter 7).

The adverse consequences of exposure to acute and intense or chronic stressors are well known in humans and animals and include physical and physiological damage such as reduced longevity, immunosuppression, reduced growth rate, and a range of disorders including gastric ulceration and sleep pattern disruption. Cognitive effects of the activation of physiological stress responses include, for example, impairments in memory formation. It should be noted that environmental challenges that lead to activation of the HPA axis are not always bad

and activation of stress responses can relate to highly positive events such as sexual activity (see Dawkins 1998). The pleasurable or distressing emotional context of an event that causes a stress response is a key to determining whether an environmental challenge may impinge on the mental and physical health of animals.

Questions relating to the experience of emotion are at the heart of discussions over the mental welfare of laboratory animals. The ability to experience emotions determines whether animals are able to experience profound, or prolonged, negative or unpleasant subjective states that make up some forms of mental distress. One recent guideline definition of animal distress published by the US Government's National Research Council (NRC) clearly emphasizes the emotional context of distress as encompassing

> the negative psychologic states that are sometimes associated with exposure to stressors, including fear, pain, malaise, anxiety, frustration, depression and boredom. These can manifest as maladaptive behaviors, such as abnormal feeding or aggression, or pathologic conditions that are not evident in behavior, such as hypertension and immunosuppression. (Institute for Laboratory Animal Research 2003)

What is the scientific basis for the claim that animal species used in laboratory research experience the kinds of emotions that humans would find distressing and that would impinge on their mental well-being? How can we determine when an animal is experiencing emotional distress? Do situations exist within the laboratory that might create such states?

EMOTIONAL DISTRESS AND MENTAL HEALTH IN LABORATORY ANIMALS

The topic of laboratory animal mental health is controversial. Only recently have animals been viewed by the scientific community as able to experience pain and thus given analgesic treatment following invasive experimental protocols like surgery (Kitchen et al. 1987, Rollin 1990). Mental suffering that might be precipitated by anxiety has been viewed as a solely human trait by some in the scientific community (cf. Rowan 1988), yet if animals *do* have mental experiences, the possibility exists that animals may experience forms of distress that are currently poorly understood. Such distress may not be taken into account during research, thus potentially leaving animals to suffer. For example, many rodents used in research perform abnormal, highly repetitive behaviors when housed in laboratory conditions. Some laboratory-housed primates demonstrate repetitive behaviors such as rocking and pacing and may also injure themselves through self-biting and other mutilations. Do such behaviors suggest a state of mental suffering? As noted above, we have difficulty assessing what another individual human experiences. Because animals cannot provide verbal accounts of their inner experiences, we require other methods to learn about their internal states.

We first need to ask whether animals need to be able to think or have complex cognitive faculties to have a state of well-being for which humans should be morally concerned. Which mental capabilities matter for welfare—the ability to communicate perhaps, or to remember? Furthermore, why worry about mental welfare—are concepts of physical health not sufficient to ensure that a laboratory animal is not in distress?

Historically, animals were viewed simply as stimulus-response organisms. For example, in the seventeenth century, the philosopher Descartes and some of those who came later (especially Malebranche) considered animals to be incapable of thinking, feeling pain, or having the sensations that humans experience. Thus, in such a worldview, there was no need to be concerned about animal welfare. If an animal was subjected to an invasive surgical procedure while conscious and it vocalized or struggled, this would be explained as being because of mechanistic and automatic processes in their body (as a rusty gate might squeal when opened), rather than representing an internal, deeply unpleasant experience of pain. In the early- to mid-twentieth century, animals were still widely viewed— by influential academics such as the behaviorist Watson—as organisms that did not think or feel, and consciousness was denied to animals on the basis that it could not be proved scientifically. In behaviorism's view, animal behavior was determined by what was learned through trial and error, and animals were conditioned to approach or avoid certain things by association if these were repeatedly presented contingently with basic positive stimuli such as food, or negative stimuli such as an electric shock.

Animals were thus seen as blank slates whose behavior was reinforced by association with these stimuli; however, studies began to show that animals could use tools, hold internal mental representations of objects, use complex problem solving strategies, and communicate in ways that demonstrated a range of features similar to human language. In other words, these were not just biological organisms programmed by experience to respond; these animals were able to mentally process complex information, generating novel solutions and interacting with their environments (see Griffin 1984, 2001).

But if animals are able to think, does this mean that they can suffer or experience distress? Certain aspects of cognitive processing might be important for the ability to experience distress. For example, a good memory might be important, as it would mean the animal could remember a greater number of stimuli or situations that had caused it harm or danger in the past. An animal species that had the concept of a "future" might be able to contemplate things that were going to happen that were harmful, a bit like a person contemplating an upcoming trip to the dentist.

The physician Eric Cassell, who has written extensively about the meaning of "suffering" in the context of human medicine (see, for example, Cassell 1982), also wrote an article on animal suffering (Cassell 1989). In the article, Cassell argued that only beings with a sense of the future (anticipation) and a sense of self are capable of experiencing suffering. Some animals do appear to have a sense of self (e.g., chimpanzees and the other great apes) and a sense of the future, or at least, they seem to be able to anticipate and reflect on future events. How far such abilities extend through the animal kingdom would necessitate a detailed analysis.

Neither of these aspects of cognitive capability matter, however, if the animal cannot experience these things as "good" or "bad," pleasant or unpleasant. In human terms, the emotional experience associated with an upcoming trip to the dentist is about contemplating possible pain that makes us anxious or fearful. Yet, in comparison to ourselves, we do not worry about whether computers can feel things as good or bad, even if they have the latest, most complex microchip inside and can do the most astoundingly efficient information processing. Are animals the kind of organisms that can feel, or, as Descartes proposed, are they without minds and just biological mechanisms? The one necessary mental capacity for animals to have states of mental well-being is the ability to experience, to be aware of their own bodily sensations, as the welfare of animals relies specifically on the ability of animals to experience states emotionally as pleasant or unpleasant. Can laboratory animal species do this?

Human processing of emotion utilizes certain areas of the brain, notably the limbic system, amygdala, and the nucleus accumbens (Gray & McNaughton 2000). Rodent species, which make up the vast majority of animals used in research, have similar areas of the brain, which are activated during evaluation of the nature of environmental stimuli such as food or the presence of social conspecifics, or aversive stimuli such as electric shocks. Other species such as monkeys and primates also demonstrate similar neurophysiological processing in these areas similar to that of humans. Even birds demonstrate brain functions that are homologous to human emotional processing (Cheng et al. 1999; Seibert, this volume). Note that although the basic neurophysiological "wiring" that underlies emotional processing in humans is also present in animals, this does not mean that animals necessarily experience exactly the same emotional states as humans. It has been argued that animal species such as rodents are incapable of emotional distress on the supposition that they cannot have "experiences." The reasoning states that they may process information in their brains in similar ways to humans but that they are not aware of the consequences of that processing—they do not *feel* the emotion.

Two reasons are given for this theory. First, it is argued that animals do not possess a sufficiently developed neocortex to experience human-type emotions. Second, it is argued that animals do not have a concept of "future" and thus cannot contemplate what will happen to them. They are thus presumed to be unable to experience emotions such as anxiety, grief, or loss (Cassano 1983). The science of animal consciousness is not sufficiently advanced to answer these questions definitively or to determine whether language capabilities or neural processes found only in humans are necessary for conscious experience (Dawkins 2001, Kirkwood & Hubrecht 2001). Some argue, however, that the ability to experience emotions is an essential adaptive trait that has developed through normal and gradual evolutionary processes across a range of species and that its effects can be observed through its influence on animal behavior (Dawkins 1998, Rolls 2000, Griffin 2001).

The claim is that animals have evolved emotions to help them evaluate rewarding and dangerous environmental events and to guide highly flexible behavioral strategies. Neuroscientist Antonio

Damasio (1994) argues that emotional processing is an essential component of human decision making and that without its primary selective function, we are incapable of setting priorities (among the hundreds or thousands of possible options) for our actions. It is not suggested that all animal species have human-quality emotions. It is possible that some complex human emotions such as grief require higher-order cognitive processing. However, it seems evident that simple emotions, such as fear or those associated with pain, appear across a broad range of the phylogenetic spectrum, including the common species used in laboratories such as rodents, rabbits, birds, cats, dogs, and primates.

These emotions may feel quite different in other species than in humans because of species differences in the social and environmental contexts of their evolution. However, the key issue that links human and animal emotions is that they serve the same evolutionary function—aversive subjective states are experienced as unpleasant so as to guide the animal away from harm, and pleasurable states motivate the animal to seek out whatever causes that pleasure (Dawkins 1998). Animals that have a strong emotional experience, such as fear when confronted by a predator, for example, respond rapidly and appropriately and remove themselves from the danger. The emotional experience guides and predisposes what motor behavior is performed. If the choice is guided by trial-and-error learning or the use of fixed rules, the individual might in the former instance be exposed repeatedly to risky situations with an increased probability of injury or death or, in the latter, be too limited in the type of behavioral choices available (Dawkins 1998, Rolls 2000). Emotional valence also increases memory formation and encoding, increasing the likelihood that the event would be available for recall from memory in future.

As animals are unable to report their emotional states verbally, methods that use theories from human economics of consumer demand have proved useful starting points to discuss the costs perceived ("felt") by an animal in its search for a resource or its escape from an aversive environment (see Mendl 2001). A wide range of costs such as pushing open a weighted door, lever pressing, or more "naturalized" costs such as asking rodents to enter an open or brightly-lit space to escape from a stimulus (a common method used for studies of anxiety) can be imposed. In these situations, the open area is something that the animal would avoid in its evolutionary environment, and the cost incurred is the exposure to the aversive environment to gain a resource or escape a situation. These methods have begun to be used to determine animals' priorities to obtain or avoid a range of aspects of housing and husbandry.

One further piece of evidence strongly suggests that laboratory animal species may experience emotions: These animals are often the primary models for the study of human emotion and its neurophysiological basis. Also, the development of psychopharmacological drugs used in the treatment of human mental disorders (e.g., anxiety and depression) rely on the use of animal models of these conditions to assess the effects of putative drugs on emotion-related animal behavior.

ANIMAL MODELS OF MOOD DISORDERS: ANXIETY, FEAR, AND DEPRESSION

The study of human emotions and their dysfunctional states, termed mood disorders, relies on the use of laboratory animals as models of the human state (see Feldman et al. 1997).

FEAR

Fear is defined as a state of intense, unpleasant agitation, apprehension, and/or dread in the presence of something perceived as presenting extreme danger. It is a potent motivator to action, often causing extreme responses in terms of flight from the environment in which the danger exists or freezing to minimize detection and potential harm or death. In itself, fear can be an extremely unpleasant acute experience. Inescapable and chronic fear can be highly debilitating to humans, leading to significant stress and an inability to respond adaptively or functionally. In animals such as dogs, chronic exposure to inescapable fear stimuli can lead to an immobile state, termed learned helplessness, in which the individual no longer attempts to escape but passively submits to repeated exposure to the stimulus, even though it is still deeply unpleasant, and even when an escape route is subsequently made available (Seligman 1975). A wide range of species have been shown to demonstrate fear responses, including domestic chicks, rodents, dogs, and primates. Some fears are considered to have an innate basis, such as the fear of heights, or fear of snakes shown by both humans and monkeys (see, for example, Cook & Mineka 1989).

The amygdala is strongly implicated in the neurophysiological processing of fear in both humans

and laboratory animal species such as rats and primates. When animals are trained to associate an electric shock with a sound, lesions of the amygdala reduce the extent of fear response when the sound occurs in a test situation (LeDoux 1994, 1995, 1996). Different neuronal pathways from the amygdala are associated with specific physiological and behavioral manifestations of fear, including heart rate, endocrine (stress hormone) responses, and freezing behavior.

Studies of fear and its neurophysiological mechanisms often use protocols that expose animals to stimuli strongly associated with pain, such as electric shocks or noise. The fear-potentiated startle test is frequently used to screen pharmacological agents for their ability to reduce fear. In this experimental procedure, a rat is placed in a test cage and exposed to a sudden loud noise, which causes sudden startle movements. Following this, the animal is trained to associate a light coming on and an electric shock occurring simultaneously, the electric shock causing fear. When the animal is tested, the light and the noise are presented together, and the fear state causes the startle response to be heightened. The pharmacological agent can then be assessed for its effectiveness in reducing the fear-related startle response. Treatment with anxiolytics such as the benzodiazepine drugs limits the increase in fear response (see, for example, Treit 1991). These animal models of fear are by no means foolproof and have shown notable variation among laboratories, species, and individual protocols.

ANXIETY

The notion of anxiety is closely associated with that of fear. Although fear is induced by an identifiable object, anxiety typically is associated with a state of agitation and apprehension in which there is no obvious object. Anxiety is an everyday feature of life but is typically described by humans as an unpleasant state. Intense or prolonged anxiety can be extremely debilitating and prevent the performance of ongoing activity. Anxiety disorders in humans manifest in a range of forms, including states of panic and "free floating," or generalized, anxiety disorders. All these states have a feature in common, however: They all involve states of extreme and unpleasant arousal.

Science has only recently come to accept that animals may be able to experience anxiety, although the notion is by no means universally accepted. Tannenbaum (1995), in his landmark text on veterinary ethics, states "it simply does not follow . . . that dogs in veterinarians' offices—much less cows, sheep, chickens or laboratory animals—have a sufficient sense of self or of the future, or are capable of sufficient dread about their own predicaments to justify the attribution of anxiety."

Scientific findings challenge this view. It has begun to be realized that the endocrine, neurophysiological, and behavioral events that occur in animals placed in anxiogenic situations are very similar to the responses of anxious humans (Ninan et al. 1982). These behaviors include motor reactivity and tension, such as shaking and "jumpiness"; hyperactive autonomic responses such as sweating and heart pulse and respiration rate increases, urination, and diarrhea; responses that indicate anticipation of aversive events; and hyperattentiveness, with rapid and repeated monitoring of the environment. The neurophysiological basis of anxiety in humans and animals also demonstrates homology. Many anxiolytic drugs such as alcohol, barbiturates, and benzodiazepines act via the same neuronal receptor sites in humans and animals (Richards & Mohler 1984) and produce the same reduction in overt signs of anxiety. Animals are widely used to research anxiety states and to screen drugs for anxiolytic efficacy, and the results have then been successfully applied to treat human anxiety. Furthermore, anxiogenic agents, such as betacarbolines, that increase anxiety in humans produce the same behavioral and physiological effects in animals (Ninan et al. 1982, Dorow et al. 1983). Evolutionarily, anxiety has been described as a "behavioral inhibition system" that functions to reduce the likelihood that animals will stumble blithely into danger (Gray 1982).

Two primary types of tests examine anxiety in the laboratory—tests of conditioned fear and conflict responses and tests that mirror evolutionarily anxiogenic situations. In conditioned fear response tests, the animal learns to associate a behavior, such as lever pressing or licking, with a food or liquid reward. After this initial training phase, the animal is then exposed to another stimulus such as a light, and during the time this stimulus is activated, the lever press or lick will produce an electric shock. The animal rapidly learns to suppress or inhibit its behavior during this time. Exposure to anxiolytic drugs limits the suppression of the response in a dose-dependent manner. However, these tests involve artificial situations and require lengthy training periods. It is possible, instead, to develop test situations that use their innate "behavioral inhibition system." Mice are thigmotaxic—meaning that they tend to stay close to walls and solid objects and away from open and brightly lit areas. The extent to which mice or rats will move into an open, well-lit area correlates very closely with the effectiveness of anxiolytic and anxiogenic agents (see Feldman et al. 1997).

The tests used to assess the pharmacological effect of anxiolytic drugs can be turned on their heads to examine whether certain environments or experimental procedures cause anxiety (see, for example, Sherwin & Glen 2003, Sherwin & Olsson 2004). The animal can be placed in an environment that is being assessed for its anxiogenicity, such as an environment in which the animal is handled or where the animal is exposed to dominant conspecifics in the home cage. The animal's behavior can then be compared between the control situation and following administration of a known amount of anxiolytic drug. If the animal is less anxious following drug consumption, it will spend more time investigating the conspecifics or will show reduced escape responses to handling. Self-selection tests may also be useful to determine the anxiogenicity of a procedure. In this case, the animal is given two flavors of liquid—one containing water, the other containing water plus the anxiolytic drug. The animal learns to associate the flavor with the drug effect. The animal is then exposed to the procedure or environment that is being assessed and presented with a choice of the two fluids. The assumption is that the animal will consume more of the anxiolytic water if the test situation causes greater anxiety. A number of controls are required for these types of drug self-administration experiments, but the experiments have worked well in assessing otherwise-hidden distress such as pain in animals and birds (see, for example, Danbury et al. 2000) and may be useful for identifying unexpected causes of anxiety in the laboratory.

Fear and anxiety have clear evolutionary adaptive advantages when they are proportional to the extent of risk that is being contemplated; however, in laboratory environments, fear and anxiety responses will reduce welfare and may also affect experimental outcomes. Both direct and indirect aspects of experimental protocols may induce anxiety, or fear if repeated, and certain cues such as the technician's clothing or scent may become associated with an anxiogenic event and thus generalize to other situations in which that cue is present, such as everyday cleaning routines. As yet, very little data is available for us to determine which features of standard laboratory practice are anxiogenic.

DEPRESSION

Like anxiety, depression is a common human mental health issue. As with other mood disorders, it becomes a concern when the intensity or pervasiveness of the state begins to disrupt normal activity and pleasurable (hedonic) behavior. Depression in humans is characterized by diverse features such as a low mood, tiredness and fatigue, disordered sleep, an inability to enjoy previously pleasurable experiences such as food or sex (anhedonia), and a pessimistic perspective on the likely outcome of events. Depression may occur co-morbidly alongside other negative mood states such as anxiety. Does a concomitant state exist in animals? Again, we can look to neurophysiology, pharmacology, and behavior for evidence.

Depressive states involve the dopaminergic and serotonin systems in both humans and animals (see Feldman et al. 1997). The oldest animal model of depression was produced by administering a dopamine antagonist, reserpine, to block dopamine-mediated neural transmission in the brain. Animals exposed to this drug displayed the inactivity and anhedonia typical of depressed people. Other screening models include behavioral despair syndrome, in which the mouse or rat is placed in a tank filled with opaque water and forced to swim without escape. As occurs in the state of learned helplessness, the animal eventually gives up. The time until swimming stops is the dependent variable in these studies.

Some studies have shown that laboratory animals maintained in standard housing display behaviors similar to those of the animal models of depression outlined above. The inactivity and anhedonia in these situations can be improved with antidepressant medication. In these situations, one may also observe obviously abnormal behaviors such as increasing self-focused behavior, including self-mutilation. These behaviors not only lead to threats to physical welfare but may also indicate psychiatric dysfunction.

One recent study has demonstrated a novel behavioral-challenge approach to determining animal perspectives and indicates that some standard laboratory housing conditions may lead to signs of depression in the rodents, even when the animals appear to behave normally. Harding et al. (2004) trained their rodents by first playing two tones—one of which predicted an unpleasant noise while the other predicted a food reward. Harding and colleagues then tested the animals by playing them a sound halfway between the two previously played tones and assessed, by the elicited behavior, which of the two original tones the animals thought was being played. Two groups of animals were tested; one group had been reared in a stable environment while another had been housed in unpredictable conditions. The animals' responses indicated that those individuals reared in unstable conditions were more likely than those reared in stable environments to expect the neutral situation to be associated with a negative outcome. This test is a first hint that standard laboratory housing may lead to cognitive states that look like depression in laboratory rodents.

KEEPING THE MIND ALIVE: BOREDOM, VARIABILITY, ENVIRONMENTAL CHALLENGE, AND EXPLORATION.

The differences between laboratory cage environments and those in which species evolved may have quite profound implications for the mental health of research animals. In recognizing that animals are cognitive and social beings, science has grasped a nettle: Are there aspects of housing, routines, or other stimuli that research animals need to maintain mental health? The captive environment provides significantly reduced diversity of resources and environmental variability. Francoise Wemelsfelder has proposed that animals may need a certain amount of environmental challenge in terms of variation and diversity and that the absence of sufficient variation may lead to boredom and understimulation (Wemelsfelder 1993, 1997, this volume; Wemelsfelder & Birke 1997).

Does the need for environmental diversity imply that the animal is "bored?" This is not necessarily the case. Rather, the animal may need certain kinds of environmental challenge appropriate to its species (Mench 1998). Environmental stimulation that is relevant to the animal will maintain levels of vigilance and physiological arousal as well as increase opportunities for functional behavior. The key here is to find the resources that matter to the animal itself; it is of little benefit to the animal to have a resource in the cage that initially provides novelty but is then just ignored. The evolutionary environment provides the initial guide to the type of environmental features that the animal might need (Olsson & Dahlborn 2002, Olsson et al. 2003), including physical objects such as shelters or nests, dimmed illumination, or social stimuli from the presence of conspecifics. For example, mink will push more than three times their body weights to get access to water for swimming and demonstrate strong physiological stress responses reflective of frustration when access is then denied (Mason et al. 2001). As discussed earlier, consumer demand studies are beginning to demonstrate priorities for particular species. Much more information is still needed about the resource requirements of laboratory animal species.

Much is made of the concept of environmental enrichment in the laboratory. "Enrichment" describes the modification or addition of resources that facilitate behavior within the cage, ideally for the benefit of animal welfare. Such enrichment does not mean constructing a fully natural environment. By relying on evidence of animal priorities, alongside a range of other behavioral and physiological measures to determine the animal's welfare (see King 2003), enrichment studies do not aim to build "gilded cages," but rather attempt to identify the key resources that the animal needs to maintain good mental and physical welfare (Olsson & Dahlborn 2002). This idea of environmental enrichment links directly with scientifically derived concepts of psychological well-being, which in turn mirror closely the WHO's definition of mental health for humans outlined earlier.

In attempting to address the Animal Welfare Act amendments of 1985, which required laboratories to promote the psychological well-being of any primates in their care, the Institute for Laboratory Animal Research (1998) identified a range of features that comprise psychological well-being, specifically

- the ability to cope effectively with day-to-day changes in the social and physical environment
- the ability to engage in beneficial species-typical activities
- the absence of maladaptive or pathological behavior
- the presence of a balanced temperament and the absence of chronic signs of distress

Features of the laboratory environment that may influence psychological well-being include social companionship and aggression, opportunities for species-typical behavior, housing design, human-animal interactions with technicians and investigators, restraint, and experimental use in studies involving diverse protocols such as multiple survival surgery and infectious disease (Institute for Laboratory Animal Research 1998).

MANAGEMENT OF AND CHALLENGES TO PSYCHOLOGICAL WELL-BEING IN THE LABORATORY

So far, we have provided a theoretical basis for understanding the psychological states of laboratory animals. Evidence from behavioral studies, neurophysiology, and psychopharmacology has begun to demonstrate that animal species used in research may experience emotional distress.

Methods for assessing aversion and anxiety in laboratory animals are only now beginning to be used for purposes of measuring applied animal welfare. Also very useful are consumer demand indices, which are based in economic theory and assess the importance that the animal places on gaining, avoiding or escaping from a resource or situation (see Rushen 1986, Dawkins 1990). As an example, a simple preference test has provided important evidence about the experience of anesthesia and euthanasia agents in laboratory animals (Rushen 1986; Leach et al. 2002a, 2002b). In this experiment, laboratory-bred rodents were exposed to the various concentrations of anesthetic and euthanasia gases in a test chamber that they were able to enter and leave at will. Aversion, assessed by measuring initial withdrawal time and total dwelling time in the test chamber, revealed that CO_2 is highly aversive when compared to other gases. It should be noted that some experimental manipulations may influence the animal's ability to respond in the test situation. For example, barbiturates and benzodiazepines slow rates of responding and can reduce cognitive capabilities. Animal subjects may be slower to move and take longer to escape because of confounding physiological effects. Investigators must be careful to control for such side effects when assessing behavior.

Many primate species are highly social and perform a multitude of social communications and interactions including mutual grooming, play behaviors, and sexual activity. Social contact is essential in apes for the normal development of behavior and later social interactions (see, for example, Fritz & Howell 1993). Deprivation of early social contact can lead to the development of self-biting, abnormal stereotypic swaying and rocking behaviors, and abnormal social interactions such as increased aggression and dysfunctional affiliative behavior in adulthood. Without social experience, maternal behavior can also be impaired, leading to neglect of offspring or unusual and potentially harmful aggression. The dynamics of the social group, influenced by sex ratio and age of conspecifics as well as their individual developmental histories, may also require consideration. The stability of dominance relationships between individuals can influence access to resources such as food, water, and sleeping areas, as well as the likelihood of aggression and injury. The benefits of social housing are profound, however, and may be augmented by provision of particular resources to facilitate play or exercise behaviors. Simple resources such as ropes can increase activities like chasing, and raised platforms can provide areas of escape for subordinate animals. Some research protocols require the primates to be housed singly, for example, where the animal is subject to stereotaxic surgery and device implantation and may be exposed to further damage and infection if housed with conspecifics. In these cases, it is important that the animal have at least visual and aural contact with conspecifics.

Social contact is not just limited to interactions with conspecifics; indeed, for primates and monkeys, the caregiver and other humans may also be sources of positive social interaction. For human-animal interactions to be beneficial, however, it is important that the animal be habituated to the caregivers and associate them with positive experiences, otherwise fear and anxiety may result. Rhesus macaques, widely used in biomedical and neurophysiological research, are often seen as highly aggressive and are consequently housed singly and restrained during handling (Bernstein et al. 1974). Single housing is associated with an increased incidence of self-inflicted injury, but aggression may well be a response to the fearful and aversive situation of, for example, being placed in a crush cage for blood sampling. Yet when given positive rewards during handling, many of the monkeys could be trained to voluntarily offer limbs for venipuncture, thus reducing the need for restraint and associated stress and potential for injury as well as allowing the animal some control over its involvement in the procedure (Reinhardt 1991, 1997, 2002). In practical terms, positive human-animal interactions can also be a source of professional and morale development for research workers and minimize health and safety risks associated with animal handling.

Social interactions are also important aspects of the laboratory environment for other species (Patterson-Kane et al. 2002, Patterson-Kane 2003). Rats are social creatures and in the wild often live in large groups made up of related individuals. Mice also form dominance relationships and utilize a range of social cues to gain information about their environment, such as the location of territory boundaries and food sources. Much information is conveyed through olfactory cues such as urine scent-marks around territories and valued resources. In addition, the scents of other mice provide information about relatedness and dominance status between males. Social dominance can influence a wide range of factors in animal well-being, such as endocrine responses, growth rate, immune function, and even behavior during experimental protocols such as the open field test (see, for example, Gerlai & Clayton 1999). Cage cleaning is an important aspect of maintenance of hygiene and physical health of research animals; however, it also disrupts scent markings within the laboratory cage. These marks are important messengers of information about the accessibility of resources, familiarity of conspecifics, and the social position of individuals, so their disruption has the potential to increase aggression and dangers within the cage.

Social factors are also important in the physical and behavioral development of rodents, even before they are born. Exposure of gravid females to stressful events can influence the growth rate, propensity for aggression, and sexual behavior of their offspring later in their adult lives. Laboratory rodents subjected to stress during pre- and neonatal periods demonstrate enhanced responses to stressful stimuli. The presence of parents and caregivers in the nest, as well as the number of littermates, influences food intake, which in itself can have dramatic effects on growth and responses to stress in adulthood (see Braastad 1998, Latham & Mason 2004).

Evolutionary factors may also influence human-animal interactions such as handling during experimental procedures and cage cleaning. For a mouse or a bird, handling by a human may well induce a state of considerable fear and anxiety. It may be possible to habituate the animal to the experience; however, in some cases, the reverse may happen, where the animal or bird's response becomes sensitized and even generalized to other caregivers (see, for example, Jones 1994). Some authors have suggested that, for laboratory rats, handling should be either frequent and predictable, or minimized (Patterson-Kane 2003).

The housing of laboratory animals, in terms of cage space, specific resources, and environmental aspects like illumination and aural stimuli, can have diverse influences on animal well-being, some of which may have a great impact on mental health. Rodent housing often includes only minimal resources compared with the diverse and highly variable environments in which laboratory mouse (*Mus musculus*) and rat (*Rattus norvegicus*) strains have their origins (Sherwin 1996). Laboratory mice demonstrate a range of unusual behaviors that are not observed in the wild environment, and these may have important consequences for behavioral development and flexibility (Balcombe 2004).

The effect of laboratory animal housing on welfare, cognition, behavior, and psychiatric dysfunction is only now becoming a topic for research. Historically, scientific protocols have been designed to standardize the housing and husbandry arrangements of laboratory animals as much as possible so that all animals experience similar conditions and extraneous environmental variables can be minimized or eliminated. However, this standardization leads to a diminution of environmental complexity in laboratory housing. Scientific research is beginning to show that laboratory housing standardization may have had the opposite effect; it may have caused greater variation between individual animals because of varying production of abnormal behavior.

Such individual differences and abnormalities only became fully apparent when researchers began to take an ethological approach to the laboratory rodent and assess its behavior when the animal was most active, which is during nighttime (Wuerbel 2001a). During their waking phase, many mice were observed to perform strange repetitive behaviors such as leaping at the cage roof or following very exact paths around the cage. Others gnawed at the cage bars and did so in a strangely predictable manner, following closely a tight timing and placement of movements that was repeated again and again. These repetitive-type behaviors rang alarm bells. They are also seen in some humans who have experienced head injuries, learning disabilities, mental disorders, and susceptibility to amphetamine psychosis. These behaviors have also been seen in other captive animals outside the laboratory, such as in zoo-housed tigers and polar bears as well as fur-farmed mink (Mason et al. 2001, Clubb & Mason 2003). Other studies have demonstrated that these "stereotypies" are associated with intense frustration or occur when particular resources needed by the animal to perform specific behaviors were not provided (Mason 1991a, 1991b; Mason et al. 2001).

Interestingly, specific resources were found to reduce or remove the laboratory rodents' stereotypic behavior. Provision of tunnels or other materials which the rodents could use to make burrows

proved to be very important (see Wuerbel 2001a). In other tests, laboratory rodents also show preferences and, in some cases, demand for shelters and nesting material (see Patterson-Kane 2003). These stereotypies take many different forms, and often, the original behavior from which they developed can be seen in the etiology of the behavior. For example, jumping and gnawing stereotypies may arise from attempts to escape and stereotypic digging from attempts to create a burrow (Wiedenmayer 1997).

The consequences of stereotypic behaviors in laboratory animals are much broader than individual animal welfare and have both ethical and scientific ramifications. Recent research suggests that the performance of stereotypic behavior is strongly correlated with the presence of psychiatric dysfunctions similar to those demonstrated by autistic individuals. It is possible that the animals displaying such behavior have experienced permanent mental damage. It is important that functional behavior provides an ability to respond flexibly and appropriately to changes in environmental stimuli.

Animals reared in standard laboratory conditions were observed to determine how much stereotypy they performed (Garner & Mason 2002; Garner et al. 2003a, 2003b). They were then tested in a task that measured whether they could respond flexibly to changes in their environment. The animals were trained to recognize that by making a particular response (e.g., pressing a lever or pecking a key), they gained a small food reward. In the test, when the reward changed to a different lever, "normal" animals would soon learn this and change their response accordingly. Those animals that demonstrated more stereotypy did not change their behavior; they continued to make the wrong response even though it was no longer rewarding. This may indicate an underlying neural deficit in which the animals' neural connections have become altered in such a way that they do not make the switch to produce a different type of motor behavior. If this is the case, it has major implications for both ethics and science, as it may mean that by being housed in standardized conditions, laboratory animals may become permanently altered. For any scientific results that rely on testing an animal's behavioral responses, it also suggests that these animals may not be able to behave properly when tested. It may also explain how stereotypic behavior seen in laboratory rodents becomes emancipated or, in other words, performed in situations where the original stimuli that caused it are no longer present. It may also explain why some stereotypies are so hard to change when enrichment is introduced in the animals' adulthood (see, for example, Cooper et al. 1996).

It should be noted that the performance of stereotypy does not necessarily mean the animal is impaired. In some cases, the performance of stereotypies themselves has been found to be rewarding. Other scientists argue further that in some cases, it should also raise concern if the animals do not perform the stereotypies when reared or housed in conditions that are known to evoke these behaviors, as they still lack the opportunity to behave functionally to get the resources they need (Mason & Latham 2004). It seems that understanding the environment in which an animal has evolved and then determining which aspects of that environment are important to the animal itself may go a long way toward ensuring that the mental health of laboratory animals is not compromised (see Olsson et al. 2003).

One question that often arises regarding laboratory animal species pertains to whether they are at all like their wild ancestors. Would it not seem reasonable that the many generations of selective breeding have altered the animals' behaviors and behavioral needs so they simply do not need these resources in the laboratory cage? Certainly, selective breeding can have dramatic effect on behavior and resulting consequences for optimal welfare conditions. For example, broiler meat chickens have been so strongly selected for growth that they develop painful leg weaknesses and also are more efficient foragers, thus reducing the amount of activity they need to perform to obtain food. Egg-laying hens have been selected against broodiness (the propensity to sit on their eggs) to such an extent that this behavior is now relatively rare. In one strain of laboratory dogs, selection caused dramatic differences in responses to humans, with one resulting strain showing extreme fear and anxiety at human interaction while the other strain, remained unconcerned (Reese 1979).

That an animal does not perform a diversity of behaviors in the laboratory cage, however, does not mean it has "lost" those behaviors. In an innovative experiment, Manuel Berdoy and his colleagues at Oxford University took adult laboratory rats and filmed their return to the wild (Berdoy 2003). The rats rapidly adapted to their new conditions and showed a huge diversity of natural behaviors including foraging, digging burrows, building nests, and social behavior such as territoriality. They demonstrated the same responses to novel foods and unfamiliar stimuli as their wild counterparts. These

behaviors clearly had not been bred out of the laboratory strain. The film account of this study, sponsored by the UK Government's research regulators, has become an award-winning educational tool for understanding both animal behavior and laboratory rodent management.

The effect of environmental conditions and human handling has been shown to have notable effects on animal experiments, not just in terms of the subjects' behavior but also in physiology and disease progression. In one experiment assessing the progress of Huntington's disease in rodents, supplying basic environmental enrichment in the form of cardboard tunnels (the readily available insides of rolls of toilet paper) altered the progression of the disease such that it more closely mimicked the human form of the disease (Hockly et al. 2002). In a study of atherosclerosis in rabbits, the effect of the quality of human interactions with the animal subjects was profound. The group of rabbits that were given gentle positive human contact (e.g., holding, petting, talking to) by a caregiver every day developed far less atherosclerotic lesions on an atherogenic diet compared to the group that received standard laboratory handling (Nerem et al. 1980).

These results suggest two conclusions. First, the concept of standardization can lead one to a false sense of comfort; environments that are standardized simply by limiting the provision of facilities to the basic life needs of the animals can and do have unexpected effects on both welfare and experimental results (Wuerbel 2001a, 2001b). As laboratories around the world are likely to use different practices, this has implications for the replicability and interpretation of scientific data. Second, if we are to understand the implications of housing, husbandry, and experimental procedures for laboratory animal well-being and scientific data, studies on animal well-being have to be undertaken and should occur alongside the basic scientific research, which results in these animals being in the laboratory in the first place.

The dualistic idea that mental and physical health are separate aspects of well-being is beginning to be challenged. It is already known that emotional context influences the subjective experience of pain and that mental well-being can influence disease progression in both humans and animals. The effects of stressors impact the whole animal in terms of emotion, cognitive performance, health, and growth. The understanding that animals have mental lives may require that the consequences of experiments for animals in terms of injury, pain, sickness, and disease are evaluated so as to consider the effect of these conditions not just in terms of their physical harm but also of their mental harm. As the experience of well-being is mediated in mental terms, it is possible that the mental suffering associated with animal use in research is currently underestimated.

SUMMARY AND FUTURE DEVELOPMENTS IN LABORATORY ANIMAL MENTAL HEALTH

We are only beginning to understand the emotional states of species used in research. However, emotional responses appear to be integral aspects of an animal's adaptive response to its environment and as such must be integrated into concepts of animal welfare and considered when evaluating the impact of research on the animals. Situations exist within the laboratory environment that appear to be mentally distressing to a substantial or prolonged extent. Evidence of fear and anxiety exists in many laboratory situations; however, much more information is needed to identify the costs of research on its subjects' well-being. Ideally, the performance of research for the sake of applied animal welfare should be piggybacked on existing research protocols so as to prevent further animal suffering and to maximize correspondence between data in biomedical research and the effects of an animal's mental well-being in terms of experimental controls (King 2003). Growing evidence also exists for psychiatric dysfunction in some laboratory animals, as indicated by the presence of abnormal behavior in lab animal populations. These behaviors may have implications for the quality of research data as well as for animal welfare.

An understanding of the ethological basis of animal behavior can allow design of laboratory environments that more closely fit the mental and emotional needs of laboratory animal species. Simple environmental modifications can reap notable rewards for laboratory animals' mental welfare, such as reducing extraneous sources of ultrasound in rodent laboratories, providing areas of cover in brightly lit cages, providing tunnels and shelters for some rodent species, and providing positive rewards and interactions to train rather than force primates to participate in experimental procedures.

Some aspects of mental well-being are only just beginning to be understood, such as the role of environmental stimuli in maintaining arousal and preventing understimulation and possible emotional consequences such as depression. Also needing much further investigation is the role of psychiatric dysfunction in the performance of abnormal stereotypic behavior. As mental well-being is now considered to be a part of animal welfare, we may be able to develop a greater understanding of the linkages between the physiological and emotional content and consequences of disease conditions, sickness behaviors, and pain related to injury or surgery (see, for example, Gregory 1998, Rutherford 2002). In so doing, we may gain information of benefit to our understanding of the mental mediation of disease and recovery, for the benefit of both animals and humans. It is now widely recognized that pain is a significant and deeply unpleasant state and that emotional processing mediates the quality and extent of the experience of pain. This increases the importance of considering emotional aspects of laboratory animal experience in analgesic management.

Mental distress is not the opposite of mental health. Conditions for the housing and husbandry of laboratory animals should meet the animals' minimum behavioral needs; however, scientists studying animal welfare have recently argued that this is not enough—that mental well-being is about states of contentment and happiness and not just an absence of unpleasant experiences. This approach notably echoes the human conceptualization of mental health as defined by the WHO. Animal "happiness" is currently a much more difficult subject of study, but in keeping with public concern for animals used in research, may become a priority for research in the future (see McMillan, this volume, Chapter 16).

Other factors in the development of biomedical research may influence future concerns for mental well-being. One of these is the exponential rise of the use of transgenic rodents as models for biomedical conditions. These animals are genetically altered so as to express certain genes or are gene "knockouts" where the effect of a particular gene is removed. The effect of preventing the expression of certain genes on a wide range of aspects of welfare that may influence mental health is diverse and unpredictable and emphasizes the need for thorough evaluation and recording of phenotypic expression and welfare profiles including humane endpoints for these animals (Morton 2000, Jegstrup et al. 2003).

The effects of gene knockouts on welfare include possibilities for behavioral limitations or increased pain due to overgrowth of body parts such as teeth and cognitive impairments preventing functional interactions (Morton 2004). Models of psychiatric disorders are of particular concern for mental welfare and the ethics of animal research, as these animals may be created to be predisposed to mental dysfunction. The breeding of animals for particular behavior and temperament or "personality" traits is not new. The breeding of fighting cockerels for aggression, the selection for strains of beagle dogs for their docility for use in research, and the presence of particular traits in certain strains of dogs for social anxiety during human-animal interactions (see, for example, Reese 1979) are examples of how humans have selected, manipulated, and amplified traits found in nature. The difference in transgenic research is the unpredictability of outcomes in the creation of knockout models and the sheer scale of their production. It is possible that the breeding and use of laboratory mice may have soared to as high as 100 million (from around 20–25 million) in the past decade in the United States. Research into gerontology and the neurological basis of aging-related diseases like Parkinsonism and Alzheimer's disease may also increase the numbers of primates used in research in future years, leading to renewed concerns for the mental well-being of these cognitively and emotionally advanced species.

Our understanding of the mental health of laboratory animals may be only in its infancy, but it is an integral part of our attempts to understand the animals' welfare and the costs these animals experience in laboratory housing and as subjects of research. The phylogenetic sphere of ethical concern is also expanding as we begin to understand the richness of the mental lives of a wider array of species. Such studies are changing the way we view our moral responsibilities to a wider array of species such as the laboratory rodents. Furthermore, new studies suggest that even those species that have previously been considered incapable of basic experiences such as pain—for example, fish—may also "feel" pain (Sneddon 2003, Sneddon et al. 2003). We owe it to those animals to ensure they are given full consideration. Finally, a better understanding of the mental health of animals used in laboratories will give us better scientific data and better insight into the complex products of modern biomedical research.

REFERENCES

Balcombe J. 2004. Laboratory routines cause animal stress. *Contemp Top Lab Anim*: in press.

Berdoy M. 2003. The laboratory rat: A natural history. Accessed 4/30/04 from www.ratlife.org

Bernstein IS, Gordon TP, Rose RM, et al. 1974. Factors influencing the expression of aggression during introductions to rhesus monkey groups. In: Holloway RL (ed), *Primate aggression, territoriality and xenophobia*. New York, Academic Press:211–240.

Braastad BO. 1998. Effects of prenatal stress on behaviour of offspring of laboratory and farmed animals. *Appl Anim Behav Sci* 61:159–180.

Broom DM, Johnson KG. 1993. *Stress and animal welfare*. London: Chapman and Hall.

Cassano GB. 1983. What is pathological anxiety and what is not. In: Costa E (ed), *The benzodiazepines: From molecular biology to clinical practice*. New York, Raven Press:287–293.

Cassel EJ. 1982. The nature of suffering and the goals of medicine. *New Engl J Med* 306:639–645.

Cassel EJ. 1989. What is suffering? In: Guttman HN, Mench JA, Simmonds RC (eds), *Science and animals: Addressing contemporary issues*. Bethesda, MD, Scientists Center for Animal Welfare:13–16.

Cheng MF, Chaiken M, Zuo M, et al. 1999. Nucleus taenia of the amygdala of birds: Anatomical and functional studies in ring doves (*Streptopelia risoria*) and European starlings (*Sturnus vulgaris*). *Brain Behav Evolut* 53:243–270.

Clubb R, Mason G. 2003. Captivity effects on wide-ranging carnivores. *Nature* 425:473–474.

Cook M, Mineka S. 1989. Observational conditioning of fear to fear-relevant versus fear-irrelevant stimuli in monkeys. *J Abnorm Psychol* 98:448–459.

Cooper J, Odberg F, Nicol CJ. 1996. Limitations on the effectiveness of environmental improvement in reducing stereotypic behavior in bank voles (*Clethrionomys glareolus*). *Appl Anim Behav Sci* 48:237–248.

Damasio AR. 1994. *Descartes' error: Emotion, reason and the human brain*. New York: G. P. Putnam's Sons.

Danbury TC, Weeks CA, Chambers JP, et al. 2000. Self-selection of the analgesic drug carprofen by lame broiler chickens. *Vet Rec* 146:307–311.

Dawkins MS. 1990. From an animal's point of view—motivation, fitness, and animal welfare. *Behav Brain Sci* 13:1–61.

Dawkins MS. 1998. Evolution and animal welfare. *Q Rev Biol* 73:305–328.

Dawkins MS. 2001. Who needs consciousness? *Anim Welfare* 10:S19–S29.

Dorow R, Horowski R, Paschelke G, et al. 1983. Severe anxiety induced by FG7142: A beta-carboline ligand for benzidiazepine receptors. *Lancet* 2:98–99.

Feldman RS, Meyer JS, Quenzer LF. 1997. *Principles of neuropsychopharmacology*. Sunderland, MA: Sindauer.

Fritz J, Howell S. 1993. Psychological wellness for captive chimpanzees: An evaluative program. *Humane Innovations Alternatives* 7:426–433.

Garner JP, Mason GJ. 2002. Evidence for a relationship between cage stereotypies and behavioural disinhibition in laboratory rodents. *Behav Brain Res* 136:83–92.

Garner JP, Mason GJ, Smith R. 2003a. Stereotypic route-tracing in experimentally caged songbirds correlates with general behavioural disinhibition. *Anim Behav* 66:711–727.

Garner JP, Meehan CL, Mench JA. 2003b. Stereotypies in caged parrots, schizophrenia and autism: Evidence for a common mechanism. *Behav Brain Res* 145:125–134.

Gerlai R, Clayton NS. 1999. Analysing hippocampal function in transgenic mice: An ethological perspective. Trends Neurosci 22:47–51.

Gray JA. 1982. *The neuropsychology of anxiety*. New York: Oxford University Press.

Gray JA, McNaughton N. 2000. *The neuropsychology of anxiety*, 2nd ed. Oxford, UK: Oxford University Press.

Gregory NG. 1998. Physiological mechanisms causing sickness behaviour and suffering in diseased animals. *Anim Welfare* 7:293–305.

Griffin DG. 1984. *Animal thinking*. Cambridge, MA: Harvard University Press.

Griffin DG. 2001. Animal minds: Beyond cognition to consciousness. Chicago: University of Chicago Press.

Harding EJ, Paul ES, Mendl M. 2004. Animal behavior: Cognitive bias and affective state. *Nature* 427:312.

Hockly E, Cordery PM, Woodman B, et al. 2002. Environmental enrichment slows disease progression in R61/2 Huntington's disease mice. *Ann Neurol* 51:235–242.

Humane Society of the United States. 2002. Taking animal welfare seriously: Minimizing pain and distress in research animals. Website: Accessed 7/17/04 from http://hsus.org/ace/11425?pg=1.

Institute for Laboratory Animal Research. 1998. *The psychological well-being of nonhuman primates*. Washington, DC: National Academies Press.

Institute for Laboratory Animal Research. 2003. Guidelines for the care and use of mammals in neuroscience and behavioral research. Washington, DC: National Academies Press.

Jegstrup I, Thon R, Hansen AK, et al. 2003. Characterization of transgenic mice—a comparison of protocols for welfare evaluation and phenotype characterization of mice with a suggestion on a future certificate of instruction. *Lab Anim* 37:1–9.

Jones RB. 1994. Regular handling and the domestic chicks fear of human-beings—generalization of response. *Appl Anim Behav Sci* 42:129–143.

Kemerling G. 2001. Ludwig Wittgenstein: Analysis of language. Accessed 4/30/04 from http://www.philosophypages.com/hy/6s.htm

King LA. 2003. Behavioral evaluation of the psychological welfare and environmental requirements of agricultural research animals: Theory, measurement, ethics, and practical implications. *ILAR J* 44:211–221.

Kirkwood JK, Hubrecht R. 2001. Animal consciousness, cognition and welfare. *Anim Welfare* 10:S5–S17.

Kitchen H, Aronson AL, Bittel JL, et al. 1987. Panel report on the colloquium on recognition and alleviation of animal pain and distress. *J Am Vet Med Assoc* 191:1186–1191.

Latham N, Mason G. 2004. From house mouse to mouse house: The behavioural biology of free-living *Mus musculus* and its implications in the laboratory. *Appl Anim Behav Sci*: in press.

Leach MC, Bowell VA, Allan TF, et al. 2002a. Degrees of aversion shown by rats and mice to different concentrations of inhalational anaesthetics. *Vet Rec* 150:808–815.

Leach MC, Bowell VA, Allan TF, et al. 2002b. Aversion to gaseous euthanasia agents in rats and mice. *Comparative Med* 52:249–257.

LeDoux JE. 1994. Emotion, memory and the brain. *Sci Am* 270:32–39.

LeDoux JE. 1995. Emotion: Clues from the brain. *Annu Rev Psychol* 46:209–235.

LeDoux JE. 1996. *The emotional brain*. New York: Simon and Schuster.

Mason GJ. 1991a. Stereotypies and suffering. *Behav Process* 25:103–115.

Mason GJ. 1991b. Stereotypies—a critical review. *Anim Behav* 41:1015–1037.

Mason GJ, Cooper J, Clarebrough C. 2001. Frustrations of fur-farmed mink. *Nature* 410:35–36.

Mason GJ, Latham N. 2004. Can't stop, won't stop: Is stereotypy a reliable animal welfare indicator? *Anim Welfare* 13:S57–S69.

Mench JA. 1998. Environmental enrichment and the importance of exploratory behavior. In: Shepherdson DJ, Mellen JD, Hutchins M (eds), *Second nature: Environmental enrichment for captive animals*. Washington, DC, Smithsonian Institution:30–46.

Mendl M. 2001. Animal husbandry—assessing the welfare state. *Nature* 410:31–32.

Moberg GP, Mench JA. 2000. *The biology of animal stress: Basic principles and implications for animal welfare*. New York: CAB International.

Morton DB. 2000. A systematic approach for establishing humane endpoints. *ILAR J* 41:80–86.

Morton DB. 2004. Personal communication. University of Birmingham, Birmingham, UK.

Nerem RM, Levesque MJ, Cornhill JF. 1980. Social environment as a factor in diet-induced atherosclerosis. *Science* 208:1475–1476.

Ninan PT, Insel TM, Cohen RM, et al. 1982. Benzodiazepine receptor-mediated experimental anxiety in primates. *Science* 218:1332–1334.

Olsson IAS, Dahlborn K. 2002. Improving housing conditions for laboratory mice: A review of 'environmental enrichment'. *Lab Anim* 36:243–270.

Olsson IAS, Nevison CM, Patterson-Kane EG, et al. 2003. Understanding behaviour: The relevance of ethological approaches in laboratory animal science. *Appl Anim Behav Sci* 81:245–264.

Patterson-Kane EG. 2003. Shelter enrichment for rats. *Contemp Top Lab Anim* 42:46–48.

Patterson-Kane EG, Hunt M, Harper D. 2002. Rats demand social contact. *Anim Welfare* 11:327–332.

Reese WG. 1979. A dog model for human psychopathology. *Am J Psychiat* 136:1168–1172.

Reinhardt V. 1991. Training adult rhesus male monkeys to actively cooperate during in-homecage venipuncture. *Anim Technology* 42:11–17.

Reinhardt V. 1997. Training nonhuman primates to cooperate during handling procedures: A review. *Anim Technology* 48:55–73.

Reinhardt V. 2002. The myth of the aggressive monkey. *J Appl Anim Welf Sci* 5:321–330.

Richards JG, Mohler H. 1984. Benzodiazepine receptors. *Neuropharmacology* 23:233–242.

Rollin BE. 1990. The unheeded cry: Animal consciousness, animal pain and science. Oxford, UK: Oxford University Press.

Rolls ET. 2000. Precis of the brain and emotion. *Behav Brain Sci* 23:177–234.

Rowan AN. 1988. Animal anxiety and animal suffering. Appl Anim Behav Sci 20:135–142.

Rushen J. 1986. The validity of behavioural measures of aversion: A review. Appl Anim Behav Sci 16:309–323.

Rutherford KMD. 2002. Assessing pain in animals. Anim Welfare 11:31–53.

Seligman MEP. 1975. Helplessness: On depression, development and death. San Francisco: Freeman.

Sherwin CM. 1996. Laboratory mice persist in gaining access to resources: A method of assessing the importance of environmental features. Appl Anim Behav Sci 48:203–213.

Sherwin CM, Glen EF. 2003. Cage colour preferences and effects of home cage colour on anxiety in laboratory mice. Anim Behav 66:1085–1092.

Sherwin CM, Olsson IAS. 2004. Housing conditions affect self-administration of anxiolytic by laboratory mice. *Anim Welfare* 13:33–38.

Sneddon LU. 2003. The evidence for pain in fish: the use of morphine as an analgesic. *Appl Anim Behav Sci* 83:153–162.

Sneddon LU, Braithwaite VA, Gentle MJ. 2003. Do fishes have nociceptors? Evidence for the evolution of a vertebrate sensory system. *P Roy Soc Lond B Bio* 270:1115–1121.

Tannenbaum J. 1995. *Veterinary ethics*. St. Louis, MO: Mosby.

Treit D. 1991. Anxiolytic effects of BDZsand 5-HT1A agonists: Animal models. In: Cooper SJ, Rodgers RJ (eds), *5-ht1a agonists, 5-ht3 antagonists and benzodiazepines: Their comparative behavioural pharmacology*. New York, John Wiley & Sons:107–131.

Wemelsfelder F. 1993. The concept of animal boredom and its relationship to stereotyped behaviour. In: Lawrence AB, Rushen J (eds), *Stereotypic animal behaviour: Fundamentals and applications to welfare*. Wallingford, UK, CAB International:65–95.

Wemelsfelder F. 1997. Life in captivity: Its lack of opportunities for variable behaviour. *Appl Anim Behav Sci* 54:67–70.

Wemelsfelder F, Birke L. 1997. Environmental challenge. In: Appleby MC, Hughes BO (eds), *Animal welfare*. Wallingford, UK, CAB International:35–48.

Wiedenmayer C. 1997. Causation of the ontogenetic development of stereotypic digging in gerbils. *Anim Behav* 53:461–470.

World Health Organization. 2001. Accessed 4/30/04 from http://www.who.int/mediacentre/factsheets/fs220/en/print.html

World Health Organization. 2003. Accessed 4/30/04 from http://www.who.int/about/definition/en/

Wuerbel H. 2001a. Ideal homes? Housing effects on rodent brain and behaviour. *Trends Neurosci* 24:207–211.

Wuerbel H. 2001b. Behaviour and the standardization fallacy. *Nat Genet* 26:263.

20
Animal Well-Being
and Research Outcomes

Hal Markowitz and Gregory B. Timmel

INTRODUCTION

Historically, a gap has existed between the methods employed in behavioral ecology and those utilized in some laboratory animal research. The application of knowledge concerning the behavior of animals in nature is necessary to ensure captive studies in which animals serve as the best research models possible. Laboratory researchers and animal care staff have become increasingly aware of this fact. However, it is important that those of us who are involved with animal studies keep this at the forefront of our minds to ensure research and teaching methodologies that take into account the natural behaviors of our animal subjects.

This may be challenging due to the compartmentalized way in which many of us have been taught research techniques. Those interested in studying the effects of independent variables on experimental outcomes are appropriately taught the importance of "controlling" variables other than the critical stimulus, the effects of which we hope to assess. For example, most of us who do laboratory research clearly know that it would be foolish to allow room heat, light, or noise to fluctuate in an uncontrolled way when we are trying to study the effect of some new drug on the metabolism of animals. The paradox lies in the fact that our efforts to ward off all *uncontrolled* variables may lead to the production of research conditions in which the controls employed *produce* unintentional and unwanted outcomes. The most apparent of these is the fact that isolation and lack of variability in the environment are *in themselves* conditions that may greatly affect the behavior and physiology of the experimental subjects.

A number of researchers such as Danny Lehrman (1953, 1958) and Frank Beach (1950) have called our attention to the prevalence and importance of species-specific and species-typical behavior in a variety of animals. This has led to the understanding that we should search for appropriate animal models in our selection of subjects to serve in biomedical and other laboratory research. It is important that we consider the emphasis that these same researchers have placed on constituents of natural *environments and social circumstances* when developing our research protocols.

We must continue to be vigilant in our efforts not to allow our animal subjects to become inappropriate "models" of their own species and, furthermore, to ensure that they are appropriate models to assess probable similar outcomes when these techniques are employed in humans. Because a laboratory animal species may be genetically similar to humans does not allow us to automatically presume that the effects of a particular drug in alleviating sickness in that species will produce identical results in humans. What we should recognize is that the failure of human trials to show the same outcomes as those seen in trials employing nonhuman subjects may result from the artificially controlled environments of the nonhumans. Stated more simply, laboratory animals are better models for predicting outcomes of some manipulation in humans if the animals are employed in natural, species-typical environments.

Herein lies our most important point in this chapter; the careful establishment of appropriate environments for the well-being of captive animals can in itself largely determine experimental outcomes. Placing a nonhuman primate in a human test environment in which the animal is singly housed may be of interest to those wishing to assess the extent to which these animals can mirror human behavior. It may also satisfy some who wish to argue that their controlled environment reduces the chance of extraneous variables affecting outcomes. But it will not allow us to assess how mentally healthy nonhuman primates are affected by changes in their natural circumstances. One might assume that such a behaviorally complex animal will be a superior experimental model if provided with a more species-typical social environment rather than an artificially isolated one.

SOME RESEARCH EFFORTS EVALUATING ENRICHMENT

Some research in our own laboratories has specifically focused on the effects of everyday living conditions on experimental outcomes for research animals. Currently, we are assessing the effects of providing variable housing materials and exercise regimen on the results of typical methods used to produce and alleviate amyotrophic lateral sclerosis (ALS)-like symptoms in mice. Although the studies and analysis of data are currently still in progress, our initial data show that the provision of opportunity for exercise may significantly affect the recovery of mice from the disease signs (Sorrells et al. 2003). Although researchers may see this as obvious, even a brief review of the literature in research on ALS models will show that this variable is often only considered in articles where it is the *focus* of the research. That is, if investigators wish to focus on the effects of exercise on recovery from ALS, of course they manipulate it or provide opportunity for exercise. But *what if they do not consider this one of their experimental variables?* It is still apparent that the caging in which the animals are routinely housed when provided, for example, with running wheels may cause significant differences in the measured outcome of the research. We include this example to illustrate the important effect that routine husbandry procedures can have on experimental outcomes.

Earlier extensive work conducted at the California Regional Primate Research Center (CRPRC) and the University of California at San Francisco (UCSF) using primates as subjects has demonstrated that the effects of routine caging may have significant effects on the behavior and physiology of research primates (Line et al. 1989c, 1989d, 1990; Markowitz & Line 1989b). Some of this work sought to explore the extent to which things that were routinely considered enriching from an anthropomorphic viewpoint had measurably positive effects on nonhuman primates in laboratory housing (Line et al. 1989a, 1991b). This work found that

simple toys that may have satisfied institutional requirements for enrichment or were thought to enhance the psychological well-being of primates actually had no measurable effects on mature rhesus macaques. It was further shown that giving animals social opportunities advocated by many for enrichment might be lethally dangerous if not carefully accomplished (Line 1987) and that routine husbandry techniques utilized in many primate facilities had surprisingly significant effects on typical measures of behavioral and physiological stress such as heart rate and blood cortisol levels (Line et al. 1987b, 1989b). Recently, researchers such as Boinski et al. (1999) and Schapiro (2002) have performed similar studies in both New World and Old World nonhuman primates and have arrived at similar conclusions.

Most importantly, in our estimation, it was also demonstrated that giving animals the opportunity to control even limited aspects of their environments served to significantly reduce or eliminate the measurable effects of routine environmental stressors (Markowitz & Line 1989a). This fact is extensively addressed in the chapter by Markowitz and Eckert in the current volume. Hence, we would emphasize that there is unquestionable importance to providing animals some control over aspects of their surroundings if we wish them to be appropriate animal models and if we wish to provide them with truly enriched environments.

ENVIRONMENTAL ENRICHMENT AND WELL-BEING

Work conducted as early as 30 years ago (Markowitz 1982, Schmidt & Markowitz 1977) illustrated that for a wide variety of captive mammals and birds, health diagnoses were clearly facilitated when animals were provided active behavioral opportunities. Recent work by Roughan and Flecknell studying the use of behavioral changes to identify discomfort in laboratory animals reaffirms this premise (Roughan & Flecknell 2001).

Animal well-being, as measured by the production of species-typical behavior and activity levels, was also enhanced. A good example of this is the case in which a previously undetected chronic diaphragmatic hernia in a serval became apparent when the cat attempted to leap for food in its captive environment. At hearing this case presented, few researchers seemed to recognize that a cat, who in the wild might flush birds out of the bush and capture them on the fly, might languish in the absence of stimulation for species appropriate exercise

(Markowitz & Gavazzi, 1995, 1996; Markowitz et al. 1978; Schmidt & Markowitz 1977).

As pressures on elected officials from humane groups began to increasingly lead to mandates for *enrichment* of captive animal living conditions, greater emphasis in meetings was placed on discussions of *well-being* of animals used in nature education and entertainment venues. It became more readily accepted that an animal's condition might decline in the absence of responsive environments. Unfortunately, much greater emphasis was placed on making captive environments *look* natural and inviting to humans than was placed on enhanced stimulation for species-appropriate behavior. Billions of dollars have been spent on providing facilities that look appealing to visitors. What remains amazing is that a miniscule fraction of this amount has been invested to evaluate scientifically whether measurable improvements in terms of animal use of the architecturally appealing edifices exist.

WHY ARE WE SPUTTERING IN EFFORTS TO IMPROVE ANIMAL WELL-BEING?

Today, a clear recognition exists of the importance of providing enriched environments for captive animals. This can be easily seen by looking at any of the recent editions of *The Shape of Enrichment* newsletter or by attending one of the international conferences on environmental enrichment. However, pervasive reluctance remains on the part of zoo designers and administrators, and laboratory researchers and administrations, to place extensive *budgetary* emphasis on providing measurable, well-researched improvements in facility design or husbandry techniques that enhance animals' well-being. It is critical that funding be made available to support additional research to determine what form of enrichment is best for a given species in a given situation. Data collected from such ongoing work will help justify potential husbandry and environmental changes to those responsible for making budgetary decisions.

It may be instructive to review some of the historical and contemporary reasons for this lack of funding emphasis on enrichment. Looking first at contemporary research facilities, we can clearly see that a continual competition exists to obtain adequate funding for even the most important research efforts. Researchers correctly identify that providing more funding for environmental enrichment means expanding their budgets. This may in turn

mean that the probability of funding their research may be reduced because budgets do not appear competitive with other laboratories conducting similar research. One way to alleviate this problem is to make it the responsibility of the institution to provide for appropriate environmental enrichment. We recognize that a number of institutions are already active in their efforts to do their best in this regard, but without adequate funding for appropriate research and implementation, this can be challenging.

Some difficulties have been seen in the expansion of requirements for facilities to promote the "psychological well-being" of animals in their care. Unfortunately, although Congress has mandated some of these requirements for institutions that receive federal funding, it has not mandated that funding agencies provide the dollars to accomplish the task of providing improvements that are truly *measurably enhancing the well-being of research animals*. With inadequate funding and incomplete knowledge as to what constitutes well-being in each species, researchers may inadvertently choose enrichment strategies that may not be appropriate for their animals.

We suggest that continued scrutiny should be made of devices and strategies that may "look enriching" from an anthropomorphic or common sense viewpoint. Instead of relying on the latter viewpoint, we should require demonstrations that devices or husbandry changes genuinely constitute *measurable improvements in the animals' well-being* before they are institutionally mandated or governmentally required. Environmental enrichment strategies should be based on sound scientific studies. If changes to a research animal's environment are made in a random manner, a risk exists that the changes will be ineffective and will interfere with the outcome of the study itself. Support for research in this area is an obvious necessity.

Further, as we have suggested elsewhere in this chapter, it may be possible to integrate important improvements in husbandry and housing as part of the experimental design. Researchers wishing to investigate treatments for illness utilizing animal models should, for example, show that the manner in which the animal is housed and cared for may have significant effects on their experimental outcomes. With careful grant writing, these improvements in animal care may then be seen by funding agencies as essential components of the research itself.

A researcher armed with the knowledge that promoting opportunities for his or her research animals to maintain healthy states of activity may have significant measurable effects, for example, on their recovery from disease with administration of a drug being evaluated, can show that this is a critical, fundable part of his or her work.

Another recommendation is that the National Institutes of Health once again actively fund laboratory animal training programs that include training for graduate veterinarians in techniques for evaluating the efficacy of environmental enrichment strategies. Such programs should include instruction in research methods appropriate to the field. This approach could help to stimulate additional research pertaining to psychological well-being and, in addition, would encourage the dissemination of awareness regarding its importance to laboratory animals and researchers.

The vast majority of researchers that we know personally are sincerely concerned about the well-being of animals that serve in their research efforts. Many worry over the fact that they do not have larger budgets to improve the lot of animals in their care. Most are willing to employ husbandry improvements as long as they are assured that the techniques will not interfere with their research efforts. What we hope to convey in this chapter is that providing measurably improved opportunities for animals can actually enhance research.

The use of animals in entertainment and educational facilities faces similar financial problems. Unlimited budgets are rarely available, and only the richest of zoos and aquariums have devoted personnel budgets for environmental enrichment. We refer readers to the chapter by Markowitz and Eckert in this volume to see expanded rationale for the provision of exhibits and husbandry procedures that measurably improve the lot of captive animals.

WHY COMMON SENSE DOES NOT ALWAYS WORK BEST

One problem that we have frequently encountered in giving advice both to those who use animals in their work and to governmental regulatory agencies is the tendency for many of us to believe that we know from empathy alone what would be most rewarding for other animals. Here we will explore just a few examples of why this common sense notion may lead to difficulties for the animals we wish to protect.

In examining the individual caging typically provided for research animals, the first thing that seems apparent is that if we were in their places, we would like to have more room. With this in mind for non-

human primates, the government regulatory agencies required that the minimum size of all primate cages be increased for any institutions that receive federal funding. No money was simultaneously appropriated by Congress to pay for the required change. Also, no research existed to show that the increase in cage size would lead to improvements in the well-being of the primates housed therein.

When dollars *were* forthcoming for us to do some systematic studies in this area, we found, much to our own surprise and the chagrin of others, that no measurable change occurred in the activity levels or physiological states of the primates. This was true when measures were made comparing paired groups of rhesus monkeys individually housed in old standard caging, new required-size caging, and caging twice the standard size (Line et al. 1989d, 1990, 1991a). We did, however, find measurable differences when the same primates were provided simple activity opportunities with which to amuse themselves in their cages, regardless of cage size (Line et al. 1987a, 1991a).

In retrospect, we can easily come to another "common sense" conclusion in an admittedly anthropomorphic fashion. If one of us were allowed to live in a space approximately 1/3 larger than our traditional space but still had no active opportunities in which to employ ourselves, it would not make a great deal of difference. Most of us are willing, however, to confine ourselves to remarkably limited areas to interact with computers that we may use to type out chapters such as this to try to convey our ideas to others. It is the ability to control aspects of the environment and to be productive that gives individuals comfort and helps to mitigate the effects of confined quarters.

A FEW SUGGESTIONS FOR FURTHER READING ABOUT ANIMAL WELL-BEING EFFORTS FOR RESEARCH ANIMALS

Space precludes identifying the work of hundreds of colleagues who have devoted much of their lives to truly improving the lot of research animals. Here are just a few representative examples to illustrate that this is a field ripe for exploration by readers of this chapter.

The work of Victor Reinhardt and his colleagues has placed much emphasis on the importance of providing social opportunities for research animals. He, too, has called for greater emphasis on scientifically measurable improvement for animals provided new equipment or procedures claimed to be enriching (Reinhardt 1987, 1989a, 1989b, 1990a, 1990b, 1991, 1998). This body of work emphasizes the importance of social opportunities to the physical and mental well-being of captive nonhuman primates. Reinhardt and his colleagues have done a great deal to show that pair and group housing of primates can be safely accomplished provided that the caretakers involved are methodical and patient in their approach. Reinhardt advocates methods that allow animals to be introduced to one another gradually, thus reducing the risk of antagonistic encounters and unsuccessful outcomes. Furthermore, Reinhardt has demonstrated the importance of social hierarchy to the successful pairing of previously single-housed macaques.

Kathryn Bayne has devised a number of well-researched, ingenious, cost-effective ways to provide foraging opportunities for primates. Her efforts have been especially useful where budgetary constraints do not allow for production of expensive equipment. Some institutions have, for example, been able to use inexpensive foraging boards that are easily cleaned and maintained by volunteers when paid staff time is not available (Bayne 1991; Bayne et al. 1992, 1993a, 1993b). Bayne's work demonstrates the effectiveness of different types of relatively simple enrichment devices that focus on giving macaques the opportunity to search for food treats. She has also shown that if such a device is removed from the animal's environment, the result may be the reappearance of previously observed abnormal behaviors (Bayne & Dexter 1992). In addition, Bayne is an advocate of using a variety of approaches to environmental enrichment in nonhuman primates, including social opportunities, foraging devices, simple toys, and opportunities for exercise. Finally, Bayne believes in the importance of the human-animal bond to the welfare of both human caregivers and research animals (Bayne 2002).

In Europe, the Universities Federation for Animal Welfare (UFAW) has been active in promoting the well-being of animals in a large variety of venues including research facilities, zoos, and farms. Trevor Poole has published extensively on this work, which includes the seventh edition of the UFAW Handbook on the Care and Management of Laboratory Animals (Poole & English 1999). This book contains many references pertaining to the physical and psychological care of laboratory animals. Examples include the importance of "vertical space" to nonhuman primates, the benefits of positive-reinforcement training to the welfare of labora-tory animals, and general husbandry recommendations for a variety of captive animal species.

Steven Schapiro has focused his efforts on exploring the effects of enrichment on the behavior and physiology of macaque monkeys (Schapiro et al. 1993, 1998, 2001). In a recent review article (Schapiro 2002), he discusses the significant effects that manipulation of the environment can have on measurements of immune function in rhesus macaques and the importance of recognizing this when designing experiments using these animals as models.

In conclusion, we believe that it is undeniable that the manner in which research animals are housed and maintained has an effect on research outcomes. It is well past time that we should actively acknowledge this fact and incorporate in all of our research protocols descriptions of how captive circumstances may bear on results. In addition, we must continue our efforts to research how best to enrich the environments of different species in different captive situations. Thus, can we improve the applicability of our research to the ultimate targets for which it is intended.

REFERENCES

Bayne K. 1991. Alternatives to continuous social housing. *Lab Anim Sci* 41:353–359.

Bayne K. 2002. Development of the human-research animal bond and its impact on animal well-being. *ILAR J* 43:4–9.

Bayne K, Dexter S. 1992. Removing an environmental enrichment device can result in a rebound of abnormal behavior in rhesus monkeys. *Am J Primat* 27:213–224.

Bayne K, Dexter SL, Hurst JK, et al. 1993a. Kong toys for laboratory primates: Are they really an enrichment or just fomites? *Lab Anim Sci* 43:78–85.

Bayne K, Dexter SL, Mainzer H, et al. 1992. The use of artificial turf as a foraging substrate for individually housed rhesus monkeys (*Macaca mulatta*). *Anim Welfare* 1:39–53.

Bayne K, Dexter SL, Strange GM. 1993b. The effects of food treat provisioning and human interaction on the behavioral well-being of rhesus monkeys (*Macaca mulatta*). *Contemp Top Lab Anim* 32:6–9.

Beach FA. 1950. The snark was a boojum. *Am Psychol* 5:115–124.

Boinski S, Swing S, Gross T, et al. 1999. Environmental enrichment of brown capuchins (*Cebus apella*): Behavioral and plasma and fecal cortisol measures of effectiveness. *Am J Primatol* 48:49–68.

Lehrman DS. 1953. A critique of Konrad Lorenz's theory of instinctive behavior. *Q Rev Biol* 28:337–363.

Lehrman DS. 1958. Induction of broodiness by participation in courtship and nest-building in the ring dove (*Streptopelia risoria*). *J Comp Physiol Psych* 51:32–36.

Line SW 1987. Environmental enrichment for laboratory primates. *J Am Vet Med Assoc* 190:854–859.

Line SW, Clarke AS, Ellman G, et al. 1987a. Hormonal and behavioral responses of rhesus macaques to an environmental enrichment apparatus. *Lab Anim Sci* 37:509.

Line SW, Clarke AS, Markowitz H. 1987b. Plasma cortisol of female rhesus monkeys in response to acute restraint. *Laboratory Primate Newsletter* 26:1–3.

Line SW, Markowitz H, Morgan KN, et al. 1989a. Evaluation of attempts to enrich the environment of single-caged nonhuman primates. In: Driscoll JW (ed), *Animal care and use in behavioral research: Regulation, issues, and applications*. Beltsville, MD, Animal Welfare Information Center National Agricultural Library:176–213.

Line SW, Markowitz H, Morgan KN, et al. 1991a. Effect of cage size and environmental enrichment on behavioral and physiological responses of rhesus macaques to the stress of daily events. In: Novak MA, Petto AJ (eds), *Through the looking glass: Issues of psychological well-being in captive nonhuman primates*. Washington, DC, American Psychological Association:160–179.

Line SW, Morgan KN, Markowitz H. 1991b. Simple toys do not alter the behavior of aged rhesus monkeys. *Zoo Biol* 10:473–484.

Line SW, Morgan KN, Markowitz H, et al. 1989b. Heart rate and activity of rhesus monkeys in response to routine events. *Laboratory Primate Newsletter* 28:9–12.

Line SW, Morgan KN, Markowitz H, et al. 1989c. Response of rhesus monkeys to routine laboratory events. *Am J Primat* 18:153 (Abstract).

Line SW, Morgan KN, Markowitz H, et al. 1989d. Influence of cage size on heart rate and behavior in rhesus monkeys. *Am J Vet Res* 40:1523–1526.

Line SW, Morgan KN, Markowitz H, et al. 1990. Increased cage size does not alter heart rate or behavior in female rhesus monkeys. *Am J Primatol* 20:107–113.

Markowitz H. 1982. *Behavioral enrichment in the zoo*. New York: Van Nostrand Reinhold.

Markowitz H, Gavazzi A. 1995. Eleven principles for improving the quality of captive animal life. *Lab Anim* 24:30–33.

Markowitz H, Gavazzi A. 1996. Definitions and goals of enrichment. In: Burghardt G, Blelitzki J, Boyce D, et al. (eds), *The well-being of animals in zoo and aquarium sponsored research*. Greenbelt, MD, Scientists Center for Animal Welfare:85-90.

Markowitz H, Line SW. 1989a. Primate research models and environmental enrichment. In: Segal EF (ed), *Housing, care and psychological wellbeing of captive and laboratory primates*. Park Ridge, NJ, Noyes Publications:43–61.

Markowitz H, Line SW. 1989b. Primate research models and environmental enrichment. In: Segal EF (ed), *Housing, care and psychological wellbeing of captive and laboratory primates*. Park Ridge, NJ, Noyes Publications:202–212.

Markowitz H, Schmidt MJ, Moody A. 1978. Behavioural engineering and animal health in the zoo. *International Zoo Yearbook* 18:190–194.

Poole T, English P. 1999. *The UFAW [Universities Federation for Animal Welfare] handbook on the care and management of laboratory animals*, 7th ed. Oxford, UK: Blackwell Science.

Reinhardt V. 1987. Advantages of housing rhesus monkeys in compatible pairs. *Scientist Center for Animal Welfare Newsletter* 9:3–6.

Reinhardt V. 1989a. Behavioral responses of unrelated adult male rhesus monkeys familiarized and paired for the purpose of environmental enrichment. *Am J Primatol* 17:243–248.

Reinhardt V. 1989b. Re-pairing caged rhesus monkeys. *Laboratory Primate Newsletter* 28:19.

Reinhardt V. 1990a. Social enrichment for laboratory primates: A critical review. *Laboratory Primate Newsletter* 29:7–11.

Reinhardt V. 1990b. Time budget of caged rhesus monkeys exposed to a companion, a PVC perch and a piece of wood for an extended time. *Am J Primatol* 20:51–56.

Reinhardt V. 1991. Social enrichment for aged rhesus monkeys that have lived singly for many years. *Anim Technol* 43:173–177.

Reinhardt V. 1998. Pairing *Macaca mulatta* and *Macaca arctoides*. *Laboratory Primate Newsletter* 37:2.

Roughan JV, Flecknell PA. 2001. Behavioural effects of laparotomy and analgesic effects of ketoprofen and carprofen in rats. *Pain* 90:65–74.

Schapiro SJ. 2002. Effects of social manipulations and environmental enrichment on behavior and cell-mediated immune responses in rhesus macaques. *Pharm Biochem Behav* 73:271–278.

Schapiro SJ, Bloomsmith MA, Kessel AL, et al. 1993. Effects of enrichment and housing on cortisol response of juvenile rhesus monkeys. *Appl Anim Behav Sci* 37:251–263.

Schapiro SJ, Nehete PN, Perlman JE, et al. 1998. Effects of dominance status and environmental enrichment on cell-mediated immunity in rhesus macaques. *Appl Anim Behav Sci* 56:319–332.

Schapiro SJ, Perlman JE, Boudreau B. 2001. Manipulating the affiliative interactions of group housed rhesus macaques using positive reinforcement training techniques. *Am J Primatol* 55:137–149.

Schmidt MJ, Markowitz H. 1977. Behavioral engineering as an aid in the maintenance of healthy zoo animals. *J Am Vet Med Assoc* 171:966–969.

Sorrells AD, Eckert KA, Fahey AG, et al. 2003. Differential effects of environmental enrichment for mice. *Contemp Top Lab Anim* 42:113–114.

21
Mental Health Issues
in Captive Birds

Lynne Seibert

Mental states in birds involve a wide range of cognitive abilities and emotions. Due to the popularity of psittacine birds as pets, a need exists for an understanding and further scientific study of their emotional needs. Psittacine birds do not have the extensive history of domestication that many other species that are kept as pets, such as dogs and cats, have experienced. At the most, some of these birds are only a few generations removed from the wild, with some pet birds being directly wild-caught.

Emotional well-being in pet birds is affected by additional unique challenges. Many psittacine species have the capacity to live as long as humans, requiring lifelong commitments on the parts of their caregivers. Unlike dogs and cats in the United States, most pet birds remain reproductively intact, which creates behavioral challenges, especially at puberty and during breeding seasons when new behaviors appear. The intelligence of psittacine birds has been documented in numerous studies and illustrates the importance of providing intellectual challenges for these highly intelligent species (Pepperberg 1987, 1994).

Understanding the behavioral and emotional needs of psittacine birds has important applications. First, we can improve the conditions for birds kept in captivity and provide for the expression of species-typical behaviors. We can reduce the incidence of behavior problems in pet birds, such as screaming, feather mutilation, and aggression. Inadequate attention to birds' mental health is an important welfare issue as it can lead to emotional suffering and poor quality of life. Boredom and social deprivation are examples of the negative influences on birds' mental well-being.

A better understanding of the emotional requirements of psittacine birds could enhance the success of captive breeding programs for endangered psittacine species. Parrots possess the largest number of threatened species of any bird family. At least 90 psittacine species are at risk for extinction (Collar & Juniper 1992). The *Psittacidae* family contains more threatened species than would be expected by chance, with an increased extinction risk with increasing body size and decreasing fecundity (Bennett & Owens 1997). Threats include habitat destruction, live bird trade, introduced species (cats and rats), persecution, being hunted for food, and fluctuations in environmental conditions.

This chapter discusses the importance of mental health and well-being in captive birds, with practical recommendations for bird owners and caregivers to maximize the mental wellness of birds in their care.

SPECIES DIVERSITY

The large variety of psittacine species presents an important limitation to generalizing about their behavioral needs and mental health. There are three families within the order Psittaciformes: *Psittacidae, Cacatuidae,* and *Loriidae.* The family *Psittacidae* is the largest, including approximately 280 species of parrots, macaws, parakeets, rosellas, and lovebirds. The family *Cacatuidae* includes more than 20 species of cockatoos and a single species of cockatiel. *Loriidae* includes more than 50 species of lories and lorikeets (Forshaw 1989).

Psittacine birds exhibit considerable range in appearance, with wide variations in size (from 10 g to >1500 g), structure (crested or non-crested), and coloration. Some species are sexually dimorphic. Some are primarily arboreal (yellow-winged Amazon, *Amazona aestiva xanthopteryx*), and others are terrestrial foragers (budgerigar, *Melopsittacus undulatus*).

Psittacine birds occupy diverse habitats, living anywhere from tropical rain forest to dry savannah. Tropical and subtropical lowland forested areas offer the most species diversity. Psittacine birds are neither sedentary nor migratory but mobile within a geographical area. Many travel substantial distances between roosting and feeding sites.

Social behavior varies among the species as well. Some appear to be solitary (kakapo, *Strigops habroptilus*), but most species are highly social. With so much variation in habitat and life history, recommendations for maintaining emotional health would need to be specific for the species and individuals involved.

MENTAL STATES AND EXPERIENCES OF BIRDS

It is important for us to recognize both positive and negative mental states in birds. Unfortunately, very few published ethograms for psittacine birds exist. Studies are needed that illustrate the meanings of various postures and actions of captive birds so that caregivers can more accurately assess mental and physical well-being. Fear or anxiety in captive birds is generally associated with increased vocalizations, defensive postures (such as crouching or flight intention movements), avoidance, frantic behaviors, displacement behaviors (such as preening), aggression, or escape attempts.

In a study evaluating neophobia, or latency to approach a novel object, Mettke-Hofmann et al. (2002) found that the natural ecology of the species influences neophobia. Sixty-one parrot species with different habitat preferences were studied in aviaries. The species with the shortest latency and longest duration of exploration were species inhabiting complex habitats and species that fed on seasonal foods (nectar, fruit, and nuts). The species with the longest latency and shortest duration of exploration were seed eaters. This study documents behavioral differences in captive species based on their natural habitats that must be considered when providing ideal captive environments.

In clinical situations, caregivers often report fearful behaviors with no known etiology. Fears can develop as a result of classical conditioning, in which the bird associates the owner with an aversive event. This situation has been reported in a case study of a Goffin's cockatoo (*Cacatua goffini*) that developed a persistent fear response toward its owner following an episode of fear-evoking construction noises (Seibert et al. 2001).

IMPORTANCE OF SOCIAL INTERACTIONS

The importance of providing some forms of social companionship must be considered for pet birds. Psittacine birds often form flocks. The benefits of flock membership include improved defense against predators, increased competitive ability, increased feeding efficiency, and access to mates (Wilson 1975).

Feeding together in organized flocks may be advantageous to the individual, who is able to benefit from the collective knowledge of the group. By following the flock, an individual has a better chance of locating adequate amounts of food when resources are unpredictable. Small foraging groups are better able than individual birds to exclude competitors from feeding sites. Some evidence indicates that birds with more limited fasting ability—smaller birds—are more likely to flock than larger birds (Gill 1995).

Indefensible areas also promote flocking behavior in birds. There is increased security in a large group, with individuals nearest the center of the flock having the least chance of becoming the victim of a predator. Flocking improves the efficiency of predator detection, allowing the individual more time for other activities. Alarm calling is common among flocks and serves to alert other members of the group to possible danger.

South and Pruett-Jones (2000) studied feral flocks of Monk parakeets in their natural environment. The birds formed foraging groups of 1–31 birds (mean < 10). Individual vigilance declined with increasing flock size, indicating that the flock serves an important function for predator detection.

The number of birds in the flock appears to be very important to the breeding success of large macaw species. Only a portion of the flock will be engaged in breeding activity during any one season, with the non-breeding birds appearing to form a buffer zone of territorial defense (Harrison 1994).

PAIR BONDING

Pair bonding is defined as a mutually beneficial relationship between sexually mature female and male birds (Doane & Qualkinbush 1994). Wilson (1975) defines pair bonding as a close and long-lasting association between a male and a female, serving the primary function of cooperative rearing of young. Pairs are characterized by allopreening, courtship feeding (also called allofeeding), pair participation in agonistic encounters, and close spatial associations (Levinson 1980).

Allopreening has been cited as the most important behavior for maintenance of social bonds. Close spatial associations are also evidence of a bond. Among bonded pairs of canary-winged parakeets (*Brotogeris v. versicolurus*), mates maintained very close proximity and were usually touching (Arrowood 1988). Many psittacine species maintain pair bonds throughout the year.

In captive environments, many birds do not have the opportunities to form close social bonds with conspecifics. In other situations, social pairings between birds can increase stress because of incompatibility. Captive environments should provide some opportunities for the expression of social behaviors and the maintenance of healthy social relationships with humans or other birds.

Meehan et al. (2003) evaluated the influence of isosexual pairing of orange-winged Amazon parrots (*Amazona amazonica*) on the development of abnormal behaviors. Paired parrots used inanimate enrichment devices more than singly-housed cohorts. Paired parrots also spent less time screaming and preening, and were more active. Parrots housed in pairs did not develop stereotypic behaviors, were less fearful of human handlers, and had reduced latency to approach a novel object.

PREDICTABLE ENVIRONMENTS

The general daily activities (feeding, maintenance, and roosting behaviors) of flocks of orange-fronted parakeets (Hardy 1965) and white-fronted Amazons (Levinson 1980) were highly predictable. Two activity peaks were commonly observed—one in the early morning and one in the late afternoon. During the periods of high activity, the birds engaged in feeding, agonistic behaviors, increased mobility, and increased vocalizations.

Pet birds are often exposed to unpredictable environments. Feedings, photoperiods, baths, attention, exercise, and social interactions are often provided based on the varying schedules of the caregivers. This unnatural state of affairs does not allow the bird to develop a sense of control or the skills for coping with stress and challenges. McMillan (2002) has discussed the adverse effects of unpredictability on the mental well-being of animals.

DEVELOPMENTAL FACTORS

Many psittacine offspring have relatively long infancies, with weaning taking up to a year in some

species, increasing the requirements for parental care (Doane & Qualkinbush 1994). The detrimental effects of early maternal deprivation on neural development and adult functioning are well-documented in primate species (Ruppenthal et al. 1976, Suomi et al. 1976).

Captive psittacine breeding programs often involve removal of the newly hatched bird from its parents and hand weaning by humans, due to the notion that this practice produces better-quality pet birds. The rearing of baby birds by human surrogates, however, may not be sufficient for the development of healthy adult coping skills and stress responses. The justifications for the practice of hand weaning are beginning to be questioned, and alternatives considered.

Aengus and Millam (1999) studied the effects of neonatal handling of parent-raised orange-winged Amazon parrots. One group was handled daily for 10–30 minutes from day 10 to fledging. The birds in the control group were handled only to obtain their weights. Significant differences in tameness existed between these groups, documenting that tameness toward humans is possible for parent-raised birds that are exposed to human handling. Sensitive periods for socialization to humans need to be determined.

There may be effective interventions for individuals that were deprived of maternal care. Bredy et al. (2003) evaluated the effects of environmental enrichment in rats that were deprived of early maternal care and found that peripubertal enrichment did compensate for some of the effects of early maternal deprivation. Francis et al. (2002) also found that environmental enrichment helped to compensate for the negative effects of postnatal maternal separation in rats.

FORAGING OPPORTUNITIES

Psittacine flocks generally maintain separate foraging and roosting sites. Levinson (1980) observed separate roosting and feeding areas in white-fronted Amazon parrots. In their observations of sulphur-crested cockatoos (*Cacatua galerita*), Lindenmayer et al. (1996) noted that the birds traveled considerable distances between roosting sites and areas where foraging occurred. Orange-fronted parakeets (*Aratinga canicularis*) in natural habitats maintained separate roosting and feeding sites one mile apart (Hardy 1965).

Pet birds are often fed commercially prepared diets on a free-choice feeding schedule, drastically reducing the amount of time spent in feeding behaviors. Meal feeding has been suggested to simulate natural feeding behavior more closely. In addition, captive birds may prefer foraging devices that require them to perform work for food (Coulton et al. 1997). Opportunities to forage have been shown to reduce feather picking behavior in Amazon parrots (Meehan et al. 2003). Foraging enrichments required the subjects to manipulate objects with openings, chew through barriers for food, sort through inedible materials, and open containers. In addition to preventing the development of feather-chewing behaviors in the enriched group, the same enrichments were used to reverse the development of feather picking in control birds. In this study, the foraging enrichments were used more than physical enrichments, which provided perching, swinging, and climbing opportunities.

PHOTOPERIOD, LIGHTING, AND SLEEP DEPRIVATION

Sleep deprivation can have detrimental effects on the mental health of captive birds. Most psittacine species are diurnal prey species, with an acute sense of vision and hearing. These characteristics present avian caregivers with the challenge of providing for an adequate amount of uninterrupted rest for the birds in their care. Pet birds are often housed in common areas of the home and covered when the caregivers retire for the evening, or at dusk. Given the level of vigilance and reactivity that is characteristic of prey species, it is highly unlikely that the birds receive adequate sleep in these environments. In addition to the stress associated with sleep deprivation, exposure to lengthy photoperiods (increased daylight or artificial light) can increase the incidence of undesirable reproductive behaviors.

Wilson (1999) has discussed sleep requirements for pet birds. It is generally accepted that natural photoperiod variation is ideal for the mental and physical health of pet birds. A two-cage system including a sleeping cage in a quiet room provides pet birds with a quiet, secluded sleeping area.

In addition to the proper amount of light, the type of lighting can also affect a bird's sensory experience. Evidence exists that birds' perceptive abilities extend into the ultraviolet range (Bennett & Cuthill 1994, Hausman et al. 2003). Hausman et al. (2003) found that 68 percent of psittacine birds surveyed had fluorescent plumage. A bird housed in a room with windows that block ultraviolet light has a more limited sensory experience than one that is exposed to full-spectrum or natural lighting.

CONSEQUENCES OF POOR MENTAL HEALTH

Emotional suffering and poor quality of life are evidenced by the prevalence of behavior problems in pet birds and the reduction or absence of species-typical behaviors. Abnormal behaviors include feather picking, barbering and self-mutilation, screaming, aggression and biting, misdirected sexual behaviors, and phobic disorders (Davis 1991).

FEATHER PICKING AND SELF-MUTILATION

Feather picking disorder, also called behavioral or psychogenic feather picking, is one of the most common behavior problems seen in captive psittacine birds (Lawton 1996). It is characterized by feather removal, feather damage, and/or soft tissue trauma with no apparent medical or physical explanation.

Boredom, defined as a lack of stimulation (Rushen et al. 1993) or a lack of opportunity to interact with the environment (Wemelsfelder 1993), is often presumed to be the cause of feather picking disorder. This presents an overly simplistic view of the disorder. Many of the individual birds presented for feather picking problems do not meet the criteria for boredom; they play with toys, interact with humans and other birds, and some are even in breeding programs and allowed free-flight opportunities. Successful treatment of feather picking disorder will need to incorporate a broader approach, evaluating early developmental deficiencies, the needs of individual birds, neurochemical correlates, and species-specific interventions.

Excessive preening may be evidence of conflict. Conflict-induced displacement behaviors are behavioral patterns that appear to have no contextual relevance and result from the ambivalence of a conflict situation (Wilson 1975). Orange-chinned parakeets exposed to stressful situations increased preening, head scratching, ruffling of the plumage, bill wiping, and flight intention (repeated crouching and leaning forward on perch) (Power 1966). Inappropriate housing conditions, frustration, stress, sexual behavior, attention-seeking behavior, overcrowding, separation anxiety, and changes in routines have also been implicated as causes of feather picking behavior (Rosenthal 1993, Welle 1999). Feather picking disorder may result from management conditions that do not allow the bird to engage in species-typical behaviors or do not provide appropriate target stimuli for these behaviors (Jenkins 2001).

Feather picking disorder has been compared to a condition in humans affecting impulse control, with noted behavioral similarities (Bordnick et al. 1994). Trichotillomania, an impulse-control disorder of humans, is characterized by removal of hair resulting in alopecia. Additional characteristics of the disorder include hair twirling, chewing or mouthing the hair, trichophagia, and skin picking (Stein et al. 1995). Avian practitioners have observed oral manipulation of removed feathers by psittacine birds with feather picking disorder.

Obsessive-compulsive disorder is characterized by obsessions, intrusive thoughts or images, compulsions, and repetitive behaviors, performed in an attempt to reduce anxiety. Hand washing is an example of a compulsive behavior in humans, which may share similarities with repetitive grooming behaviors in animals, including feather picking in birds (Grindlinger & Ramsey 1991, Stein 1996). Identifying similarities between avian disorders and human conditions may contribute to our understanding of the etiology of the disorder and the negative emotional experiences of the affected individual.

In addition to feather picking disorder, captive birds engage in a variety of nonproductive, repetitive behaviors (stereotypies) that are often interpreted as evidence of poor welfare or poor mental health. Stereotypic behaviors observed in captive birds include pacing, spot pecking, beak wiping, perch running, repetitive vocalization, head shaking, head bobbing, weaving, and flight intention movements (crouching, posing) (Sargent & Keiper 1967). Dilger and Bell (1982) postulated that the stereotypic head movements seen in some birds might be an early sign of neurosis, which could eventually lead to further behavioral abnormalities. The importance of stereotypic behaviors in captive birds as an indicator of poor emotional health is currently unclear and warrants further study.

SCREAMING AND EXCESSIVE VOCALIZATION

Because many parrots are noisy and communicate vocally, excessive vocalization is a common complaint of avian caregivers. Intense calling and vocalization is typical when arriving or departing from roosting sites. It is generally considered normal for pet psittacine birds to vocalize loudly several times a day (Harrison & Davis 1986). However, there are species differences in noisiness and differences in caregivers' tolerance of noise. Excessive vocalizations are often made worse when the caregiver responds directly to the noisy bird, providing positive reinforcement for the behavior. Birds lacking environmental enrichment may be predisposed.

Although screaming is often evidence of normal or exuberant behavior, it can also be a symptom of an environmental or emotional deficiency, indicating fear, undesirable changes to the environment, boredom, or frustration. It is important to determine the temporal patterns, eliciting stimuli, housing conditions, and opportunities for social interaction, as well as other potential causes for excessive vocalization, before recommending any interventions.

Contact calling occurs in avian species when they are separated from flock members. In some cases, it will be appropriate for the caregiver to answer the bird when it vocalizes, but in other cases, this intervention will be ineffective.

Captive birds may present with fear or stress-induced screaming. Alarm vocalizations have been measured in wild birds, showing similarities across species in responses to flying predators and other threats (Jurisevic & Sanderson 1994). Captive birds may also vocalize to indicate distress or injury. It is crucial that safe housing and accessories be provided and that pet birds be treated like curious toddlers, with attention paid to bird-proofing the environment.

Treatment considerations for excessive vocalization should target the needs, both physical and emotional, of the individual bird. It is helpful for the caregiver to keep a diary of excessive vocalization behavior, including date, time of day, location, duration of screaming without intervention, and persons and stimuli present during the episodes. If a pattern to the behavior exists, feeding, play time, or training sessions can be scheduled just before the bird's "loud times." Enriching the environment and rewarding appropriate behaviors can lessen the severity of screaming problems. The environment should be modified to maximize stress reduction, which might include the provision of environmental sounds, exposure to other birds and household activities, hiding places, quiet times, predictable schedules, and reduced confinement. When necessary, a time-out or removal of attention (a form of punishment) can be used to discourage screaming.

AGGRESSION PROBLEMS

Aggression problems are reported in pet birds, although not as commonly as feather picking and screaming. The relatively heavy jaw musculature allows parrots to crack seeds and nuts and inflict injuries. Psittacine birds have evolved flexible necks that allow rapid movement and detection of predators, and along with the beak, allow the bird to rapidly inflict injury during restraint. Parrots also tend to use their beaks as "hands" to explore the environment.

The causes of intraspecific and interspecific aggression in psittacine birds have not been systematically classified. The author uses a similar classification system as that used for other species, with some modifications for species differences (Beaver 1983, Overall 1993). Possible causes of human-directed aggression in birds include territorial defense, fear, intolerance of petting, sexual aggression, redirected aggression, play, attention seeking, lack of learned bite inhibition, and inappropriate mouthing.

Territorial Aggression

A territory is defined as an area occupied exclusively by an individual by means of repulsion through overt defense (Wilson 1975). Many avian species establish, maintain, and protect access to particular areas in their natural habitats. However, the prevalence of territorial behavior among psittacine species has not been determined. Territorial defense may involve defense of feeding areas, roosting positions, or nesting sites. Nest defense should be differentiated from mate guarding—close association with mates to ensure paternity—a common feature of the early stages of nesting in some species.

Aggression may be directed against any intruder, regardless of familiarity. Pet birds with territorial aggression may be fine when taken away from the vicinity of their cages. Treatment involves working in a neutral area on command training with positive reinforcement, and gradually moving training sessions closer to the cage area (desensitization and counterconditioning).

Fear Aggression

Many situations can predispose a pet bird to a fear-induced aggressive episode: inconsistent use of reprimands or punishment by the caregiver, confinement to restrictive areas (cages) that do not allow escape, inappropriate housing conditions contributing to stress, absence of flock support, inadequate socialization to humans, and unstable perching surfaces. Aggressive responses can be modified by learning over time (negative reinforcement of aggressive displays), such that aggression becomes the distance-increasing behavior of choice any time the bird feels threatened.

Redirected aggression occurs when the caregiver is present, the bird is exposed to an offensive stimulus, and the caregiver becomes the recipient of aggression. Redirected aggression can occur when strangers approach the cage, during veterinary visits, or during exposures to unfamiliar environmental stimuli. Through classical conditioning, the bird can learn an association between the caregiver and the fear-evoking stimulus, resulting in persistent fear of the caregiver and aggression whenever that person is present.

The treatment of fear-induced aggression involves avoiding fear-evoking situations, gradual desensitization and counterconditioning, and favorite treats and toys provided only when the feared individual is present (Seibert et al. 2001).

Play Aggression, Inappropriate Mouthing, and Lack of Bite Inhibition

Play behaviors, seen most commonly in juveniles, imitate essential adult activities without consummating any serious goals (Wilson 1975). Juveniles of several psittacine species have been observed to engage in social play in the wild (Levinson 1980). Play behaviors include clawing, play biting, and mock fighting.

During play with conspecifics, young birds would presumably learn the maximum amount of beak force that can be applied without injuring their playmates. Restricted early contact with clutch mates could jeopardize this early learning, resulting in excessive mouthing of human caregivers. Inappropriate responses to this behavior by human caregivers can cause fear.

Young birds should be provided with chew toys and opportunities for locomotor, object, and interactive play. Simply discontinuing interactions when the bird's mouthing becomes excessive will teach the bird to inhibit mouthing behavior.

Reproductive Causes of Aggressive Behavior

Problems may arise as pet birds reach sexual maturity, with reports of behaviors that seem to indicate that the bird is misdirecting sexual behaviors toward a human caregiver. Undesirable behaviors include attempts to allofeed (regurgitate), masturbation, excessive contact seeking or calling, aggressive attempts to drive away other members of the family, and defense of the cage as a nesting site (Harrison & Davis 1986). The onset of these behaviors may coincide with the natural breeding season, increasing day length, or excessive artificial photoperiods.

Treatment may require that other family members assist with feeding and maintenance care while a healthier relationship between the bird and its primary caregiver is cultivated. Reproductive behaviors can be diminished by decreasing the photoperiod, removing nesting areas, and avoiding handling that may be stimulating for the bird. Desensitization and counterconditioning have been successful when the bird is with the preferred caregiver and others gradually approach them.

Dominance in Psittacine Birds

The term "dominance" has been grossly misused in the field of avian behavior. Dominance is not synonymous with aggression, and in fact, the formation of stable dominance hierarchies is associated with a reduction in aggression. Stable flock membership requires mutual recognition of members and a system for allocation of group resources. Within a dyadic encounter, a dominance relationship exists when the individuals behave with predictable assertive or submissive responses based on previous experiences with each other. By using ritualized postural signalling, the birds avoid overt aggression. Once relationships are established, consistency of the social interactions exists, resulting in fewer or less intense aggressive assertions of dominance (Bernstein 1981). With the exception of one study of captive cockatiels (*Nymphicus hollandicus*), few studies have systematically measured dominance relationships in psittacine birds (Seibert & Crowell-Davis 2001).

Assuming that all aggression is dominance-related is counter-productive and sometimes harmful. No direct evidence exists that psittacine birds aggressively challenge the social status of their human caregivers. Most of the aggression observed in psittacine birds does not meet the criteria for a dominance-related problem—specifically, aggressive challenges by socially mature birds accompanied by species-specific dominance postures, which are not location or stimulus-specific. Cage- or resource guarding is not definitive evidence for a dominance-related problem. Frightened birds will often aggressively defend their spaces. Attempts by caregivers to "establish dominance over their birds" are likely to increase stress and induce fear responses.

A relationship between perch height and dominance status has not been established for any psittacine species. If a relationship does exist, species differences are likely based on variations in natural habitats and ecology. An inverse relationship between perch height and dominance status may exist, with lower-ranking birds preferring higher perches. Many birds prefer higher perching sites, which is more likely to be a safety issue than a dominance-related issue. Likewise, difficulty removing a bird from the top of its cage does not necessarily indicate a dominance problem. Lowering cages and perches for a problem bird may result in increased anxiety. For any behavior problem, including aggression, it is crucial to identify and understand the causative factors, take a detailed behavioral history, make a specific behavioral diagnosis, and develop a treatment plan based on accepted practices of behavioral medicine.

ENHANCING THE QUALITY OF CARE FOR CAPTIVE BIRDS

Potential bird owners should be advised not to purchase a psittacine bird unless they are prepared for a life-long commitment. Veterinarians and aviculturists can assist in the selection of the appropriate species and individual, taking into consideration longevity, exercise requirements, disease susceptibility, cost to purchase and maintain, and social needs. It is important to locate a reputable source for the bird and purchase a healthy bird that has already been weaned. Providing quality preventive health care and nutrition is critical for maintaining health and emotional well-being.

Early socialization experiences are important for young birds, and caregivers should expose their birds to a variety of people, stimuli, and situations without causing fear or risking disease exposure. Avian playgroups and social gatherings are commonly available in many communities. Well-socialized birds can take car trips, visit friends, and participate in animal-assisted therapy programs.

Evans (2001) has reviewed housing requirements for pet birds. Enclosures should address the needs of the bird, be constructed of non-toxic materials, provide the appropriate bar spacing, and be large enough to allow a full range of movements. Cages need to provide privacy and security, such that one side of the cage is placed against a wall or is partially covered.

The position of the enclosure is also important. Varying the location may be beneficial for some birds. Some birds may require an area with more activity, and some may require a quieter area of the house. Enclosures should be positioned at eye level of standing family members with varying perch heights. The position of the enclosure should also provide exposure to fresh air and natural sunlight but avoid drafts. Birds should never be exposed to pesticides, aerosols, scented oils, or cigarette smoke.

Birds should be allowed out of their cages regularly, with appropriate supervision, and given opportunities to exercise. This can be accomplished by using playpen stands, tree stands, freestanding perches, cage-top gyms or activity centers, hanging perches, or caregiver handling. Harness training allows flighted birds safe access to outdoors and opportunities for flight.

The benefits of enrichment interventions for psittacine birds are well-documented (Coulton et al. 1997, Vanhoek & King 1997, Meehan et al. 2003). A stimulating environment can improve emotional well-being and prevent aberrant behaviors. Recommendations include providing stimulating toys without overcrowding the enclosure and rotating them regularly. Caregivers must be certain that any toy offered to the bird is safe, nontoxic, and will not be consumed. Some toys, such as wooden ice cream sticks, plain cardboard, paper towel rolls, whiskbrooms, rawhide pieces, pieces of nontoxic wood, or alfalfa cubes should provide the bird with an opportunity to chew. A variety of commercially available toys exist for birds, and individual preferences may require the caregiver to offer several varieties before identifying the most favorable objects. Unique color preferences of individual birds can influence their choices of toys and foods. Less-confident birds may initially avoid novel items, so gradual or repeated introductions of novel items and foods may be necessary.

A variety of perching materials of variable diameters is recommended for healthy feet and for behavioral enrichment purposes. Nontoxic, chemical-free, natural branches provide birds an opportunity to chew, and the perch diameter variation that is recommended for optimal pedal health. Other perching options include manzanita wood, PVC pipe, concrete, braided sisal, and cotton rope.

Maintaining a natural-to-semi–natural photoperiod variation will provide adequate rest and prevent the onset of undesirable reproductive behaviors. Day length can influence hormonal cycles. Providing a sleeping cage in a quiet room will give the bird a quiet, undisturbed sleeping area during dark hours. A minimum of 10 hours per day of sleeping time has been recommended (Evans 2001).

Avian caregivers should set a regular and somewhat predictable schedule for daily activities. Scheduled feeding times simulate natural foraging habits. Foraging enrichments include providing chew foods and using food puzzles or toys to hide food and promote searching behavior. Many psittacine species also enjoy bathing. Baths can be provided by misting, taking the bird into the shower, or providing a water bowl.

Avian caregivers often serve the functions of a flock member and should talk to the bird, interact with the bird, play with the bird, preen the bird, and involve it in family activities. Some birds respond favorably to hearing familiar sounds, especially in the caregivers' absence, such as tape recordings of family activities, other birds, nature sounds, or music.

Pet birds should be taught basic commands using positive reinforcement, such as a highly palatable food treat, praise, a favorite toy, or attention. Command training can teach the bird appropriate behaviors and can be used to redirect inappropriate behaviors. Birds should be encouraged and rewarded for playing by themselves, for sitting quietly, and for chewing on appropriate objects. Ignoring undesirable behaviors will prevent inadvertent reinforcement of the behaviors. After a pause in the undesirable behavior, the bird can be redirected to obey a command that has been previously taught. Physical punishment is never appropriate for psittacine birds. Simply leaving the room, withholding attention, or placing the bird in a time-out cage for a few minutes when it misbehaves are often effective interventions.

An understanding of the native behavior of psittacine birds is essential to the prevention and treatment of behavioral disorders of birds in captivity and for optimizing emotional health. The importance of flock social interactions for various species and the effects of isolation on welfare are also pertinent issues. Recognizing that psittacine birds have evolved as prey species should alert caregivers to the importance of environments that provide a sense of security and predictability, particularly in the absence of a flock. Caregivers should also be aware that the sensory experiences of birds will be different from those of humans because of the birds' specialized visual capabilities. The intellectual capacity of psittacine birds should not be underestimated and should motivate avian caregivers to provide intellectual stimulation for the birds in their care.

REFERENCES

Aengus WL, Millam JR. 1999. Taming parent-reared orange-winged Amazon parrots by neonatal handling. *Zoo Biol* 18:177–187.

Arrowood PC. 1988. Duetting, pair bonding, and agonistic display in parakeet pairs. *Behavior* 106:129–157.

Beaver BV. 1983. Clinical classification of canine aggression. *Appl Anim Ethol* 10:35–43.

Bennett AT, Cuthill IC. 1994. Ultraviolet vision in birds: What is its function? *Vision Res* 34:1471–1478.

Bennett PM, Owens IP. 1997. Variation in extinction risk among birds—chance or evolutionary predisposition. *Proceedings of the Royal Society of London Series B*:401–408.

Bernstein IS. 1981. Dominance: The baby and the bath water. *Behav Brain Sci* 4:419–457.

Bordnick PS, Thyer BA, Ritchie BW. 1994. Feather picking disorder and trichotillomania: An avian model of human psychopathology. *J Behav Ther Exp Psy* 25:189–196.

Bredy TW, Humpartzoomian RA, Cain DP, et al. 2003. Partial reversal of the effect of maternal care on cognitive function through environmental enrichment. *Neuroscience* 118:571–576.

Collar NJ, Juniper AT. 1992. Dimensions and causes of the parrot conservation crisis. In: Beissinger SR, Snyder NFR (eds), *New world parrots in crisis*. Washington, DC, Smithsonian Press:1–24.

Coulton LE, Waran NK, Young RJ. 1997. Effects of foraging enrichment on the behavior of parrots. *Anim Welfare* 6:357–363.

Davis CS. 1991. Parrot psychology and behavior problems. *Vet Clin N Am-Small* 21:1281–1288.

Dilger WC, Bell J. 1982. Behavioral aspects. In: Petrak ML (ed), *Diseases of cage and aviary birds*. Philadelphia, Lea and Febiger:123–141.

Doane BM, Qualkinbush T. 1994. *My parrot, my friend: An owner's guide to parrot behavior*. New York: Macmillan.

Evans M. 2001. Environmental enrichment for pet parrots. *In Practice* 23:596.

Forshaw J. 1989. *Parrots of the world*, 2nd ed. Melbourne: Lansdowne Press.

Francis DD, Diorio J, Plotsky PM, et al. 2002. Environmental enrichment reverses the effects of maternal separation on stress reactivity. *J Neurosci* 22:7840–7843.

Gill FB. 1995. *Ornithology*, 2nd ed. New York: W.H. Freeman.

Grindlinger HM, Ramsey E. 1991. Compulsive feather picking in birds. *Arch Gen Psychiat* 48:857.

Hardy JW. 1965. Flock social behavior of the orange-fronted parakeet. *Condor* 67:140–156.

Harrison GJ. 1994. Perspective on parrot behavior. In: Ritchie BW, Harrison GJ, Harrison LR (eds), *Avian medicine: Principles and application*. Lake Worth, FL, Wingers Publishing:96–108.

Harrison GJ, Davis C. 1986. Captive behavior and its modification. In: Harrison GJ (ed), *Clinical avian medicine and surgery*. Philadelphia, W. B. Saunders:20–28.

Hausmann F, Arnold KE, Marshall NJ, et al. 2003. Ultraviolet signals in birds are special. *Proceedings of the Royal Society of London B Biological Sciences* 270:61–67.

Jenkins JR. 2001. Feather picking and self-mutilation in psittacine birds. *Vet Clin N Am-Exotic* 4:651–668.

Jurisevic MA, Sanderson KJ. 1994. Alarm vocalizations in Australian birds—convergent characteristics and phylogenetic differences. *Emu* 94:67–77.

Lawton MPC. 1996. Behavioral problems. In: Beynon PH, Forbes NA, Lawton MPC (eds), *BSAVA manual of psittacine birds*. Ames, Iowa State University Press:106–114.

Levinson ST. 1980. The social behavior of the white-fronted Amazon (*Amazona albifrons*). In: Pasquier RF (ed), *Conservation of new world parrots. Proceedings of the ICBP Parrot Working Group Meeting*. Washington, DC, Smithsonian Institution Press:403–417.

Lindenmayer DB, Pope MP, Cunningham RB, et al. 1996. Roosting of the sulfur-crested cockatoo (*Cacatua galerita*). *Emu* 96:209–212.

McMillan FD. 2002. Development of a mental wellness program for animals. *J Am Vet Med Assoc* 220:965–972.

Meehan CL, Garner JP, Mench JA. 2003. Isosexual pair housing improves the welfare of young Amazon parrots. *Appl Anim Behav Sci* 81:73–88.

Meehan CL, Millam JR, Mench JA. 2003. Foraging opportunity and increased physical complexity both prevent and reduce psychogenic feather picking by young Amazon parrots. *Appl Anim Behav Sci* 80:71–85.

Mettke-Hofmann C, Winkler H, Leisler B. 2002. Significance of ecological factors for exploration and neophobia in parrots. *Ethology* 108:249–272.

Overall KL. 1993. Canine aggression. *Canine Pract* 18:29–31.

Pepperberg IM. 1987. Acquisition of the same/different concept by an African grey parrot (*Psittacus erithacus*): Learning with respect to categories, of color, shape, and material. *Anim Learn Behav* 15:423–432.

Pepperberg IM. 1994. Numerical competence in an African gray parrot (*Psittacus erithacus*). *J Comp Psychol* 108:36–44.

Power DM. 1966. Agonistic behavior and vocalizations of orange-chinned parakeets in captivity. *Condor* 68:562–581.

Rosenthal K. 1993. Differential diagnosis of feather picking in pet birds. Proceedings of the Annual

Conference of the Association of Avian Veterinarians, Nashville, TN:108–112.

Ruppenthal GC, Arling GL, Harlow HF, et al. 1976. A 10-year perspective of motherless-mother monkey behavior. *J Abnorm Psychol* 85:341–349.

Rushen J, Lawrence AB, Terlouw EMC. 1993. The motivational basis of stereotypies. In: Rushen J (ed), *Stereotypic animal behavior: Fundamentals and applications to welfare*. Wallingford, UK, CAB International:41–64.

Sargent TD, Keiper RR. 1967. Stereotypies in caged canaries. *Anim Behav* 15:62–66.

Seibert LM, Crowell-Davis SL. 2001. Gender effects on aggression, dominance rank, and affiliative behaviors in a flock of captive adult cockatiels (Nymphicus hollandicus). *J Appl Anim Behav Sci* 71(2):155–170.

Seibert LM, Sung W, Crowell-Davis SL. 2001. Animal behavior case of the month. Fearful behavior in a Goffin's cockatoo. *J Am Vet Med Assoc* 218:518–520.

South JM, Pruett-Jones S. 2000. Patterns of flock size, diet, and vigilance of naturalized Monk parakeets in Hyde Park, Chicago. *Condor* 102:848–854.

Stein DJ. 1996. The neurobiology of obsessive-compulsive disorder. *Neuroscientist* 2:300–305.

Stein DJ, Simeon D, Cohen LJ, et al. 1995. Trichotillomania and obsessive-compulsive disorder. *J Clin Psychiat* 56(S4):28–35.

Suomi SJ, Collins ML, Harlow HF, et al. 1976. Effects of maternal and peer separations on young monkeys. *J Child Psychol Psyc* 17:101–112.

Vanhoek CS, King CE. 1997. Causation and influence of environmental enrichment on feather picking of the crimson-bellied conure (*Pyrrhura perlata perlata*). *Zoo Biol* 16:161–172.

Welle KR. 1999. Clinical approach to feather picking. Proceedings of the Annual Conference of the Association of Avian Veterinarians, New Orleans, LA:119–124.

Wemelsfelder F. 1993. The concept of animal boredom and its relationship to stereotyped behavior. In: Lawrence AB, Rushen J (eds), *Stereotypic animal behavior: Fundamentals and applications to welfare*. Wallingford, UK, CAB International:65–96.

Wilson EO. 1975. *Sociobiology*. Cambridge: Belknap Press.

Wilson L. 1999. Sleep: How much is enough for a parrot? *Pet Bird Report* 43:60–62.

Index